Start Strong,

Finish Strong

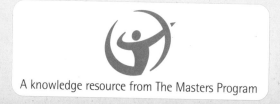

A knowledge resource from The Masters Program

AVERY

a member of

Penguin Group (USA) Inc.

New York

Start STRONG,
Finish STRONG

PRESCRIPTIONS FOR A LIFETIME OF GREAT HEALTH

Kenneth H. Cooper, M.D., MPH

Tyler C. Cooper, M.D., MPH

with William Proctor

Published by the Penguin Group
Penguin Group (USA) Inc., 375 Hudson Street, New York, New York 10014, USA · Penguin Group (Canada),
90 Eglinton Avenue East, Suite 700, Toronto, Ontario M4P 2Y3, Canada (a division of Pearson Canada Inc.) · Penguin
Books Ltd, 80 Strand, London WC2R 0RL, England · Penguin Ireland, 25 St Stephen's Green, Dublin 2, Ireland
(a division of Penguin Books Ltd) · Penguin Group (Australia), 250 Camberwell Road, Camberwell, Victoria 3124,
Australia (a division of Pearson Australia Group Pty Ltd) · Penguin Books India Pvt Ltd, 11 Community Centre,
Panchsheel Park, New Delhi–110 017, India · Penguin Group (NZ), 67 Apollo Drive, Rosedale, North Shore 0632,
New Zealand (a division of Pearson New Zealand Ltd) · Penguin Books (South Africa) (Pty) Ltd, 24 Sturdee Avenue,
Rosebank, Johannesburg 2196, South Africa

Penguin Books Ltd, Registered Offices: 80 Strand, London WC2R 0RL, England

First trade paperback edition 2008

Most Avery books are available at special quantity discounts for bulk purchase for sales promotions, premiums, fund-raising,
and educational needs. Special books or book excerpts also can be created to fit specific needs. For details, write Penguin
Group (USA) Inc. Special Markets, 375 Hudson Street, New York, NY 10014.

The Library of Congress catalogued the hardcover as follows:

Cooper, Kenneth H.
    Start strong, finish strong : prescriptions for a lifetime of great health / Kenneth H. Cooper,
Tyler C. Cooper, with William Proctor.
    p.   cm.
    Includes bibliographical references and index.
    ISBN 978-1-58333-282-5
    1. Exercise.   2. Physical fitness.   3. Self-care, Health.   4. Health.   I. Cooper, Tyler C.
II. Proctor, William.   III. Title.
    RA781.C623   2007   2007022469
    613.7—dc22

ISBN 978-1-58333-318-1 (paperback edition)

Printed in the United States of America
10   9   8   7   6

Book design by Meighan Cavanaugh

To Clark Cooper

and Ridge and Tenley Estes,

with the hope that the information contained in this book will
help these young children live long, full, and healthy lives

ACKNOWLEDGMENTS

In producing this manuscript, we owe thanks to many people, including:

Our editor, Megan Newman, who has patiently and expertly guided our work to publication.

Our agent, David Hale Smith, whose advice, perseverance, and sensitivity to the publishing process have helped us shape the final product.

Cynthia Grantham, who, as usual, has oiled the administrative machinery necessary to help us communicate and collaborate effectively and efficiently.

Kathryn Miller, a registered dietitian at the Cooper Clinic, who has provided invaluable insights and information relating to the nutritional sections of the book.

Todd Witthorne, president of Cooper Concepts, as well as cohost and executive producer of our nationwide radio program, *Healthy Living Radio from the Cooper Aerobics Center,* who has made essential contributions to our chapter dealing with supplements.

Nina Radford, M.D., director of the cardiovascular medicine department at Cooper Clinic, who has provided important insights on the latest medical understanding about the efficacy of functional foods designed to lower levels of "bad" LDL cholesterol.

Jenna Adams, whose research abilities have enabled us to identify and organize the necessary scientific support for the manuscript.

David Atkinson, director of program development at Cooper Ventures, who has exercised his considerable creative skills in helping to prepare photo illustrations for exercises in the book.

Rebecca Behan, assistant editor on the Avery editorial staff, who has handled with aplomb many editorial and administrative matters related to the manuscript.

Pam Proctor, whose diligent editing was instrumental in helping to shape the initial draft of the manuscript.

Angie and Millie Cooper, whose advice and emotional support have kept us going through the months required to complete this effort.

Bill Proctor, whose writing and research skills have once again played an essential role—as they have with a dozen previous "Cooper books."

Of course, many others have contributed to the final version of *Start Strong, Finish Strong*, including editors and staff at Avery and the Penguin Group; the staffs at the Cooper Clinic, Cooper Institute, Aerobics Center, and Wellness Center; and the staff at the DHS Literary Agency. They have given us a strong start—one that we trust will culminate in a strong finish for all those who need to jump-start their health and fitness.

Kenneth H. Cooper, M.D., MPH
Tyler C. Cooper, M.D., MPH

CONTENTS

Part Three

Strategies for Finishing Strong

PREFACE

Because one of us is thirtysomething and the other is in his seventies, we believe we're in a unique position to offer a broad range of intergenerational health advice. Of course, like any other pair of strong-minded physicians—who also happen to be father and son—we don't always agree on all the details of each problem and solution. But in the interests of full disclosure, when we do part company seriously on an issue, we'll let you know in no uncertain terms through a series of doc-to-doc dialogues and personalized boxes strategically positioned throughout the text.

Also, we'll occasionally speak to you in the first-person singular when we recount personal experiences one or the other of us has had in developing our respective medical understanding and philosophy. But the point of view in most of our narratives will be conveyed in the first-person plural, in part because most of the time, especially with regard to the latest scientific findings, we are in full agreement.

Many times, the names and identifying characteristics of patients we refer to have been altered to protect privacy and confidentiality. Other times, including those situations where the facts and names have been published elsewhere, we have used real names. In all cases, the basic framework of different illustrations and cases is factual.

INTRODUCTION

Dr. Ken Cooper probably saved my life.

Specifically, he and his colleagues at the Cooper Clinic have used their cutting-edge screening procedures to identify various red flags in my health profile, such as gradually rising cholesterol and an unexpected, and probably genetic, tendency to develop coronary artery plaque at a certain age. Strategic prescriptions and recommendations have corrected the problems and dramatically improved my risk profile.

But our friendship didn't get started in the examination room. I first met Ken in 1980 on a professional basis when I became the writer for his *Aerobics Program for Total Well-Being,* published in 1982. That collaboration, which helped me establish my own set of energy- and health-enhancing aerobic exercise habits, led to a twenty-six-year working relationship, during which we've produced more than a dozen books, including this current project, which breaks significant new ground with his son, Tyler, as coauthor.

Of course, it's been exciting for me to see the Cooper books spreading around the globe, being translated into forty-one languages and

Braille, with more than 30 million copies sold. But I feel especially fortunate that I've been in a position to be cared for as his patient at the Cooper Clinic. In the process, my odds of maintaining high physical functionality as I age have increased—a benefit that he and Tyler call "squaring off the curve" of life (see Chapter 2).

Nor am I alone in reaping these benefits. In fact, I'm just one of millions whose lives have been changed by the preventive medicine revolution sparked by Dr. Kenneth H. Cooper more than forty years ago.

So how exactly did this medical revolution get started?

It all began when Ken received his M.D. from the University of Oklahoma School of Medicine and then earned his master of public health degree (MPH) from the Harvard School of Public Health while an air force flight surgeon stationed in Texas. In the process, he received one of the earliest certifications from the American Board of Preventive Medicine.

The air force was Ken's experimental laboratory for developing the aerobics concept. During his thirteen years of military service, he designed a series of unique fitness programs, including the twelve-minute and 1.5-mile fitness tests and the Aerobic Points System. The Aerobic Points System (see Chapter 8) assigns point values to various endurance exercises to rate their relative value as aerobic conditioning vehicles. In general, those who accumulate sufficient Aerobic Points on a regular weekly basis can expect to enjoy a much higher quality of life and a marked decrease in their risks for dying from any cause, including cardiovascular disease or cancer.

After Ken's identification of the aerobic exercise concept, many others have built on—and extended—his work with such popular movements as aerobic dance and various cardio programs. Also, his historic aerobic fitness innovations and definitions are used by scientists as the standard to evaluate the impact of exercise on health and mortality. As a testament to the foundational quality of his research, Ken's original fitness tests and other aerobic programs are also still employed by a variety of organizations, including the U.S. military, other governmental agencies, foreign military commands, FIFA (the international soccer association), many U.S. and foreign corporations, and more than a thousand universities and public schools.

Rising to the rank of lieutenant colonel, Ken also served as director of the Aerospace Medical Laboratory (Clinical), in San Antonio, and helped the National Aeronautics and Space Administration (NASA) condition America's astronauts for space. But after his aerobics research found its way into his 1968 megaseller *Aerobics,* he left the air force, moved to Dallas, and turned his energies toward the practical application of preventive medicine in the population at large.

During the 1970s, he founded the Cooper Clinic, the Cooper Institute, and the Cooper Aerobics Center in Dallas and eventually became widely acclaimed as the world's leading authority on fitness and preventive medicine. Now known as the "father of aerobics," he has been recognized as the leading pioneer of aerobic exercise by the *Encyclopaedia Britannica,* the *Oxford English Dictionary,* and other authorities.

As president and CEO of the Cooper Aerobics Center, Dr. Ken Cooper is supported by a 650-person staff in carrying out his mission to educate and encourage optimum health in as many segments of the population as possible. The thirty-acre Cooper Aerobics Center campus in Dallas features the world-renowned Cooper Clinic, the Cooper Fitness Center (with more than three thousand members), a guest lodge with luxury rooms for more than a hundred travelers, and the nonprofit Cooper Institute.

Programs at the Cooper Clinic include not only the famed one-day Cooper gold-standard medical examination, but also special programs to train professional athletes, coaches, law-enforcement officers, and other government officials. An intensive live-in program, the Cooper Wellness Program, offers sessions ranging from four to thirteen days for total wellness assessment and lifestyle modification—including nutritional counseling.

In many ways, my own health practices have been influenced by what I've been exposed to as I've worked on the Cooper books. For example, in *Running Without Fear* (1985), I was deeply impressed by the late running guru Jim Fixx's fatal fitness flaw of failing to get regular comprehensive gold-standard preventive-medicine exams. To guard against this danger, I make sure that I'm evaluated regularly by competent physicians. Then, in our *New York Times* best seller *Controlling Cholesterol* (1988), and in the sequel, *Controlling Cholesterol the Natural Way* (1999), I learned exactly what I had to do to improve my own lipid profile.

As my son Mike got involved in sports in kindergarten and elementary school, we both benefited from my work on *Kid Fitness* (first published in 1991 and later revised as *Fit Kids!* in 1999). Mike went on to play varsity basketball at Amherst College and to pass the demanding physical and mental screening that has enabled him to become a U.S. Marine Corps pilot. My personal supplement program even received a needed corrective nudge from *Antioxidant Revolution* (1994) and *Advanced Nutritional Therapies* (1996). In short, the original Cooper focus on aerobic exercise now embraces all of preventive medicine, and millions have benefited—including my own family.

Bringing the Cooper message into the new millennium in January 2000, Ken launched the radio show *Healthy Living with Dr. Ken Cooper,* which is now syndicated nationally. Stretching his international reach, he not only has published many books and articles in foreign venues, but also has lectured in more than fifty countries. His impact has been so great that in Brazil, running is called "coopering" or "doing the cooper," and the *cooperteszt* is the national fitness test in Hungary.

More recently, as a result of his work with Frito-Lay and other major corporations, the *Wall Street Journal* and other leading news organizations have recognized Ken as the nation's major physician-advocate for eliminating trans fats from the American diet. He has also worked closely in the "functional food" area with Johnson & Johnson to test the company's cholesterol-lowering spread, Benecol. On another front, the Cooper Concepts division has tested and produced its own special line of Cooper Complete vitamin and mineral supplements, which are now being used worldwide.

In the research arena, the Cooper Institute's 1989 landmark study, which was published in the *Journal of the American Medical Association* and still garners kudos from the medical community and mass media, established a direct relationship between fitness and mortality in 13,600 patients. Other major research findings at the institute are regularly published each year by leading medical journals.

Now, as Ken passes the mantle of preventive medicine leadership to Tyler, the Cooper health-and-fitness vision is extending to promote a total lifestyle revolution in the twenty-first century. In addition to shouldering a patient practice in the tradition of his father, grandfather, and numerous other past "Doctors Cooper," Tyler works directly with Cooper Life at Craig Ranch. This planned community north of Dallas features full-size versions of the Cooper Clinic and Aerobics Center and offers residents extensive health facilities and services. Benefits include full regular medical exams by the Cooper Clinic staff; a wide variety of athletic facilities, such as tennis courts, swimming pools, and running trails; lectures by the Cooper Institute experts; and even elite athletic training.

A graduate of Baylor University (BBA in management and marketing), the University of Texas Medical School at San Antonio, and the Harvard School of Public Health, Tyler is well-equipped to shoulder his expanding responsibilities. Among other accomplishments, he has created Cooper Ventures, a division of the Cooper Aerobics Center that performs management and service analysis of national and international medical clinics and health clubs. Cooper Ventures also seeks to expand the reach of the Cooper Aerobics Center into other communities.

A former elite collegiate athlete himself, Tyler also understands the importance of serving as a personal fitness model for the thousands who come through the Cooper programs and facilities each year. In a kind of "basic training" for fitness leadership, he served as captain of both the track and cross-country teams at Baylor University, with meet performances that earned him All-Southwest Conference status. His academic work placed him on the All-Southwest Conference Academic Honor Roll, and his cross-country team was the Southwest Conference Champion in 1992. In addition, he was a Division I National Championship Qualifier.

Even though his days of college competition are behind him, Tyler still recognizes the importance of leadership by example. He can be seen most days at the Cooper Fitness Center exercising side by side with patients and club members on the running tracks, in the pools, and in the indoor gyms. The results of this kind of fitness leadership are evident in the relationships he has developed—including his role in the remarkable story of Rick Salewske (see Chapter 15).

As for me, like many Cooper Clinic patients outside the Dallas area, I maintain a regular relationship with a personal physician near my home. But to increase my odds of transforming my "strong start" into a "strong finish," I continue to make regular pilgrimages to the Cooper Clinic. In my daily life at home, I follow the "Cooper gospel," the revolutionary message that both Doctors Ken and Tyler Cooper preach and practice so effectively in the pages of *Start Strong, Finish Strong*.

William Proctor
Vero Beach, Florida

Part One

Finding Your Special Inner Drive

One

■ How to Jump-start
■ a Stubborn Body

On her forty-eighth birthday, Christine experienced one of those "fitness epiphanies"—a devastating flash of self-recognition that may trigger panic or depression in even the most self-possessed middle-aged man or woman. It was a sunny Saturday morning, and her middle-school daughter, an avid basketball player, had asked her to spend a few minutes in the driveway playing one-on-one defense as the girl practiced a few feint-and-drive moves her coach had been teaching her.

At first, Christine declined the invitation. But then her daughter resorted to taunts: "So what if you're forty-eight! You may be old, but you don't have to move. Just stand in front of me as I practice."

That was all it took to get Christine into her sneakers and outside on the pavement. Actually, she felt pretty confident because she had been playing some tennis doubles once a week, and her weight wasn't that much heavier than it had been five or so years before. In any event, she certainly wasn't going to play the statue and stand still as her daughter dribbled around her. Just a year or so ago, she had been pretty adept at keeping up with the girl.

Christine lasted only ten minutes before she felt a muscle go in her left calf. "I've got to quit," she told her daughter.

She knew from experience that if she kept playing, she could be out of action for days if not weeks. So she hobbled upstairs, removed her clothes, and took a close look at herself in the full-length mirror in her bathroom. She was shocked at what she saw. She realized that somehow, even though she looked at herself in the mirror every day, she had apparently been fooling herself during the last few years. She had been seeing herself as she had been—or as she wished she was—rather than as she *really* looked.

Although it was no surprise to see the extra wrinkles and the little sagging that had begun on her face, the *shape* of her body startled her. The youthful curves had started to flatten out around her waist more than she had ever been willing to admit. And the rolls of fat that she had known were accumulating on her stomach and hips—but that she had chosen to ignore or deny—now somehow seemed quite prominent.

Continuing to contemplate her image, Christine asked herself, "What am I going to look like in two more years, when I'm fifty? And what about fifty-five, or sixty . . . ?"

The painful calf and an overall feeling of fatigue and stiffness added to her anxiety. Perhaps for the first time in her life, Christine began to feel mortal and physically vulnerable—and she realized that her neglect of her body had to end immediately. Otherwise, she knew she would almost certainly be caught in a nosedive in her ability to function energetically not only with her active daughter, but also in her many other life activities.

USING CHRISTINE'S TEST

Christine's experience suggests an uncomfortable personal "test" that just may change your life:

Find a nice, big mirror and take a good, close look at yourself. Forget what you looked like ten, twenty, or thirty years ago. Throw away those rose-colored memories and observe yourself honestly, as you are *right now.*

Mirror, Mirror on the Wall . . . Perhaps you see a little extra fat around the middle. Maybe the muscle tone in your arms or legs has lessened just a bit. Check to see if there's more than a trace of extra loose flesh on the back of your upper arms—flab that won't firm up or disappear when you flex your biceps. Also, check whether you can pass the "jiggle test": turn sideways or jump up and down to see if anything shakes or shimmies more than you'd like.

Now, look closely at your forearms and wrists: do they seem a tad smaller or less substantial than they did when you were younger? And your face—does it look a little more washed out or tired than you'd like?

As uncomfortable or even painful as this process may have been, you've now completed a crucial few seconds contemplating the way you *actually* look on the *outside*. Next, let's move *inside*.

Consider the way your body currently feels and works. Move your arms up over your head and back down to your sides, and then twist your torso back and forth, to the right and to the left. Do you feel any discomfort or stiffness? Next, bend over from your waist, knees straight, and see how far down you can reach with your fingertips. Maybe—like Christine—you once could touch your toes or at least come close, but now do you find your fingertips far off the old mark?

Staying with this self-examination, reflect back on your activities during the past few days. Did your legs get fatigued when you climbed a particular flight of stairs? Did you become winded as you walked fast to make an appointment on time, or as you were lugging some bags in an effort to catch a plane?

Did some unaccustomed work around the yard or house make your muscles unusually sore? At the end of a typical day, do you tend to feel "wiped out" earlier than you did a decade ago? In general, do you lack energy more than you think you should?

Finally, ponder for a few moments how you feel *deep* inside.

Are you basically a happy and optimistic person—or are you feeling down about as often as you are up? Do you experience general feelings of inner peace and well-being most of the time—or do you sense a fair amount of inner turmoil? During a typical day, do you find yourself worrying excessively about money, or a family member, or your health, or the health of a loved one? Is the stress in your life mostly under control—or is it too often out of control?

If you're like most adults moving into their forties, fifties, or beyond, the chances are that your answers to many of these questions are not as positive as you would like. But even if you're not as slim, toned-up, optimistic, or full of life as you had once hoped to be at your present age, you're not alone—nor are you doomed to a state of steadily deteriorating health and well-being.

Our goal is for you to enjoy your life—and be able to do the many things you want to do. Yet surprisingly, reaching this goal isn't as hard as you might think. You just need first to face a few hard facts about yourself and the aging process—and then *start strong* with a well-designed "youth recovery" program that will make you look forward to your next birthday rather than dread it.

Facing a Few Hard Facts

Beginning in the mid- to late thirties, we *all* face the onset of a wave of disturbing physical and mental changes that accompany natural aging. But those who are physically unfit experience this decline more extensively and rapidly than those who are in good shape. In other words, they "rust out, not wear out."

But whether slowly or quickly, the unattended human body begins to fall apart after a certain age. That's a fact of life as certain as death and taxes. More specifically, scientific studies show that those who enter the second half of life without a wise personal health strategy can expect:

- *Steady loss of total bone mass*—2 percent every two years. (In fact, at age twenty-five you can expect to start losing more bone than you make!)[1]

- *Regular loss of muscle mass*—1 percent per year.
- *Decline in aerobic (endurance) capacity*—1.5 percent per year, including a tendency to huff and puff more during shorter periods of exertion.
- *Lower energy levels*—with a tendency to run out of steam earlier in the afternoon, or to fall asleep before the TV at night.
- *Impaired physical functioning*—the average American suffers at least one seriously limiting health problem, such as a chronic heart condition or back ailment, long before the end of life.
- *Weakened immune function*—including more infections.
- *Loss of mental functioning*—including memory problems.
- *Reduced life span*—typically, a loss of at least ten to twenty years off your maximum possible life span.

But even though time and chance eventually overtake us all, a number of studies have revealed that only about a third of the natural processes of aging are beyond our influence. In other words, about *two-thirds* of that steady deterioration of mental acuity, physical strength, and stamina *can be slowed down, stopped—or even reversed.*

The essential message of the Start Strong, Finish Strong program is that, beginning right now, you can take some rather easy but extremely important steps to counter the natural physical and mental decline occurring in your body. These include a few adjustments in your personal health practices, physical activities, diet, and inner life—simple changes that will help you alter your life forever.

The Start Strong, Finish Strong Promise

The basic promise of our program can be summarized like this:
If you take seven simple start-up steps, namely . . .

Step #1: Quit putting off that gold-standard physical exam;

Step #2: Launch a realistic fitness plan;

Step #3: Begin eating a longevity diet;

Step #4: Follow a wise supplement strategy;

Step #5: Do serious smoke control;

Step #6: Counteract creeping substance abuse; and

Step #7: Engage in effective mind-spirit practices . . .

. . . you'll blast off to a strong start in a new life.

And if you stick with these steps so that they become ingrained health and fitness habits, you will greatly increase your chances of maintaining superior physical and mental function, maximizing your life span, and *finishing strong*. Or as we like to say, you will "square off the curve" of life by enjoying your greatest possible levels of strength, stamina, and mental acumen right up to your final breath (see Chapter 2).

Proof of the Promise

In a study spanning 1998 to 2003, Cooper Clinic President Dr. Tedd Mitchell demonstrated in practical terms how the Start Strong, Finish Strong strategy works. Using such measures as performance on stress tests, he and his research colleagues evaluated the effect of fitness—low, moderate, and high—on the quality of life of 10,331 men and women, whose health histories are on file at the Cooper Clinic.

Mitchell and his team concluded that, in twelve areas of health and fitness, there is a direct correlation between better fitness and better quality of life. Specifically, the in-shape individuals, or those in the "moderate" and "high" fitness categories, enjoyed *significantly* lower rates of these complaints:*

---

*The only problem measured by the researchers that was unaffected by fitness levels was chronic constipation. See page 10 for a chart detailing these findings.

- Unexplained fatigue
- Problematic snoring
- Frequent heartburn
- Sexual problems
- Decreased sex drive
- Male impotence
- Chronic joint or muscle pain
- Low back pain
- Frequent headaches
- Difficulty sleeping
- Depression
- Anxiety

These findings, shown in the chart on page 10, reveal the dramatic increase in benefits that occur as a person's level of fitness moves up from the lowest 20 percent (very poor fitness characterized by a sedentary lifestyle), to the next 40 percent (moderate fitness, which greatly increases health and longevity), to the top 40 percent (high fitness, which increases quality of life even further). According to the chart, as fitness increases, the percentage of those suffering various health complaints goes down.*

Now reflect for a moment on how this "well-being checklist" may apply to you personally. Do you ever have a problem with low energy levels? Insomnia or snoring? Sex drive? Joint, muscle, or back pain? Depression or anxiety?

If so, you should know that there is a very good chance that becoming more fit will make you feel and function better. But over and above these advantages, the Cooper Start Strong, Finish Strong program will open the door to a bounty of additional health and longevity benefits.

---

*Note that "fitness" as used here refers to aerobic fitness as measured by the person's ability to walk to exhaustion during a treadmill stress test, while his or her cardiovascular and respiratory functions are being monitored. See the description of the stress test and the Balke protocol in Chapter 5 page 107, and also the Appendix.

QUALITY-OF-LIFE VARIABLES BY FITNESS STATES
(10,311 Men and Women)

	Low (n = 1077) %	Moderate (n = 3555) %	High (n = 5679) %	P for Trend
Unexplained Fatigue	25.8	16.3	11.2	<0.001
Problematic Snoring	49.9	34.8	21.9	<0.001
Frequent Heartburn	30.9	22.1	12.1	<0.001
Sexual Problems	11.0	7.4	5.0	<0.001
Decreased Sex Drive	29.8	22.2	19.6	<0.001
Impotence (men only)	9.7 (932*)	7.2 (3126*)	4.6 (4910*)	<0.001
Chronic Joint or Muscle Pain	34.0	29.3	23.5	<0.001
Low Back Pain	44.8	41.5	35.4	<0.001
Frequent Headaches	16.7	15.0	12.0	<0.001
Difficulty Sleeping	28.7	24.9	21.9	<0.001
Depression	20.9	15.9	12.9	<0.001
Anxiety	20.2	16.4	13.6	<0.001

*%(n)

Source: ACLS, The Cooper Institute, January 2006

A Bounty of Benefits

There's something for everyone in the Start Strong, Finish Strong program, depending on your personal preferences for foods, exercise, and lifestyle practices. For example, different scientific studies have revealed that by following the simple guidelines in these pages you will open the door to at least ten major benefits:

#1: The longevity benefit

- You'll be 65 percent less likely to die prematurely than those who are unfit.[2]
- You'll add at least three years to your life—if you exercise briskly.[3]
- You could add ten years to your life if you're a man, and six-plus years if you're a woman—if you're a vegetarian, exercise, and don't smoke.[4]

#2: The mental-health benefit

- You'll improve your mental health, with less likelihood of depression—if you exercise more.[5]
- You'll slow age-related mental decline by 10 percent annually—by eating only one fish meal per week.[6]
- You'll enjoy better mental functioning and less cognitive decline—if you're a woman engaging in regular physical activity, such as walking.[7]

#3: The physical-function benefit

- You'll delay by at least seven years the age at which you develop even minimal disability—if you establish superior health habits.[8]

#4: The cardiovascular benefit

- You'll be 33 percent less likely to die from coronary heart disease, and 24 percent less likely to die from cancer—if you're on a Mediterranean diet, which features foods rich in olive oil, vegetables, legumes, fish, chicken, fruit, and pasta, with infrequent consumption of red meat.[9]
- You'll lower your risk by 20 percent and 15 percent, respectively, of developing two major new markers of heart disease—elevated

C-reactive protein (CRP) and homocysteine—again, if you eat a Mediterranean diet.[10]

- You'll lower your risk of irregular heartbeats, a major risk factor in heart disease—with a smart supplement program.[11]
- You'll lower your risk of dying from cardiovascular disease—if you are a man who is optimistic rather than lacking in hope.[12]

#5: The cancer-protection benefit

- You'll significantly reduce your risk of colorectal cancer—if you take regular small doses of aspirin.[13]
- You'll reduce your risk of death from colon cancer by 90 percent—if you observe proper cancer-screening procedures and treatment.[14]
- You'll lower your risk for any cancer—if you make such lifestyle changes as not smoking, avoiding the sun, eating well, and exercising.[15]

#6: The strong-bone benefit

- Whether you're a man or woman, you'll lower your risk of excessive bone loss after age fifty—if you do regular weight-bearing exercise and consume a bone-healthy diet.

#7: The pain-relief benefit

- You'll suffer 25 percent less musculoskeletal pain—if you're a runner who is fifty or older.[16]
- You may ease physical pain when you lose weight—because obese people are more sensitive to pain than nonobese people.[17]

#8: The healing benefit

- You'll experience faster healing of skin wounds—if you're an older adult who exercises regularly.[18]

#9: The fatal-accident benefit

- You'll lower your risk of being killed in a car accident—if you avoid obesity and maintain normal weight.[19]

#10: The wealth benefit

- You'll increase your wealth assets by nearly $12,000 on average— if you're a woman who reduces her BMI (body mass index) by 10 points.
- You'll increase your wealth assets by almost $13,000 on average— if you're a man who reduces his BMI by 10 points.[20]

Furthermore, you can begin to take advantage of these benefits no matter how old you are. The Start Strong, Finish Strong program will revolutionize your life, whether you're in your thirties, forties, fifties, or older.

Start Strong at Any Age

If you want proof of the ageless nature of the Start Strong program, visit the Cooper Clinic and chat with any of the thousands of our older patients who are in their seventies, eighties, and nineties. They keep coming back, sticking faithfully to their fitness regimen, because they know from experience that it works.

Or consider a 2005 Canadian study at the University of Western Ontario, London, which examined the effects of exercise training on two groups of basically healthy but sedentary adults between the ages of fifty-five and seventy-five. One group remained sedentary while the other group "started strong" by engaging in regular supervised physical exercise training.

After ten years, the active participants showed a 3.5 percent increase in fitness levels. In contrast, the couch potatoes experienced a 13.8 percent decline in their fitness.[21] Also, almost three times as many of the sedentary people had developed what's known as the metabolic syndrome—or the cluster of risk factors that includes high blood pressure, high "bad" cholesterol, low "good" cholesterol, high blood sugar, and obesity.

But as replete as this rosy picture is with benefits and promises that accompany a fitness makeover, a massive problem remains: a situation that might be called the *Great Disconnect.* That is, there is a huge difference between what we *say* we want in the way of scientifically proven health benefits, and what we're *really willing to do* to get those benefits. So how do we overcome this disconnect?

Overcoming the Great Disconnect

Most of us—84 percent, to be exact—believe there are things we can do to control the aging process.[22] Most people also think there are steps they can take to counter inferior fitness. But after failing time and time again to lose weight or stick with a fitness program, many also just give up.

Fortunately, your former fitness history isn't the end of the story. Even if you have given up many times in the effort to transform the state of your health, fitness, and general well-being, you're not stuck in your present position. No matter what your current age, physical condition, emotional status—or past record of failures—you can *start strong right now* with a life-changing fitness program. And you can also position yourself to *finish strong,* with the opportunity to function well until the very end of life. To achieve this strong start and finish, let's now examine what it really means to "square off the curve of your life."

Two

Squaring Off the Curve
of Your Life

M ost people's lives begin to curve downward when they hit their thirties. And by the time they pass fifty, that downward slope becomes very steep.

Or to put this point in terms that we've already used, the greatest challenge to your personal well-being and to the achievement of your life goals is that *after age thirty, the unattended human body begins to fall apart.*

The inevitable consequences of this process are a deterioration of physical, mental, and emotional functioning, which results in a lack of the acuity, strength, and drive necessary to achieve many important life purposes. Without a carefully designed and closely followed health and fitness program, which has been tailored to your needs and objectives in life, you'll never achieve what you set out to do.

This is what might be called the Start Weak, Finish Weak approach to life. The steady drop-off of health, fitness, and productivity in the unattended, uncared-for human body—along with a steady loss of the ability to function at a high level—can be pictured graphically by the Start Weak, Finish Weak Curve, depicted in Figure 1.

FIGURE 1.

The Start Weak, Finish Weak Curve

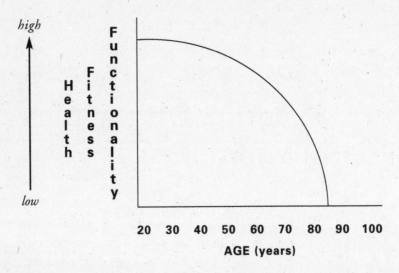

As Figure 1 shows, if you are currently operating in a relatively weak, unfit state, *or* if you grow weak as your life progresses, *or* if you allow yourself to let down and finish weak—you'll almost certainly head downhill in your ability to achieve at high levels of functionality. You'll lack the strength and stamina necessary to attain your most cherished goals at work and in your personal life. And the situation will only grow worse as you pass age fifty, sixty, and seventy.

At this point, it's worth repeating in detail the natural progression of deterioration—the steady weakening of body and mind—if you fail to embark on a preventive program to head off the natural declines associated with aging. You'll recall that this downward plunge is driven by several factors:

- *Steady loss of total bone mass*—2 percent every two years.
- *Regular loss of muscle mass*—1 percent per year.
- *Decline in aerobic capacity*—1.5 percent per year, including a tendency to huff and puff more during shorter periods of exertion.

- *Lower energy levels*—with a tendency to "run out of steam" earlier in the afternoon, or to fall asleep before the TV at night.
- *Weakened immune function*—including more infections.
- *Loss of mental functioning*—including memory and cognitive analysis problems.
- *Impaired physical functioning*—with the average American suffering at least one debilitating health problem, such as a chronic heart or a back condition, at least twelve years before the end of life.

But this downward curve in life is by no means necessary or inevitable. You may recall from Chapter 1 that it's possible for you to slow or stop about two-thirds of this "natural" deterioration of physical strength, stamina, and mental capacity. Our answer to this problem of maintaining an ongoing, high level of energy and function has been what we call "squaring off the curve" of life.[1]

Squaring Off the Curve

The Start Strong, Finish Strong strategy is the antidote to this "natural" state of affairs. In contrast to the declining health-fitness-functionality curve in Figure 1, a well-attended body and mind will be more likely to "square off the curve" of high functionality—as indicated in Figure 2.

Now look a little more closely at Figure 2. You can see that when you start strong, your personal fitness and functionality curve will spike upward to a new, better-conditioned level—as indicated on this diagram around age thirty. But don't be discouraged if you're a good bit older than thirty. If you get started at a later age, you'll simply experience your spike at that later age.

As you continue with your program, you'll typically find yourself enjoying a relatively high level of fitness, energy, and functionality over

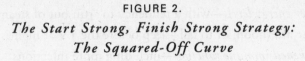

FIGURE 2.
The Start Strong, Finish Strong Strategy:
The Squared-Off Curve

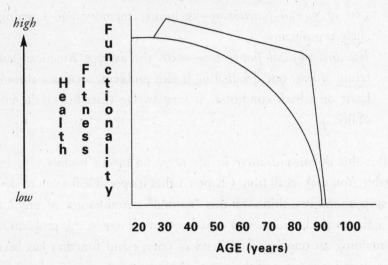

years or even decades. Of course, age will bring some decline—again, as indicated in the slightly downward-slanted straight line in Figure 2. But barring some catastrophic illness, that decline will usually be minor, in contrast to the relatively steep, long-term sloping drop that the unattended body experiences in Figure 1 (reproduced as the curve in Figure 2).

Finally, of course, your genetic makeup and the natural limits of your life span will catch up with you. But by pursuing a Start Strong, Finish Strong strategy, you'll be much more likely to shorten the inevitable low-functioning, low-energy time most people experience at the very end of life. Or to put this another way, squaring off the curve means compressing the time of senility and senescence into a brief period immediately before death.

What this means in practical terms is that, no matter what your age, your primary *physical* goal in life should be to devise and launch a wise, individually tailored preventive-medicine program *immediately* so that you'll become strong enough to fulfill all the life goals you feel driven to achieve.

Or to put this point in terms of Figure 2, you should *start strong* by embarking on a health and fitness plan that will work for the rest of your life and hold off the ravages of age as long as possible. With practically everyone—including former college athletes like the two of us, who were highly conditioned for sports competition early in life—the human body, left alone, will begin to soften and weaken. But by embarking on a start-strong strategy *right now*, whatever your current age—forty, fifty, sixty, or older—you'll maximize your chances to square off your personal health and fitness curve and *finish strong* in the latter part of your life.

Still, even though the two of us agree on this fundamental principle of squaring off the curve of life, we view that curve from widely divergent generational hilltops. After all, one of us is in his midthirties, the other his midseventies. Obviously, the health challenges that confront a young man or woman are typically quite different from those facing an older person. Furthermore, we know from personal experience and professional practice that a fitness regimen that works well for a seventy-five-year-old may not be at all appropriate for a thirty-five-year-old.

For example, we recommend that those in their thirties and forties concentrate on a proportionally heavier dose of aerobic exercise and a lighter dose of strength training. But when you pass age fifty, strength training should increase steadily, both to ward off bone loss from the aging process and to protect against loss of balance and physical functioning ability.

In any event, regardless of your age, it's important to remain keenly aware that the Great Downward Curve of Life is always lurking in the background—and that you must do all you can to counter those threats that have the power to prevent you from squaring off the curve.

The Threats to Squaring Off the Curve

Recent scientific studies have revealed a number of threats that are endangering huge numbers of adults—threats that you should take very personally because they pose a significant danger to your ability to square off the curve of your own life. To put it bluntly, if you don't stave off these threats, you won't square off your own curve—and you'll risk paying the consequences both in loss of functionality and shortened life span.

After considering each of the threats described below, you might put this book down for a moment and ask yourself, "Am I responding adequately to this threat in my own life?" To remind you, we've placed pertinent "ask yourself" questions at the end of each "threat." There are typically three possible answers to these questions: yes, no, and maybe. If you answer yes—and do so with some understanding of the issue—then you are probably on the right track. But a no or maybe answer to any of the questions indicates that you definitely need to increase your understanding of the particular issue.

The obesity threat

- About 64 percent of Americans are overweight.[2]
- On average, obesity decreases life expectancy by six years.[3]
- The surge of obesity may halt the rise in American life expectancy—causing us to live shorter, less healthy lives than our parents.[4] Obesity among our children is of particular concern because the condition increases the incidence of adult-onset (type 2) diabetes.
- Among adults thirty to seventy-four years old, excess body weight increases the risk of death from all causes.[5]
- An estimated 365,000 Americans died from being inactive and overweight in 2000.[6]

. . . yet the weight problem worsens regularly

- The percentage of overweight U.S. men rose to 71 percent in 2004.[7]
- In 2004 the percentage of overweight women in the U.S. was 62 percent.[8]
- Intake of calories rose 22 percent for women and 7 percent for men between 1971 and 2000.[9]

Ask yourself: Does my daily diet consist mainly of low-fat or no-fat foods? Do I eat at least five servings of fruits and vegetables each day? Do I avoid or partake very sparingly of alcoholic drinks? Do I limit myself to one reasonable-size portion of food per meal? Do I avoid junk food and fatty snacks?

The tobacco-and-substance-abuse threat

- The leading causes of death in 2000 were tobacco use, poor diet, physical inactivity, and alcohol consumption.[10]
- Nearly one-fifth of U.S. adults are daily smokers, and one-fifth consume five or more alcoholic drinks at a sitting at least once a year, according to government statistics.[11]
- Smokers are also putting their friends and families at risk: 10 to 15 percent of lung cancer patients are nonsmokers—a sign of the lethal danger of being exposed to sidestream smoke. Also, non-smoking women are twice as likely to get lung cancer as male non-smokers.[12]

Ask yourself: Have I quit smoking, or have I always been a non-smoker? Do I avoid restaurants or other public or private places that contain the "passive smoke" of others?

The sedentary-living threat

- Poor physical fitness has been directly linked to higher death and disease rates from all causes.[13]
- Only 20 to 30 percent of Americans do any regular physical activity.[14]

Ask yourself: Do I engage in aerobic (endurance) exercise at least three to four days per week, for at least thirty minutes each session? Do I devote at least two days a week to strength work? Do I do *some* significant physical activity every day?

The diabetes threat

- Worldwide, diabetes will soar from 117 million to 370 million by 2030—because of bad diet and exercise habits.[15]
- An estimated 21 million Americans are diabetic, and 41 million more are prediabetic. (Prediabetic refers to those with high blood sugar levels that could reach the diabetic level unless they improve their diet, exercise, and lifestyle habits.[16])

Ask yourself: Do I mostly eat foods that are low in simple sugars? Do I exercise regularly? Am I at my ideal weight—or am I carrying around some extra pounds?

The poor-sleep threat

- A lack of sleep contributes to weight gain and blocks weight loss, with 38 percent of adults sleeping less than they did five years ago.[17]
- Middle-aged men with obstructive sleep apnea are five times more likely to develop heart disease than those without this condition.[18]

Ask yourself: Do I get seven to eight hours of sleep per night? Is that sleep restful, or do I feel tired when I wake up? Do I receive reports from my spouse or others who observe me asleep that I snore heavily and/or have periods in which I stop breathing for ten to fifteen seconds? (A yes answer to this last question might indicate the condition known as sleep apnea, which has been identified as a health risk factor.)

The premature-disability threat

- Among thirty- to forty-nine-year-olds, those who could not care for themselves or do other routine tasks increased by more than half from 1984 to 2000.[19]
- Disability rates are soaring among those under sixty, with obesity being the prime suspect.[20]

Ask yourself: Are there any daily tasks I'm unable to do today but which I could do in the past? Can I perform simple strength tests, such as push-ups or abdominal crunches, as well as I did ten years ago?

The heart-disease threat

- Coronary heart disease becomes the leading killer of U.S. men when they reach forty-five years of age, and the top killer of women by age sixty-five.[21]
- About 47 million Americans have metabolic syndrome—which raises the risk for heart disease, stroke, diabetes, and kidney disease.[22]*
- Some primary risk factors for heart disease that *can* be changed include a lack of exercise, smoking, high cholesterol, high blood pressure, and obesity.

Ask yourself: Do I know my current levels of cholesterol (total, LDL, HDL, and total/HDL ratio)? Do I know my current blood pressure? Am I on a regular exercise program? Am I more than ten pounds overweight? Have I been in for a complete medical exam, with a stress test and other extensive cardiovascular screening, during the past two years?

The cancer threat

- In 2002, cancer became the number-one killer of all Americans younger than eighty-five, edging out heart disease.[23]
- Some primary risk factors for cancer that you can influence include smoking; excessive, unprotected exposure to the sun; and

---

*Those with metabolic syndrome have any three of the following conditions according to the National Cholesterol Education Program: 1) Excess weight around the waist—with waist measurement greater than 40 inches for men and 35 inches for women. 2) High triglycerides (a type of blood fat) of 150 mg/dl or higher. 3) Too little HDL (good) cholesterol—less than 40 mg/dl for men or less than 50 mg/dl for women. 4) High blood pressure—at 130/85 mm/Hg or higher. 5) High blood glucose (fasting level of 110 mg/dl or higher).

a failure to undergo regular cancer screening, including colonoscopies, fast CT scans, and prostate examinations and blood tests.

Ask yourself: Have I had a physical exam with cancer screening
during the past year?

After reflecting on this list of deadly dangers, don't be surprised if you
have found that you're in effect a kind of poster person for physical decline, a classic case study that puts flesh on the statistics. Also, if your risk
for one or more of these health conditions is high—or if you're failing to
go in for regular medical screening—you're not alone. Millions of other
men and women are in your precise situation: they are not taking adequate steps to square off the curve of their lives.

But now for the good news.

Even though you may not realize it, there's a lot you can do to correct
your current health and fitness situation. You are *not* the prisoner of your
genes or family history. In Part Two, we'll examine chapter and verse exactly what practical programs are available to help you change your life.

But what's the secret to starting—and sticking with—such a program? The absolutely essential first step is to identify a *personal passion or
conviction that will motivate you profoundly*—a *hot button* that will spark
an inner drive to enable you to maintain your body and mind in the best
shape possible.

Finding Your Hot Button

This personal fitness revolution starts in your head. Before anything
else, you must learn to *want—really* want—to improve your health and
well-being. And that means discovering an inner switch deep inside that
will turn you on regularly to achieve your maximum levels of good
health and well-being. Your underlying objective will be to find what
works for you personally—because, of course, not everyone is motivated
the same way.

So now, let's explore the answer to a basic motivational question that will enable you to jump-start even the most stubborn body: "What's my personal hot button—my inner motivational ignition switch that will make me *want* to put this book down, get off the couch, and begin to revolutionize my life?"

Three

What's Your Hot Button?

The Achilles' heel for any fitness program—the most vulnerable point, where the best intentions typically fall by the wayside—is a lack of motivation. And a failure of motivation is often associated with a very reasonable, if mistaken, set of excuses.

Getting to the Bottom of the Excuses

In the combined sixty-plus years that the two of us have spent in the field of medicine, we have seen many well-meaning people either fail to get started at all or stop shortly after beginning a fitness or weight-loss program. They give many reasons:

I don't have the time.
I can't find a good place to work out.
I can't spare the money for a club membership . . . or equipment . . .
    or . . .

I get too tired when I try to increase my physical activity.

I lose energy when I try to reduce my calorie intake.

My demands at work and my hours on the job have increased.

The new baby is just too much to handle at this point.

Regular exercise just doesn't fit into my busy schedule.

Fitness programs aren't any fun.

I lack the willpower to stay on a diet or exercise regimen.

The real reason for such attitudes is usually not the stated excuse, but, rather, a lack of *genuine* motivation. We know from practical medical experience that with a strong inner drive, excess weight can be lost—without such fitness failures as the yo-yo syndrome, where you take those extra pounds off but then put them all back on again. We also know that dramatic fitness improvement is possible for men and women of any age. But again, the main reason for falling off the exercise wagon after a few days or weeks is the lack of a powerful, life-changing impulse. Finally, there are those reports from many fitness clubs that enthusiastic new members tend to sign up in droves, but then they disappear for most of their membership contract. The reason? You guessed it—poor motivation.

In fact, many clubs appear to count on poor motivation among many of their members: according to the business plans of many clubs, the club facilities are designed to be large enough to handle only 10 to 25 percent of their actual membership!

Although it might surprise you, the same motivational problems that confront the average exerciser or would-be exerciser may also plague former competitive athletes who have trained their bodies for years and have often reached high levels of performance. Their typical problem is that they have a lot of trouble making the transition from high-profile sports events to a daily lifetime fitness routine.

From School Sports to the Real World

As former college athletes, we have both confronted the challenge of moving from a controlled sports-training environment, with ironclad workout schedules and attentive coaches, to a self-starting fitness program. So we know as well as anyone how hard it can be to shift from intense collegiate competition to a regular fitness routine in the real world.

Consider what happened to several former athletes featured in the *New York Times,* who had been in great shape as athletes in high school and college. In the decades following their competitive days, however, they went completely sedentary.[1] The athletes included:

- *Howie, age 32*—an all-state high school runner and a college athlete. But he hadn't worked out in about ten years, primarily because he knew that he would never run as fast as he once did. As a result, he couldn't see any point in donning his running shoes again. He told the *Times:* "With no goal, I find it hard to get out there. There's nothing to shoot for."
- *Karen, age 39*—an all-American college lacrosse player in college. After becoming a mother, she saw no real reason to train. Also, she lacked teammates to push her to get in shape.
- *John, age 41*—a former high school baseball player. After high school, according to the article, "he didn't know how to motivate himself. No glove, no glory."

After putting on 100 pounds and ending up with 265 pounds on a five-foot-eleven frame, John finally "felt he had run out of excuses," according to the report. So he joined a weight-loss program and started working out every day, with basketball drills, walking, and bicycling. John is still a work in progress, but at least he's confronting the problem that every unfit man and woman must face: getting past the excuses to those deepest impulses that can drive us to start and stick with a fitness program.

The underlying problem with former outstanding athletes is basically the same one that confronts most other people. We simply don't understand how to identify and harness those special inner passions that have the power to transform our lives. Or, to put this another way, we don't know how to find the particular *hot button* that will cause us to *want* to pursue superior health and fitness practices, not just for a few weeks or months, but for the rest of our lives.

So how can you discover your own special hot button?

If you're willing to engage in a little imaginative thinking, we'll show you, step by step, how to plumb your reservoirs of powerful motivation. In the process, you'll discover the inner drive that can usher you *permanently* into the Promised Land of Fitness, which so many fitness gurus and promoters of exercise gadgets have claimed can be yours for the asking.

The Promised Land of Fitness

Let's begin by painting a mental picture of this special world of fitness where you'd like to reside for the remainder of your life. In your mind's eye, imagine that you're standing outside a high wall, and Fitness Land is just on the other side. As you peek through a window on the door, you can glimpse some unusual things going on inside.

For one thing, the inhabitants of Fitness Land, regardless of their age, appear to be quite healthy and energetic, as they jog, walk, cycle, swim, or engage in other types of brisk exercise. Surprisingly, despite their activity, they really don't seem to get tired or to dislike their physical exertion. Instead, in almost every case, they appear to be quite happy, and sometimes you even catch many of them smiling at one another.

And by the way, very few of these people you're watching are involved in formal competitive sports. Not many are ranked senior tennis players or participants in master's track and field events. Rather, the large majority are ordinary people who walk, jog, cycle, or swim several times a week just to keep in shape—and they love it!

Furthermore, many of the older ones are performing physical feats you'd never expect of someone their age. Even those in their sixties, seventies, and eighties are running, lifting weights, playing racket sports, or even pole-vaulting. In the midst of this whirlwind of activity, some also manage to find time to engage in animated conversations. Overall, they seem to be enjoying a high-energy, low-body-fat, stress-controlled existence, which you grudgingly admit lies well beyond your current capacities.

You'd love to join those people on the other side of the wall, but you have a problem: the door to Fitness Land is locked tight, and you don't know how to pry it open. For a while, you try to emulate what the people on the other side of the wall are doing in the hope that you'll somehow be able to create your own little Fitness Land on your side of the wall. But no matter how hard you try, you can't seem to achieve or sustain what those people on the inside are doing. You sometimes get off to a good start, but then you lose heart and give up. Also, maybe you've spent a small fortune on exercise equipment and fitness club memberships, but the equipment sits stored away in a closet, and the memberships go unused.

Soon it becomes evident that if you're going to become anything like those people you're observing through the window, you're going to have to find a way to join them. But how can you get through that locked door?

As you contemplate the door further, you notice that it has a sign posted above it that says, KNOW YOUR MOTIVATION, and you also see a button next to the door with the letter M on it. You've tried pressing that hard, cold, lifeless button until the tip of your finger has developed a callus, but nothing has happened. For a long time you've just assumed that the device was broken—and that it was impossible to open the door and visit the Promised Land on the other side.

But gradually it dawns on you that maybe that M on the button, like the inscription above the door, refers to motivation. So perhaps if you can just find the secret to motivating yourself, you may be able to activate that button—to make it "hot"—and cause the door to swing open.

Finding Your Hot Button

Identifying the motivating forces deep inside you will require a little soul-searching. To get started, you might ask yourself a few salient questions:

What is the most important thing in my life?

What do I love to do?

What kinds of activities or situations can hold my attention for hours on end?

Do I tend to be a loner, or a person who thrives on social and group interactions?

What five qualities best describe my basic personality and character?

On this last question, you might come up with a few words that seem to capture the real you and your inner drives. Adjectives that come to mind might be "competitive," "independent," "self-sufficient," "sociable," "spiritual," "achievement-oriented," "concerned about my looks," "worried about my health," "practical," "addictive," or "unhappy about how I'm aging."

Engaging in this little exercise will draw you into the ancient Western tradition of self-exploration, an approach to life pursued by Socrates and other Greek philosophers—many of whom were inspired to look for the meaning of life by the words inscribed over the temple of the Delphic oracle in ancient Greece: "Know thyself."

After exploring your inner self for a time, you should find that you're well on your way to figuring out the exact nature of your hot button—which you'll probably find fits into one or more of the following motivational categories. As you consider these hot buttons, stay alert to those that seem to apply to you personally. Most likely, you'll find that several describe your deepest drives, and so you may want to take advantage of more than one as you design your program. After all, we all need as much motivation as we can get.

THE FEEL-GOOD HOT BUTTON

We regularly ask our patients: "What makes you continue with a regular exercise program?"

In response, the vast majority say: "It makes me feel good!"

These informal surveys confirm that the most important motivational factor that keeps regular exercisers going indefinitely—and craving their next workout—is the fact that exercise makes them feel better. People who exercise regularly are on average less depressed and less hypochondriacal, and have a much more positive attitude toward life, with fewer bodily complaints.

One of the main reasons for this phenomenon is that after a short period of exercise—typically about ten minutes for the average jogger and somewhat longer for the brisk walker—the body begins to produce "feel-good" chemicals and hormones, including neurotransmitters such as dopamine and endorphins. These neurotransmitters, which are secreted and circulated in the brain and nerve connections throughout the body, have a morphine-like effect, causing euphoria, relaxation, and a generalized sense of well-being. A kind of "positive addiction" may even occur, where the individual craves regular exercises and feels achy or out of sorts after missing a few workouts. (For more details on the science behind the Feel-Good Hot Button, see Chapter 4, page 68.)

On a personal note, both of us acknowledge that we are driven by this particular hot button because we do, indeed, feel great after a run, basketball game, strength training session, or other workout—and we feel lousy if we miss a session. On the other hand, we are quick to admit a potential problem with this hot button that may confront beginning exercisers.

If you have been completely sedentary or have engaged in little regular physical activity in recent months or years, you're unlikely to find yourself experiencing the effects of the Feel-Good Hot Button at the beginning of your exercise program. The feel-good experience, which depends on the release of various chemicals and neurotransmitters, probably won't kick in until you've developed at least a rudimentary level of fitness. In the very first part of your start-up phase, most of your focus will likely be on getting used to a higher level of activity, sticking to a regular workout schedule, and perhaps putting up with a little muscle soreness. Also, it's usual for most new exercisers to go through a biological transition period, where their biochemical and hormonal output gradually adjusts to new activity levels.

The best advice is just to be patient and keep this principle in mind: if you stick with the program, the Feel-Good Hot Button *will definitely* become a factor within the first few weeks of your new exercise regimen. But you'll have to gird yourself to make it through a short transition period before the endorphins, dopamine, and other chemicals of well-being really take hold.

In part, then, starting strong may involve a simple act of the will, where you'll fortify yourself mentally to wait a short time before the feel-good benefits of fitness become part of your life. But fortunately, you don't have to wait to be motivated from other directions: many additional hot buttons—including those mentioned below—are available right from the beginning to push you along.

Activate Your Feel-Good Hot Button: After each workout, ask, "How do I feel right now? Better than I did before my workout?"* As your fitness level begins to improve (say, after about one month into your program)—and your body's biochemicals become better conditioned to respond to a workout—this hot button will immediately activate as you walk, run, or perform other exercise.

---

* *Comment from Ken:* I've had many patients tell me, "The hardest part of a workout is putting on my shoes, and the best part is the shower when I finish."

THE COMPETITIVE HOT BUTTON

Reflect on your experiences in sports, chess, debate teams, or academics when you were younger. Did you find that you really "got going" when you were competing head-to-head with some other person or team in a particular event? If so, the Competitive Hot Button could be just the key to get you started and to keep you involved in a powerful Start Strong, Finish Strong program.

The experience of "Ann" illustrates an approach along these lines that has worked for some people. Ann had tried to start both exercise and dietary programs on a half dozen occasions, but had always failed in her attempts.

"I don't think I ever made it past the first week," she recalled.

But then she decided to call three friends and set up a "pounds-off game," which involved competing to see who could lose the most weight and the most inches from stomach, hips, and thighs during a one-month period. Every pound lost counted as one point, and every half-inch lost counted as two points. To monitor their progress and motivate one another, they set up a time each week to weigh and measure themselves and enjoy some diet snack. The winner would then be treated to a "splurge" banquet at the end of the month—and the group would decide if they wanted to continue for another month.

"The key thing was not who was the fattest at the beginning or even who won at the end of the month," Ann said. "What we really wanted to do was to inspire everybody to lose something—that way, everybody would be a winner."

In fact, that's exactly what happened. The entire group of four lost pounds and inches, and they resolved to keep the "competition" going indefinitely.

For those just beginning a fitness program, however, competition can be a two-edged sword. On the positive side, the prospect of being able to compete more effectively in your club tennis program, golfing tournaments, charity walks, fun runs, or master's events may motivate you to push through the initial phases of a conditioning program. In such a case, before you realize it, you will really begin to increase your aerobic and strength capacities—and start putting out endorphins and dopamine on a regular basis.

But if you have an overly competitive personality, you may become your own worst enemy, especially in the first phase of trying to establish a good routine. For example, we've witnessed many out-of-shape competitors try to run too hard or fast at the beginning of a new program. Then they sustain injuries, such as muscle pulls or sprains, which derail them at the very beginning—and end up sabotaging their good intentions.

Others may be like the forty-one-year-old attorney who was still impressed by what a wonderful half-miler he had been in high school, even though he had done nothing to keep in shape since then. As a result of his memories of past glory, he began his Start Strong program a little *too* strong on the jogging track at his club, trying to run without any warm-up at a pace of under seven minutes per mile. In part, he wanted to compete successfully with his younger self; and in part, he couldn't bear the sight of other runners, including women and men who were older than he was, passing him with ease.

Less than a half mile into his first workout, he pulled up on the side of the track with a violently upset stomach. After throwing up a couple of times, he managed to drag himself back to the locker room, where he took a long shower and changed into his street clothes—and resolved never to run again.

This man's reaction to an overly strenuous workout without any attempt at prior conditioning was completely predictable. Nausea frequently overwhelms men and women of any age—including young military recruits—who are thrust into highly demanding aerobic activity without being in shape. Unfortunately, this man didn't have a drill sergeant to force him to get back on the track day after day at a lower level of intensity, until he built up the aerobic capacity to run without experiencing such side effects. As it was, his excessively competitive drive got him out on the track—but then turned against him when he started trying to accomplish physical feats for which he was unprepared.

Ken on Competition

Competition—with myself and with others—has always been an important factor in helping me stay in shape. I always "rev up" the intensity of my workouts when I'm scheduled for my annual stress test. This measure of aerobic capacity always shows clearly whether I've lost ground or have progressed enough to achieve another "personal best" in the time spent walking on the treadmill.

I'll admit that my sense of pride has always caused me to fear falling below the top "superior" category of fitness for my age group (as we measure performance at the Cooper Clinic). My competitive instincts have also driven me to prepare for a number of race-walk competitions in recent years—and I've even managed to win or finish toward the top in some local events.

At the same time, I'll admit that I'm sometimes like the guy retching on the side of the track in the previous example, in that I occasionally allow my competitive impulses to get out of control. I've been known to champ at the bit when someone passes me on a running trail when I think he or she shouldn't be passing me. I've almost knocked myself out by trying to take hairpin turns on a mountain bike at too high a speed. And I've broken my leg on a downhill skiing run that I should never have attempted, in part because my level of conditioning wasn't up to par.

I guess the lesson I'd derive for myself—and for you—from my past experience is that competition can be a great motivator. But it can also become counterproductive or even dangerous if you allow it to get out of control. So compete if you're so inclined, but compete with common sense!

Activate Your Competitive Hot Button: To make the best use of your competitive juices, you might join an organized athletic program, such as a master's swimming competition, a singles' tennis league, or a community basketball team. As you look forward to competitive events, you'll be more likely to gear your daily workouts to those events, as you engage in more demanding strength and endurance training in an effort to turn in a good performance.

THE LONER HOT BUTTON

Some people find that they love the idea of doing aerobic exercise because it gives them time to be alone with their thoughts.

A number of studies, including several involving Dr. Herbert Benson of the Harvard Medical School, have shown that some of our most creative thinking can done when we work hard to solve a particular problem and then find a way to break prior thought patterns. A great way to achieve this "creative break" is to engage in the repetitive movement of your feet and arms, especially in endurance-type workouts. The change of focus and activity leads to a reordering of brain patterns and physiologic responses—and frequently results in new ideas and the solution to seemingly insoluble problems.[2]

If you happen to be in this "loner" category, as a person who prefers solitary workouts, you may well find that a one-person sport, such as long-distance running, walking, or swimming, is just what you need. Furthermore, once you begin to develop a basic level of aerobic fitness after about three weeks to one month of working out, you'll likely find that you're also drawn to your daily routine by the Feel-Good Hot Button (see the description above). But at the same time, you'll almost certainly continue to savor the opportunity to spend an extended time alone with yourself and your musings.

Activate Your Loner Hot Button: If you're the loner type, reflect on what you like to do or think while you're alone. Do you mull over hard

Ken on Solitude

Even when other runners, walkers, or cyclists are in the vicinity, I often keep to myself as I work out because the experience gives me an opportunity to clear my mind after a hard day's work. I'm not really interested in talking—because I've usually been doing a lot of talking throughout the day.

Many times, as my feet rhythmically hit the ground, I find that I enter an almost trance-like state. Far from being physically exhausting, my exercise time at the end of each day is a reenergizing and rejuvenating experience. Some of my most creative thoughts and ideas occur during or immediately following my workout.

Caution: It's advisable not to engage in certain high-risk sports, such as skiing, when you're by yourself. If you do, and you're in an accident like the one that sidelined me (see Chapter 15) in Colorado, you could find yourself without help in a dangerous situation.

problems you're trying to solve at work? Ponder personal or family issues? Pursue a hobby? Enjoy the scenery? Pray? Just let your mind go blank?

If you're in this category, plan ways to incorporate your special interests into solitary exercise sessions. You might select a business problem that you want to consider while you're out for a walk. Or you might pray as you work in your garden. Or you might just clear your mind of all thoughts and look around at the foliage or buildings you pass on your outing. As the old adage goes, "Take time to smell the roses and listen to the birds sing." The objective is to reinforce your physical workout with a compelling mental component, which will further motivate you to exercise.

THE SOCIABILITY HOT BUTTON

Some people prefer to schedule a time to work out with a friend or group of friends and then to make those outings a regular part of their

Tyler on Electronic Companionship

Although I prefer working out with other people most of the time, I also have incorporated a kind of "companionship" into solitary workouts.

For example, I may use an iPod to listen to music as I walk. Or I might listen to a downloaded audiobook or some public radio program. I might even place calls on my cell phone or buy a newspaper and glance at it as I stroll along (but not, of course, when I'm crossing a street).

If I'm working out in the gym on some equipment, such as a treadmill or elliptical machine, I may simultaneously watch the news on TV. Another of my favorites is the TV quiz show *Jeopardy!* Because the program is thirty minutes long, it's perfect for the length of run I sometimes take.

There are many options these days to make working out alone less lonely—and many can motivate me to look forward to my workout sessions.

routine. Moreover, without such companionship, they may quickly lose interest in staying on a fitness program.

One fifty-five-year-old tennis player, "Jerry," loved the game, but, even more, he loved playing it with a particular friend. They typically got together twice a week for a few rigorous sets of singles, but the sessions weren't just devoted to the sport. At some point after playing a set or two, they would take a break and enjoy a conversation about their families, their work, their deepest longings, and other common interests. Because they had known each other for a couple of decades, they never ran out of comfortable, meaningful topics to discuss—and Jerry always looked forward to those regular talks as much as he did to the tennis.

But then Jerry's friend moved to another city, and Jerry confronted a hole in his schedule and in his life. He tried signing up for some random tournaments and round-robin matches at his club and also at a local recreational site. But even though the tennis was challenging, the experience just wasn't the same. What he missed even more than the sport was the social part, the friendship.

Soon, Jerry lost interest in tennis and went through a period when he did very little exercise. Eventually, though, after urging from his wife and his doctor, he got involved in a community slow-break basketball program for older players and began to enjoy some of the social interaction that he had missed since his tennis partner had moved.

Ken on "Misery Loves Company"

On some occasions, I find it necessary to work out at home, perhaps by taking walks in the neighborhood or doing calisthenics in the bedroom. But without question, what I enjoy most about working out at the Aerobics Center is the association with other people.

It's certainly true that when I walk, jog, or do strength work at the center, I nearly always exercise alone. But the camaraderie I enjoy *before* and particularly *after* the workout in the locker room is the reason I exercise at the center more than 75 percent of the time. Far from being a situation where misery loves company, working out in the presence of others is just more fun.

As you can see, relying on others to provide your motivation to stay fit can be a risky affair if your range of friendships is too narrow. Working out with one favorite person can be a highly satisfying experience, but if you've identified yourself as an innately gregarious, sociable type, you would do well to build some backup relationships into your fitness program. Otherwise, you may find that what you thought was a powerful hot button can, without warning, lose all power to transform your life.

On the other hand, there is often a major advantage to working out with only one other person if you have set up regular times to meet for your workout. That kind of scheduling commitment can be an extremely powerful motivator because the other person is depending on you to show up. If you don't show, you not only miss your workout but you also let the other person down. In a way, this situation becomes a concrete illustration of the ancient proverb that warns, one who "ignores discipline comes to . . . shame."[3] At the very beginning of a Start Strong program, this kind of mutual dependence may become the very factor that keeps you going long enough to establish a well-ingrained habit—even on those days when you would most likely skip a workout if you were pursuing a regimen on your own.

 Tyler on Sociability

Although I can always entertain myself when I'm exercising alone, I'd much rather run with someone else. In part, I'm just responding to the way I'm made: for as long as I can remember, I've liked spending time with friends and socializing during my leisure hours. But I've also been influenced by my experience on varsity cross-country and track teams in college.

Probably this preference for teams is the reason that I always gravitate toward running with a group or playing a team sport, such as basketball. It's much, much harder for me to stay motivated to follow a regular fitness routine if I try to do it by myself. On the other hand, I've always maintained a wide circle of friends who are interested in fitness—runners, skiers, rock climbers, basketball players. This way, I know that if any of my group outlets for working out should shut down, I'll still have plenty of others to rely on as my personal hot button.

Activate Your Sociability Hot Button: Join a fitness club or a group of friends who like to walk, jog, or do other brisk exercise regularly. If you need the reinforcement of others to stay on a weight-loss diet, you might also join Weight Watchers or some other established weight-loss group.

THE GOOD-LOOKS HOT BUTTON

Exercise can be used in three general ways: for cardiovascular conditioning; for rest and relaxation (or countering stress); and for muscle-building and figure-contouring. The first two have the obvious potential to prolong life. But the third use also can play a role in enhancing health—at least to the extent it keeps you on a regular fitness regimen.

One of the most disconcerting things about getting older is watching your face and body change—and concluding that those changes are entirely for the worse. So, depending on the extent to which looks are important to you—and to one degree or another, they're important to all of us—a major motivation for a Start Strong regimen may be that the program can make you look better, even as you age.

Think back on that little "mirror, mirror on the wall" exercise we suggested at the beginning of Chapter 1, where you took a hard, realistic look at your reflection. Being totally honest with yourself is an essential early step in planning a Start Strong program. But such honesty can be excruciating for those who have placed great value throughout their lives on looking attractive and youthful.

Fortunately, a precipitous deterioration in your physical appearance isn't inevitable. After you begin your fitness and diet regimen, you'll be amazed at the extent to which you can make that extra fat disappear and begin to restore the shape you enjoyed as a youth. Of course, you won't become twenty or thirty again, but you can certainly reverse or at least hold at bay many of the ravages of aging.

Perhaps most encouraging and exciting of all, you'll begin to garner all sorts of satisfying compliments:

You've lost some weight, haven't you?

Hmm, that arm is pretty hard—you work out?

What happened to that little potbelly?

That dress looks great on you.

What's happened to you—you look so relaxed and so much younger!

Sticking with a serious fitness program for a few months, and certainly for a year or more, will most likely completely transform your body and face. Such a commitment will cause you *to look younger than your years*—and in the end that's the real objective that will satisfy almost anyone who has a normal need to look good.

Activate Your Good-Looks Hot Button: Install a full-length mirror if you don't already have one. That's one of the most powerful motivational devices for those concerned about their looks. Also, it helps to associate with friends who are free with their compliments. The motivational juices can really begin to flow when another person says, "Wow, you're getting thin," or "You really do look younger."

THE COOL-CLOTHES HOT BUTTON

How many old clothes do you keep in your closet because you hold out the hope that someday you'll slim down and fit into them again?

Some spot-checking has revealed to us that one of the most powerful motivators that makes many women, and also a number of men, want to diet and work out is the desire to fit into clothes they have outgrown (or out-expanded!). You may have a favorite skirt that just won't hook in the middle anymore. Or a pair of slacks that is so tight along the backside that the seam seems about to split. Or a perfectly fine tuxedo with a jacket that binds almost painfully in the shoulders and back—and not because of too many muscles.

Many people in such situations find that they can stay focused on their fitness program just by remembering those overly tight articles of clothing—and periodically checking on any progress that's being made in making their body fit the wardrobe again. As mundane or even trivial as such motivation may seem at first blush, just remember this: the fundamental purpose of your hot button is to get you into that Promised Land of Fitness every day of your life. If that skirt you wore as a college student or the military uniform you've packed away is your measuring stick for how you're doing, take advantage of it.

Activate Your Cool-Clothes Hot Button: Select three favorite sets of clothing that no longer fit. Then try the clothing on about once every week to ten days. When you can start buttoning buttons you haven't buttoned in decades, your desire to stay on your program will soar.

THE HEALTH-CRISIS HOT BUTTON

Perhaps you've experienced a particular health scare, such as cancer or a heart attack. Or your doctor has warned you that some current condition—such as a vague type of chest pain, high blood pressure, a high PSA reading for your prostate, or a high blood sugar reading—makes you a prime candidate for a heart attack, stroke, prostate cancer, diabetes, or some other life-threatening condition. In such a case, you begin this Start Strong experience with a built-in Health-Crisis Hot Button that is likely to motivate you to do all you can to head off the impending threat.

Many times, it may seem a good idea to combine this particular hot button with one or more of those mentioned below—such as the Please-the-Doctor or Numbers-Game Hot Buttons—and there's absolutely nothing wrong with such combinations. The hot button you design should be your most effective personal "switch," which will turn on the most powerful reservoirs of motivation you possess. So feel free to be creative as you explore those inner forces that are most likely to help you start and finish strong.

Activate Your Health-Crisis Hot Button: Closely monitor the medical measurements that relate to your health condition. If you're most concerned about cardiovascular risk—perhaps because you've had a heart attack—check your blood pressure regularly with a home monitoring device (daily wouldn't be too frequent). Also, during your checkup with your doctor, ask for copies of tests for your cholesterol, C-reactive protein, homocysteine, calcium deposits in coronary arteries, and other measurements related to your cardiovascular problem (see Chapter 5). Then compare how you're doing with the results of your last physical.

THE FEAR-OF-DEATH HOT BUTTON

The Health-Crisis Hot Button often includes a heavy dose of fear of death. But this fear is not something most people like to talk or think about. In fact, just mentioning the D word in a typical social setting can be a total conversation-stopper—for very understandable reasons: when the subject is introduced, listeners tend to experience a rise in their levels of what has been called "personal death awareness," a response that causes them to go into a state of total denial about their own death.[4]

Of course, this dread of death is by no means a recent phenomenon. The first-century BC Latin writer Publilius Syrus wrote, "The fear of death is more to be dreaded than death itself." William Shakespeare restated the same insight in his *Measure for Measure* when his character Isabella said, "The sense of death is most in apprehension."[5]

Contemporary thinkers and philosophers since Ernest Becker in his landmark, Pulitzer Prize–winning book, *The Denial of Death,* have recognized that a fear of death underlies most of our other major fears and anxieties.[6] Yet this fear—which most of us experience periodically—isn't just a psychological quirk or a figment of somebody's imagination. The older you get, the more normal and natural it is for you to become aware of your own mortality. In fact, studies show that by the time you reach age forty-five, you can expect disease to become a bigger mortality threat than accidents.[7]

In any case, if you are one of those hearty souls who can look death in the eye without blinking—and you know a major reason you want to improve your fitness is to postpone death—then by all means use this hot button. There's absolutely nothing wrong with getting involved in a fitness and weight-loss program because you want to postpone a visit from the Grim Reaper. In fact, there's much to be said for such a motivation.

As indicated in the discussion of the previous Health-Crisis Hot Button, many, many of our patients get involved in life-giving, life-sustaining Start Strong, Finish Strong programs after they discover they are at high risk for a certain disease or health condition, or after they have experienced a heart attack or some other scare. They know that after learning of their mortality risk, they don't have to lie down and give up on life. Instead, they have been given an extremely valuable opportunity to counter their genetic weaknesses, poor family history, or unhealthy lifestyles of the past. The fear of death they are experiencing is often all they need to activate an extremely powerful hot button, push open the locked door in that wall, and enter the Promised Land of Fitness.

Activate Your Fear-of-Death Hot Button: Don't aggravate the fear of death, but do learn to use it. Usually, we don't have to worry about activating this fear—it will pop up automatically. Yet most people find that when they embark on a fitness and weight-loss regimen—and become aware that increased fitness and weight loss lower their risk of mortality[8]—the fear of death remains but doesn't paralyze them.

THE PHYSICAL-FUNCTION HOT BUTTON

Almost one-third (29 percent) of Americans fear loss of physical capacity as they grow older—and rightly so.[9] A number of government studies beginning in the 1980s and continuing to the present have revealed that the average American may live the last eight to twelve years of his or her life with some chronic, debilitating health condition, such as heart disease or back or joint problems that limit mobility and normal functioning.[10]

If you have had to care for bedridden or otherwise disabled elderly relatives, you know firsthand just how devastating such a condition can be. In any case, the simple awareness from such experiences that *your own* normal functioning might be in danger in the future may be sufficient to prompt you to see your physician and launch a Start Strong program.

In the same vein, for a long time now we have been preaching the importance of "squaring off the curve" of life (see Chapter 2), or taking rigorous steps to improve your fitness so that you will be less likely to become one of those people who loses the ability to function in some major way as aging occurs. National and international government reporting agencies have taken to referring to this concept as the "healthy life expectancy"—or the number of years you can expect to live a fully functioning life. Some of the most recent figures show that the average American male born now can expect to have a "healthy life expectancy" of sixty-eight years, and the average American female, seventy-three years—even though the *actual* life expectancy for each is considerably longer. (When males and females are averaged together, the average life expectancy of a child born in 2006 is 77.9 years.)

So how might you translate these facts into an effective hot button?

The answer is relatively simple: if you are disturbed by the thought of losing your ability to function physically, you can take one of two courses of action. On the one hand, you can just worry, as many do, by doing nothing more than saying to yourself and others: "Oh, I hope I won't be one of those who ends up disabled or confined to a wheelchair in a nursing home for the last five or ten years of my life. That's the worst thing I can imagine." Or you can *do* something about your anxiety, beginning right now. The best—and perhaps the *only*—antidote to a premature failure of function in life is a Start Strong, Finish Strong fitness program, which should begin immediately!

Activate Your Physical-Function Hot Button: Begin to keep a record of your ongoing strength and endurance capacity.

In a notebook, diary, or computer folder, enter the number of minutes you spend walking or jogging a mile; the number of crunches or sit-ups you do in a typical workout; the number of push-ups you do; and so forth. Then, at least once a month, revisit your entries to see if you're improving, staying the same, or declining in your strength and endurance.

If you find you're either improving or staying the same (if you've reached a performance peak), then you're probably succeeding in warding off a loss of physical function.

THE MENTAL-FUNCTION HOT BUTTON

Many of our patients over fifty years of age begin to express concern about a slowing down or loss of mental functioning, and their experience is apparently normative. According to one national survey, nearly two-thirds of Americans (62 percent) fear losing their mental capacity as they age.[11]

Some will say, "I don't memorize as easily as I did when I was younger."

Others complain, "I'm not as quick as I used to be crunching numbers in my head."

Still others moan, "I find that when I'm making an argument, I sometimes lose track of the point I'm trying to make."

In fact, a number of studies have shown that as people age, their ability to remember long sequences of numbers diminishes. People in their late thirties or early forties may be able to remember a sequence of nine to twelve unrelated numbers, while those older than sixty or seventy may drop to five or six, or even fewer.

Yet as we already know from the previous chapter, staying physically fit can enhance your mental functioning. For one thing, you'll find that as you exercise more, your mental health will improve, and you'll be less likely to become depressed.[12] In particular, regular physical activity, such as walking, will help mental functioning and hold off cognitive decline.[13]

Also, eating a kind of brain-food diet—especially the consumption of fish—may bolster your mental functioning. One fish meal a week has been shown to slow age-related mental decline by 10 percent annually, and two fish meals a week slow mental decline by 13 percent annually, according to a 2005 study in the *Archives of Neurology*.[14] Fish-oil supplements containing high levels of omega-3 fatty acids, including EPA and DHA, also may be beneficial.

Simply on an anecdotal basis, we have found consistently that Cooper Clinic patients—including the two of us—tend to think more incisively and crisply when regular exercise is a standard part of the daily routine, along with one or two grams of omega-3 fish-oil supplements. Most likely, you'll find the same benefits, and if you do, this Mental-Function Hot Button may well become your primary motivation to stay on a fitness program.

Tyler on Mental Alertness

I've consistently found that combining exercise with intellectual activity makes me mentally sharper. When I was studying in medical school and began to get mentally fatigued, I'd take a break for a run. When I returned to the books, my mind was always clearer and my thoughts more focused.

While working on my master's from the Harvard School of Public Health, I discovered a similar benefit: I got into the habit of walking about a half hour from our apartment to class. I was always much better prepared to sit, think, and participate in class after the walks than I ever was after driving to classes.

Activate Your Mental-Function Hot Button: Just launching the aerobic phase of your Start Strong fitness program will improve your mental functioning, according to the latest research.

Also, get into the habit of doing crossword puzzles or other mental exercises. Or sign up for a course at your local college. Or embark on a memorization program—using Shakespeare's works, the Bible, or some other classic literature. You might also learn to play a new musical instrument or learn new songs for an instrument you already play. The added mental challenge will help remind you that physical fitness and mental functioning go hand in hand as you grow older.

THE SPIRITUAL HOT BUTTON

Those who have a deep religious faith may well find that their basic assumptions and convictions about life demand that they take care of their minds and bodies.

For example, those with a Christian or Jewish orientation might start out with the common understanding that all that God has made is "good"—and that includes our bodies.[15] Also, there are various passages in the New Testament that state that our bodies are the "temple of God" or the "temple of the Holy Spirit."[16]

Such views, which have analogues in Islam and other faiths, may add a strong impetus to avoiding food and beverages known to place the body or mind at risk. Sometimes, those with these beliefs may decide that eating unhealthy foods or drinking to excess (or drinking at all) "pollutes" the body and mind that God has made. The individual's own willpower then begins to conform to his or her broader belief system—and staying on a productive fitness program becomes immeasurably easier.

One forty-eight-year-old man, after contemplating his image in a full-length mirror for a few moments, found himself coming to the remarkable conclusion that "God doesn't want me to be carrying around this excess fat." For a long time he had known that he was overweight. But somehow, he had never connected the rolls around his waist to God.

Still, an important question remained: how could he translate this insight—the conviction that God didn't want him fat—to the dinner table?

He found a fairly simple, straightforward answer: recalling various admonitions from his religious tradition against gluttony and imbibing alcohol, he resolved to eat only one modest helping of food at each meal (he had been accustomed to piling on at least one extra helping every time he sat down at the table). Also, he limited himself to one glass of wine at his evening meal—and cut out cocktails before the meal. As a result, he began to lose at the rate of two pounds a week, and at the end of six months on this program, he was thirty-five pounds lighter.

Those from most of the major religious traditions have found that combining prayer and meditation with repetitive aerobic exercise, such as walking, jogging, or cycling, can enhance both the spiritual and physical experience.[17] One jogger, for instance, reported that by combining his morning meditations with his running, he had inadvertently created a double reason to stick with his fitness program:

"At the beginning of each day I can't wait to experience the encounter with God in prayer, but also I can't wait to experience the sense of well-being that always comes after the workout."

Activate Your Spiritual Hot Button: Examine closely what your own religious tradition teaches about caring for your body and mind. Then integrate your fitness workout into some spiritual discipline. For example, you might jog with a friend who likes to discuss theology. Or if you exercise alone, you might meditate on a short passage of religious or spiritual literature.

THE PLEASE-THE-DOCTOR HOT BUTTON

If your physician serves as a kind of cheerleader for his or her patients, take advantage of it. Most internists and many specialists will become deeply interested in you personally and your progress if you will just make them aware that you want to improve—and that you value their help. Also, by bringing your doctor into the equation, you'll reinforce your motivation—because most people (even physicians themselves) respond positively to recommendations made by a physician who examines them.

Remember, most patients dread visiting the doctor's office, and they can't wait to get out of the examining room. The idea of disrobing and submitting to prodding and poking and various uncomfortable tests often obscures what the exam is all about: monitoring your health and fine-tuning your improvement with appropriate lifestyle adjustments and various prescriptions and medical procedures. In dealing with your doctor, we'd suggest that you follow a strategy that includes these features:

- Ask your doctor specific questions about exactly where you stand in terms of your cholesterol, your blood pressure, and other risk factors.
- Tell him or her that you really want to improve—and ask for advice about what you can do on your own to make progress.
- Be open to the idea of scheduling more frequent visits to your doctor.

An annual physical by your family doctor is a minimum for this hot button. But if you have a problem you're trying to correct, visiting twice or three times a year or even more often could be appropriate.

- *Don't* view your doctor as an adversary, or as someone conducting distasteful tasks that you have to endure. Instead, see your physician as a *source of motivation,* who can keep you moving in the right health and fitness direction.
- *Don't* feel that you have to limit yourself to a physician for this benefit.

Sometimes, having a personal trainer, dietician, tennis or golf pro, or other "coach" who has oversight over your health or fitness will work just as well. Typically, this person will contact you several times a month to monitor your progress as you try to lose weight, stop smoking, control your alcohol consumption, stop substance abuse, or follow a physician-prescribed medication routine.[18]

The main idea is to decide whether this health or fitness "authority" is someone you would like to please—and would be very unhappy to disappoint.

Activate Your Please-the-Doctor Hot Button: See your physician more often. Once every two to four months is not too often if seeing him or her motivates you. And if you have a particular condition that's being monitored, a doctor's visit once a month may be appropriate.

If you prefer working with a trainer or other fitness professional, sessions once a week or more often may keep your motivational levels high.

THE NUMBERS-GAME HOT BUTTON

A related hot button focuses on the "health numbers" you assemble during each visit to your physician. Many patients want to become more knowledgeable about their bodies and about the meaning of blood work or other tests that may be flagged as "high" or "low." When patients understand the meaning of the various numbers and measurements, they are more likely to be motivated to do what they need to do to improve.

For example, one fifty-one-year-old woman became particularly intrigued by the challenge of lowering her cholesterol through lifestyle changes rather than through prescription drugs. Her total cholesterol number was in the 240 range, which placed her in a higher-risk category than her physician wanted. Also, a couple of her emerging markers for heart risk—C-reactive protein and homocysteine—were elevated.

The doctor told her that to help correct these problems, he would advise her to go on Lipitor, a rather expensive cholesterol-lowering drug, *unless* she could bring her numbers down below the 180 range. Most of the reduction in her total cholesterol number would have to come from a lowering of the "bad" LDL cholesterol. (Her "good" HDL cholesterol was high enough that a total cholesterol reading in the 180 range would most likely make her ratio of total cholesterol to HDL cholesterol less than 3.0—a level that would place her in a low-risk category for heart disease.)

As the physician explained the steps this patient would need to take to lower her cholesterol, he expected that she would quickly become discouraged. So he was surprised to see her eyes light up and her interest heighten when he said:

> You'll have to lose about twenty pounds. And you should increase your exercise from your current walking times of twenty minutes a day to more like forty minutes. Also, you'll have to get rid of those foods with excess saturated fat and trans fats—such as the cookies or piece of cake you like to eat for many of your desserts, and the fried foods you eat once or twice a week. Finally, and I know this is going to hurt, those stops at fast-food restaurants will have to go.

Contrary to the doctor's expectations, the patient became excited by his suggestions. Just the challenge of lowering the "bad" LDL cholesterol and raising the "good" HDL cholesterol was enough to inspire her to want to change her way of life. She said she saw the experience as a kind of game, which she would win—through bettering her health and lowering her heart risks. All she had to do was to succeed in changing her numbers significantly.[19]

Activate Your Numbers-Game Hot Button: Keep good records of the numbers that most interest you, and periodically see how you're doing. You might get into the habit of recording your weight at least once a day in a journal. Another possibility is to enter your weight in your daily schedule diary. The same approach works with cholesterol readings, blood pressure, or any other numbers relevant to your particular health concerns. Then the game becomes your challenge to lower those numbers or put them in a healthier balance.

THE MATERIAL-REWARDS HOT BUTTON

The so-called token-economy method of inducing behavior changes often works quite well, especially with children. The main idea here is to provide material rewards, such as products or even money, in exchange for improved fitness behavior.

With adults, this approach to motivation has changed the lives of many who have joined certain fitness plans offered by a growing number of employers. These companies have set up health and well-being programs that provide financial bonuses for those workers who stop smoking, lose designated amounts of weight, lower their blood pressure or cholesterol, or pursue a regular exercise program. For example, at the Cooper Aerobics Center we have had a Cooper Fit program for more than fifteen years. Members of our staff receive a monetary reward at the end of each year if they meet our Cooper Fit Standards, which include markers for weight loss, physical fitness levels, and other health-related factors. As a result, our health insurance cost is quite low.

What's the motivation for the employer to make such arrangements available? Those companies that employ this strategy have found that absenteeism goes down and their medical costs plummet—because their workforce is becoming healthier. In particular, corporations who have implemented work site wellness programs with incentives have noticed one or more of the following:

- Decrease in the cost of employee health care
- Decrease in absenteeism due to disease
- Increase in work productivity
- Increase in the company's ability to recruit the best employees in the marketplace
- Reduction in employee turnover

Because of the benefits of such programs, the majority of companies with five hundred or more employees have some type of work site wellness plan. Clearly, good physical fitness for the employee is also good "fiscal fitness" for the employer.

Apart from such a formal job-site program, this material-rewards motivation can be difficult to establish for adults. For children, the parents can control the dispensing of rewards fairly effectively. So if the child misses a particular workout, he or she doesn't get the allowance bonus or toy that is being held out as the carrot for the desired fitness behavior. But adults in charge of their own behavior find it easy to cheat; that's why having an employer in charge works so well.

Still, there are ways around this problem, particularly if you decide you're going to be completely honest with yourself. For example, you might resolve that if you lose five pounds, you'll reward yourself with a new dress. Another five pounds will qualify you for another reward, such as a massage.

To reinforce your commitment to spend the minimum time it will probably take to form new habits (see Chapter 4), you might decide that at the end of thirty straight days of following your chosen exercise and diet regimen, you'll award yourself a new tennis racket or set of golf clubs. But again, the key component of this independent token-economy approach is to be ruthlessly honest with yourself—and don't under any circumstances give yourself that reward if you haven't earned it.

If you know you'll never abide by such a reward system on your own, you might form a group and charge "dues" from each member, which goes into a pot and is distributed as various members meet attendance goals. The main objective would be consistency and faithfulness in sticking to the program. So if your goal is to work out together three times a week, at the end of each month you might reward all those who have participated in every session that month.

Numerous studies by behavioral psychologists have shown that participants in such token-economy programs—whether in a formal organization, such as a corporation, or on their own—tend to be driven initially by the material rewards. But after a month or two, the habits become ingrained and develop a self-sustaining life of their own, with no need for the dispensing of material rewards. (For a fuller discussion of how habit formation works, see the discussions in the next chapter.)

Activate Your Material-Rewards Hot Button: Act today to set up a simple set of goals—either weekly or monthly or both. Also, choose the rewards you'll give yourself if you achieve your goals. Write them down in a journal, computer folder, or other location where they'll be readily available for your reference and where there won't be any chance you'll misplace them.

A tip: For best effect, rewards should be dispensed *regularly* and *in close proximity* to the act being rewarded. So it's best for most people to plan on weekly awards *and* a monthly "grand prize," and not monthly rewards alone.

Is It Okay to Have More Than One Hot Button?

The easy answer to this question is yes—definitely yes. Also, one motivational impulse may sometimes be hard to distinguish from another.

For example, the preceding description of the Numbers-Game Hot Button may have reminded you of the Competitive Hot Button, and, in fact, the two can be quite similar. In other words, these inner "passion switches" aren't mutually exclusive, and may overlap. So you don't have to choose one and then automatically eliminate all the others. In fact, you may find that your particular hot button is a combination of several of those described earlier.

As a further illustration, you might experience your strongest surge of motivation when you link both the Numbers-Game and the Please-the-Doctor Hot Buttons. Or you might prefer to rely on a Please-the-Doctor Hot Button initially. But then you find you're more influenced by the Feel-Good Hot Button as you develop a greater aerobic capacity and experience more and more of those surges of dopamine, endorphins, and other biological sources of well-being.

Or as many of our patients do, you may rely on the Spiritual Hot Button to get you started on a program. Then you turn to the Competitive Hot Button to add excitement as you get in good shape and want to test your progress against that of others. And finally, you "press" the Sociability Hot Button to allow you to spend more time with your friends and family when they want to go out for some exercise.

By now, you're probably coming to some conclusions about what hot button, or combination of hot buttons, will work best for you. As you make your decision, keep in mind this guiding principle: the main reason to find the right motivation is to get past that high wall with the locked door and enter that Promised Land of Fitness—the exciting, high-energy world where you will be able to transform your life physically and emotionally.

But it's one thing to enter this Promised Land and quite another to make a permanent home there once you've arrived. To achieve an ongoing fitness program, which will enable you not only to *start* strong but also to *finish* strong, you'll have to learn how to employ your newfound motivation to create habits that will last a lifetime.

Because forming good habits is a scientifically based process, it seems fitting to begin our exploration of this issue with an observation by the nineteenth-century British physicist John Tyndall: "The formation of right habits is essential to your permanent security. They diminish your chance of falling when assailed, and they augment your chance of recovery when overthrown."[20]

"Right" habits, then, are more than just nice things to have. They are essential to protect us from the most challenging physical threats we may face in life, including those that accompany aging. Fortunately, once established deep in our inner nature, right habits have the power to do great good in our lives. So now, let's consider exactly how we can incorporate these important new behaviors into our own personalities.

Four

The Science of Starting
and Finishing Strong

The secret to finishing strong with a fitness program—or anything else in life—is to establish personal habits that will last a lifetime. So how can you cultivate the habits that will lead to the benefits described in the last couple of chapters?

As we all know, developing positive patterns of behavior is often not easy. But fortunately, the science that lies behind the Start Strong, Finish Strong program is solid and powerful. If you can exploit that science effectively, you'll be off to a good start in actually establishing those habits in your own life.

The Incredible Power of Habits

Good and bad habits have long been the subject of deep concern—so much so that massive social and political campaigns have arisen to eradicate various bad habits. Yet it's become evident that legal prohibitions will go only so far in correcting bad habits. In fact, many times, attempts to legislate morality fail miserably because those who have made up their minds to pursue a particular bad habit will always find some way around the law.

Furthermore, from the medical viewpoint, bad habits are often too powerful to eliminate from the outside—except in a few situations where medications may help to blunt extreme cravings for certain substances, such as alcohol, drugs, or nicotine. Usually, though, bad habits must be tackled from the *inside* if you hope to change them, and one of the best ways to achieve this transformation in personal behavior is to replace bad habits with good ones.

Of course, none of these observations is particularly new. The Latin writer Publilius Syrus beat us by more than two thousand years when he declared in the first century BC: "Powerful indeed is the empire of habit."[1] In any case, it's up to *you* to recognize that powerful forces rage deep inside, pushing you toward bad health and, ultimately, physical destruction, or toward good health and a more energetic, productive life.

But still, you have to find ways to *develop* those good habits. And for the past century or so, some very smart people in our Western scientific tradition have been sending us messages that provide at least a part of the answer we need.

One of the most innovative thinkers who began to pull all this together in scientific terms, William James, lived and worked at the end of the nineteenth century and the beginning of the twentieth. But he was a man ahead of his times. In fact, James was, in many respects, the founding father of all our modern theories of habit formation.

William James: Small Acts Lead to Big Habits

As part of a long Harvard University tradition that has explored mind-body interactions, the philosopher-psychologist-physician William James became intrigued by what it might take to develop good habits.

James, who trained and taught at Harvard, Stanford, and other leading universities, was one of the first to perceive and explore scientifically how habits are formed in the body. In the process, he came up with insights that can be extremely helpful to us today.

In his 1890 work, *Principles of Psychology,* James said that to transform ourselves, we must "make our nervous system our ally instead of our enemy. . . . We must make automatic and habitual, as early as possible, as many useful actions as we can and guard against . . . growing into ways that are likely to be disadvantageous to us."[2]

Now think about that statement for a moment. What James was calling for more than a century ago is precisely what we're calling for in this book—the building of powerful, positive behaviors. But he didn't stop just with stating a good goal. He proceeded to show the average person how to *form* good habits. To this end, he laid down some maxims that we prefer to call "habit rules," which establish this basic guiding principle for those pursuing a Start Strong, Finish Strong program: *Daily acts, no matter how small, are the key to forming permanent habits.*

In more detail, here's what James advised:

HABIT RULE #1: "LAUNCH [THE HABIT] WITH A STRONG INITIATIVE."[3]

In effect, James said "start strong" more than a hundred years ago. He advised that you should place yourself in situations that will encourage the development of the habit you want to foster. If possible, "take a public pledge" that will make it hard for you to break the habit when you're in the company of friends and colleagues.

HABIT RULE #2: "SEIZE THE FIRST POSSIBLE OPPORTUNITY TO ACT."[4]

From the first moment you act, James argued, new patterns and "grooves" will begin to form in your brain, influencing your "nerve-cells and fibers" where "molecules are counting" the acts, protecting you against a relapse. James emphasized that no matter how good your intentions, if you don't act, your body, mind, and spirit will remain entirely unaffected. "With mere good intentions, hell is proverbially paved," he said.

HABIT RULE #3: "ACT ON YOUR HABIT A LITTLE EVERY DAY."[5]

Do something, no matter how small, every single day, and preferably several times a day, to reinforce the good habit you're trying to build, James advised. He said that the action that reinforces your habit may "be the least thing in the world . . . but let it not fail to take place." Only by constant action, he added, will good wishes be "grooved by habit in the brain."

James outlined this "intention-habit-character" growth sequence:[6]

- Act frequently on your good intentions.
- As you act, your will strengthens.
- As your will strengthens, your personal character improves.
- As your character improves, your brain "grows," making it natural for you to continue to act.

Ahead of his time scientifically, James anticipated that the repetitive actions that groove habits involve changes in the brain and body, including our nervous, hormonal, and biochemical systems. Today, we know a great deal more, and some of the most significant findings continue to emerge from James's alma mater, the Harvard Medical School.

The Biology of All Sorts of Habits

William James stood at the beginning of a Harvard Medical School scientific tradition of mind-body medicine that continues up to our own day.[7] Furthermore, much of that landmark research has added substantially to our understanding of what goes on in our brains and bodies as habits become ingrained.

In the 1890s, James asked one of his top students at the university, Walter Cannon, to find all the scientific research he could dig up on human emotions and their influence on the body and brain—an experience that gave Cannon a lifelong enthusiasm for investigating the effects of the mind on the body. Perhaps most significant of all his work, Cannon is credited with identifying the fight-or-flight response—a physiologic reaction to stress that can fix many *bad* habits deep inside us.

FROM THE STRESS RESPONSE TO BAD HEALTH HABITS

During the fight-or-flight response, the body releases adrenaline, noradrenaline, cortisol, and other "stress hormones" and neurotransmitters. The original purpose of this stress response was quite positive: appropriate fear or anxiety elevates our blood pressure, heart rate, breathing rate, and various metabolic reactions so that we become better prepared to fight wild animals or other life-threatening challenges—or run away if fighting seems too dangerous.

Unfortunately, the contemporary pressures of work and personal life can cause our minds and bodies to release the stress hormones in inappropriate situations. This stress response can, in turn, encourage the development of negative physiologic responses—and related bad habits—which may result in such disastrous, health-threatening conditions as chronic high blood pressure, heart disease, obesity, chronic pain, and other stress-related ills.[8] Here are just a few types of bad health and fitness habits that may arise when we fail to plan ways to control out-of-control stress:

The overeating—or unhealthy eating—habit: Eating favorite foods causes the release of neurotransmitters of well-being, much as aerobic exercise can do. So you may overeat whenever you feel "there's nothing else to do"—and you become bored or agitated by what you perceive as a lack of other options. Or you may turn to comfort foods to ease the impact of stress or unhappiness. As we often say, "Obesity is the most common manifestation of stress." (Many people know how chocolate works in such situations.)

To counter stress, many have slipped into the habit of eating second and third helpings—or consuming huge portions of a first helping. In fact, nutritionists at New York University reported in 2002 in *The American Journal of Public Health* that the average serving of pasta is now 480 percent greater than the one-cup recommended serving size.[9] They also said that actual servings of some cookies are 700 percent larger than the recommended serving amounts.

The sedentary-living habit: You may have found that you've avoided a scheduled workout—or even an exercise program—because it seems easier to give in to less demanding diversions from exercise, such as a snack, a TV program, or a cocktail. Those distractions, which easily become ingrained habits, almost always add unnecessary calories. Or at least they prevent you from enjoying the benefits of a regular fitness program.

The poor-sleep habit: As we all know, skimping on sleep will exact a heavy price the following day. Yet often, we allow stress to creep into our lives and rob us of sleep.

Job and personal worries and preoccupations may cut into our regular physical activity, and to compensate we may turn to unhealthy "feel-good" activities, such as staying up late watching mindless TV, eating snacks, or drinking extra alcohol. The body and mind gradually become comfortable with that "bad" behavior and actually begin to crave it. Also, late eating, drinking, or dozing in a chair before the TV set—especially without exercise—will often contribute to insomnia or fitful, disrupted sleep. At one time or another, we've all lain awake in bed worrying about some person or issue that seemed unimportant or completely manageable the next morning.

The substance abuse habit: When we're under stress in our society, alcohol, drugs, and tobacco are the usual ways to counter the stress and to "feel good" quickly. Unfortunately, such substance habits lead to an array of unhealthy results, such as heart disease, cancer, liver damage, and the like.

The accommodation-to-stress habit: After falling into bad habits such as those mentioned above, the body begins its own silent, often deadly responses. Blood pressure goes up. The risk for various cancers increases. Adult-onset diabetes may appear. The brain doesn't work as well, often with a decreasing ability to concentrate and an overall deterioration of brain cells.

The constant triggering of the stress response in your life and automatically grasping for a familiar bad habit may force you into one of these ruts, with serious health consequences. Fortunately, a physiologic answer to the stress response—a kind of "antistress response" that can open the door to good fitness habits—was identified over three decades ago by Herbert Benson, a Harvard Medical School scientist and cardiologist who stands in the tradition of William James and Walter Cannon.[10]

FROM THE RELAXATION RESPONSE TO GOOD HEALTH HABITS

Herbert Benson's landmark research culminated in the late 1960s and early 1970s in the identification in humans of the "relaxation response," a biological mechanism that is the polar opposite of the fight-or-flight response.[11] Now, the experts are concluding, the relaxation response has the power to do for good habits what the stress response does for bad ones. The research by Benson and scientific teams who have collaborated with him has shown that the relaxation response works in a predictable sequence, which we believe has significant implications for the formation of Start Strong fitness habits. In a nutshell, here's how the sequence unfolds:[12]

- Actions that break the train of prior thought and emotion—including repetitive exercises such as jogging, walking, regular breathing, or silently repeating a word or phrase—trigger a release of nitric oxide in your body's cells.[13]
- This release of nitric oxide coincides with the release of various "neurotransmitters of well-being," such as endorphins and dopamine.
- As these and other "feel-good chemicals" take hold, your mood becomes positive, pains disappear, and a sense of happiness and well-being becomes dominant.

THE START-STRONG HABIT EFFECT

As this sequence proceeds, your mind and body—that is, *you*—are going to be *pulled* toward experiences that make you feel good. And it would be hard to find an experience that feels better than the endorphin-dopamine rush you get with exercise. As your fitness level increases, you'll actually find you don't have to "work up" positive feelings toward your fitness routine: they'll already be at work on their own because of the beneficial changes in your body chemistry.

Furthermore, when mental exercises that evoke the relaxation response—such as repetition of a positive phrase or word—are combined with aerobic exercise, your oxygen uptake (efficiency in processing oxygen) improves. Also, your satisfaction with the exercise tends to increase.

As exercise is combined with peaceful inner thoughts, including steady repetition of a word or phrase that is rooted into your deepest passions and motivations, the pull toward the exercise gets even stronger. Herbert Benson's research into the relaxation response and related issues makes this "magnet effect" quite clear.[14]

In the resting state after exercise—and in any resting state where the relaxation response is operative—your heart and breathing rate decrease, your blood pressure goes down, and your overall rate of metabolism is lowered. Functional MRIs conducted by Benson and his research teams have shown that when the relaxation response takes over, overall brain activity calms down—though attention and executive centers of the brain, which control attention and learning, become more active.[15]

The calming of the brain and other physiologic changes that occur with the relaxation response will actually prepare your mind and body for beneficial conditioning and learning.[16] Medical research has established that exercise itself raises levels of biochemicals and hormones "known to serve synaptic plasticity and learning."[17]

So if you work out regularly, you can expect the connections in your brain to improve and your ability to learn to expand. In a related set of findings, studies were conducted on the connection between fitness and mental performance in almost one million fifth, seventh, and ninth grade students in California in 2004. They showed a highly significant relationship between levels of fitness (as measured by our Fitnessgram designed by the Cooper Institute) and academic achievement in reading, mathematics, and English-language arts.

The mental benefits continue well into old age. Those who regularly invoke the relaxation response over a period of years actually experience an increase in the cortical thickness of their brain cells, according to the research of Benson and his colleagues. This result points to antiaging benefits for such relaxation-promoting activity as aerobic exercise— because aging involves thinning of cortical thickness.[18]

To sum up, then, as you pursue the Start Strong, Finish Strong strategies, there is solid scientific evidence that you can expect to develop fitness habits that will transform your life permanently for the better. Furthermore, you can expect those habits to become part of an overall experience that has been called "positive addiction."

The Ultimate Goal: Positive Addiction

The term "positive addiction" refers to behaviors and habits that are good for us, but that also produce certain "withdrawal symptoms" if we attempt to stop pursuing them. The psychiatrist William Glasser, who has been credited with originating the term, concluded that the long-distance runners he had studied had become addicted to the repetitive movements of their sport.[19]

In other words, "addicted" runners, as well as those involved in other types of regular aerobic exercise, typically reach a point where they feel they *have* to work out daily. Otherwise, they experience overall achiness, fuzzy-headedness, and other out-of-sorts symptoms. But unlike unhealthy addictions, the final result of this kind of addiction is *positive*, as shown by the numerous scientific studies that have proven exercise is good for health and longevity.

Over the years, those who have accepted the idea of positive addiction resulting from regular fitness activities have offered a variety of reasons for the phenomenon. But the dominant explanation has focused on an increase in the body during exercise of the natural morphine-like transmitters called endorphins. This explanation, of course, fits in nicely with the more extensive findings of Benson and other researchers that the good feelings associated with the relaxation response are linked to the various neurotransmitters of well-being, such as endorphins and dopamine.

As a caveat, there may be a point where a very strong positive addiction may have adverse effects—in particular, a phenomenon referred to as "overtraining."[20] To avoid turning a positive addiction into a negative one, you should "listen to your body," as the saying goes. In other words, monitor yourself regularly to be sure you don't experience ongoing muscle pains, fatigue, or the like. If signs of overtraining occur, cut back on the frequency of intensity of your workouts, or shift to another type of physical activity—but don't stop. You can't "store" fitness. Like many other great experiences, exercise is truly a journey, not a destination, and for maximum healthful effect it must be continued for the rest of your life.

The experimental biologist Peter Sterling has offered an intriguing explanation of how both negative and positive addictions might work to form habits. "Many behaviors . . . are driven less by the promise of reducing anxiety than by the expectation of 'reward'—some outcome that leads to a feeling of satisfaction," he said.[21]

This reward, he says, is the rush of dopamine produced by certain of our acts—regardless of whether those acts are good or bad for us. So if we can find a way to select a *healthy* activity that produces the dopamine that turns us on, we'll have the key to transforming our bad behaviors into good ones. And what activity could be healthier than exercise?

So now, we know some of the "hard" science that undergirds habit formation, but what do the psychologists have to say? One who has been very active in this area is James O. Prochaska, director of the cancer prevention and research consortium and professor of clinical and health psychology at the University of Rhode Island.

The Psychology of Habit Formation

Prochaska, who has focused on breaking such bad habits as alcohol abuse and smoking, has developed a rather simple strategy, known by the mouthful term, "transtheoretical stages of change model."[22] Simply stated, his model identifies five basic stages for transforming bad habits into good.

These include first what he calls *precontemplation,* a phase where a person really isn't thinking about changing at all. Then, he says, the individual moves to a state of *contemplation,* which involves beginning to understand that change may be beneficial. This stage may involve a period of several months where the person begins to wake up and consider seriously the benefits and drawbacks of making changes.

A stage of *preparation* comes next, which includes making small changes but still is characterized by a lack of complete commitment to change. This preparation phase appears to be primarily a transition stage, which may lead to the *action* stage. It's during this action stage that real change and the fixing of good habits begin to take hold. Typically, it's necessary for the person to be in this action mode for at least six straight months for true change to take hold. Finally, Prochaska identifies a *maintenance* stage of change, where the person continues to strengthen his or her new habits daily.

This Prochaska sequence has worked rather well in many areas of habit formation, including altering unhealthy behaviors such as smoking, alcohol abuse, or even exposing the skin to the sun without using sunscreen. But even with all the solid scientific and psychological evidence for habit formation that we've examined so far, we still need a practical motivational model that will fit the Start Strong, Finish Strong program.

The Start Strong, Finish Strong Motivational Model: How to Form Your Personal Fitness Habits

The model that we suggest you follow to establish solid fitness, dietary, and health habits can be summarized in the following seven "motivational acts."

ACT #1: MAKE A FINAL SELECTION OF YOUR HOT BUTTON.

This special motivational switch will light a fire in your life—and will cause you to *want* to start and continue to follow a life-changing fitness program. Although a number of possibilities for this hot button have been listed in the previous chapter, don't regard that list as exhaustive. If you possess a passion that hasn't been mentioned—but you believe it will get you started and keep you going—be sure to take advantage of it.

ACT #2: SET STARTING DATES.

Write them down in your daily calendar of things to do. These would include kickoff dates to start your exercise program, shop for better foods, look into a substance abuse program, and undergo a comprehensive medical exam.

ACT #3: PLAN YOUR PROGRAM.

The seven simple start-ups described in Part Two will give you all the information you need to plan your fitness and weight-loss program. Once again, here's a summary of what we'll be exploring in Part Two:

Step #1: Quit putting off that gold-standard physical exam.
Step #2: Launch a realistic fitness plan.
Step #3: Begin eating a longevity diet.
Step #4: Follow a wise supplement strategy.
Step #5: Do serious smoke control.
Step #6: Counteract creeping substance abuse.
Step #7: Engage in effective mind-spirit practices.

ACT #4: BEGIN TO ACT DAILY ON EACH PART OF YOUR PROGRAM.

Now, begin to move forward in the William James mode, with consistent small steps or acts that create those "brain grooves" that will culminate in a positive habit. Your actions can be small, but they must be consistent and regular. In this regard, it's helpful to remember the old adage "By a yard it is hard; by an inch, it's a cinch."

More specifically, when you are trying to establish habits, you should do something to reinforce those habits *every single day.* So if a low-fat diet is one of your primary objectives, your first main challenge may be to avoid buying as many foods containing trans fats or saturated fats as possible (see Chapter 9). The small but steady steps you take to alter your supermarket shopping routine will go a long way toward helping you avoid *eating* commercially prepared desserts or crackers, which are full of trans fats. And cutting back on your regular pit stop at the local fast-food joint will eliminate hundreds, if not thousands, of calories in saturated and trans fats.

Your daily action plan for your fitness program might involve this routine: let's say you walk only ten minutes a day, three or four days a week. Then, you work in the yard on a fourth day. On a couple of your nonwalking days you begin some sort of strength training, such as ten minutes of calisthenics or light weight work. As you can see, we're not talking about long, onerous time periods to help you jump-start your program. Rather, the goal at the beginning is to do something, no matter how small, to firm up your habit *every single day of the week.*

But as you build up your endurance and strength, it's certainly acceptable to allow for some flexibility within each daily objective. For example, as you increase your walking time—say, to thirty or forty minutes, three to four days a week—you may find that you can't always do it for the full time period. That's okay! But do try to get out there for a short time—even five to ten minutes. *Regular daily actions* at the outset are the key to establishing a permanent habit.

You may notice that this exercise advice is somewhat different from the common recommendation to take one or two days off each week to allow the body time to rest and repair itself from any soreness, stresses, or strains. The reason for our variation is that we're assuming that when you first launch your program, you'll be exercising at a lower intensity level than you will later. As you increase your endurance and muscle strength over a number of months, you'll probably want to jack up the intensity of your activities, a change that will most likely cause you to shift to fewer days of certain activities per week.

But at the very beginning, even if you don't do some formal exercise every day, *do* engage in some sort of physical activity, such as a longer walk to the supermarket or vigorous yard work. With the Start Strong, Finish Strong strategy your overriding objective is to develop habits that can surmount all sorts of challenges over the years. To achieve this result, your fitness behaviors should become so ingrained that they morph into permanent parts of your personality. To achieve this result, you should set and reach a series of daily health and fitness targets.

Finally, the daily actions you take with your emerging Start Strong program should be associated with your hot button. That way, you'll be much more likely to *want* to act rather than to avoid action. For example, if you've selected a Sociability Hot Button, try to act in concert with others. Or if you prefer the Competitive Hot Button, turn your actions into challenging games. Or if you are drawn to the Spiritual Hot Button, incorporate some prayerful or meditative component into your activity.

ACT #5: CONTINUE TO ACT DAILY
FOR FOUR WEEKS.

Daily actions in support of your fitness habit will become an integral part of your being after about three to four weeks. At the end of that period, you'll begin to move naturally every day toward the exercise and foods that are going to transform your life.

Caution: If you sustain an injury during this period or later in your program—or if you miss a few sessions for some other reason—don't give up. First of all, you can continue with your new dietary regimen, even if your ability to exercise has been impaired. Second, just because you are blocked from one activity—say, you can't jog because of tendinitis—you still may be quite capable of swimming, cycling, or doing strength work that avoids putting stress on the injured part of your body. Also, remember always to listen to your body and respond accordingly.

ACT #6: KEEP ON ACTING DAILY
FOR ANOTHER FIVE MONTHS.

At the end of this period, you will have devoted six straight months to fixing the new fitness behaviors in your brain and body (one month to make a strong start, and five more months to fix the habit). Most experts would regard that length of time as quite adequate for developing new habits that won't go away, even if you experience some significant distractions or relapses.

How long does it take to form a habit? In general—provided that you can find the right hot button that will enable you to jump-start your motivational juices—you can expect that most good habits will begin to become a fixed part of your mind and body after about four to six weeks of following the desired behavior.

During the initial start-up period, your body's physiologic response to physical activity—such as aerobic exercise—will tend to change for the

---

Ken on Getting Hooked on a Habit

I tell my patients that if they will stay with a fitness program for a minimum of six weeks, the chances are they will be hooked.

I've seen a number of people fall by the wayside and fail to follow an exercise program because they allow themselves to be distracted—and the program to be interrupted—after only about two to three weeks. Many times, they give up for one of the reasons listed at the beginning of Chapter 3, such as the excuse they don't have enough time or the program isn't fun.

But when patients make it past the six-week mark with their exercise regimen, few fall by the wayside. And when they make it to the four-to-six-month threshold, their success rate approaches 100 percent.

better. Instead of feeling strange or uncomfortable, you'll actually begin to crave the activity. But even with this positive shift, it will be important to fortify yourself further against a total collapse of your program—a collapse that can cause you to return to your prefitness state. To bulletproof yourself against such backsliding, it will probably be necessary to set a goal of four to six months as the minimum period to fix your habit.

Of course, certain habits may be especially hard to form or break. As

 ## Ken on Relapsing

I've been about as faithful as anyone could be with my exercise program during the past fifty years, and I must say I had a great start as a young athlete. I was a varsity track and basketball player in high school, and I went to the University of Oklahoma on a track scholarship.

But in medical school and the few years following, I completely abandoned any effort to keep in shape. As a result, my weight ballooned, and my endurance capacity and strength declined precipitously (see Chapter 9 for a fuller version of my eating problems during those days).

Fortunately, after a heart irregularity following an intense waterskiing workout, I came to my senses and embarked on a fitness regimen, which culminated in the aerobic message that I advocate around the world today. But I also realize that I was very lucky to have been scared into making the transition from high-level college sports to an ordinary fitness program. Too many former athletes are driven to stay in shape only by the next school competition or by the pressure placed on them by a coach.

When the competition and the coach are gone, they need to find another source of motivation—or risk becoming total couch potatoes. Fortunately, my own Feel-Good Hot Button and Loner Hot Button have sustained me over the past five decades and, I'm sure, will continue to do so in the years to come.

a result, there may be more of a tendency to relapse with certain behavioral changes than with others. If you're trying to quit smoking, drinking, or overeating, for example, you may find that unless you stay on a formal program, such as Alcoholics Anonymous or a clinic-run group dietary or antismoking regimen, you'll slip back into the bad habit.

But with these caveats in mind, you can assume that you'll need at least three to six weeks to begin to condition your biochemical and neurological responses in the desired way. After that, it will begin to seem "natural" to exercise and eat well. And after four to six months, you'll find it's relatively unlikely that you'll revert to a total relapse in behavior. Now, with these basic facts and guidelines in mind, let's pull it all together into a Start Strong motivational model that will work for you.

ACT #7: EXPECT TO SLIP—BUT ALSO EXPECT TO GET BACK ON TRACK.

There are many reasons for you to slip or relapse with your program. You might sustain an injury that makes it impossible to continue for a while with your chosen mode of exercise. Or you might splurge with food or drink on a particular weekend. But none of these failures should discourage you from picking yourself back up and returning to your program. There are many alternative strategies to overcoming temporary setbacks—such as the time-honored tradition of cross-training.

One way or another, a good habit should always become a "good fit" with a person's overall personality and personal makeup. In other words, even before the habit becomes an ingrained behavior, you should see it as something that will make you a better or more effective person—and as something that connects with what motivates you most deeply in life. Or, to put this in Start Strong terms, your hot button should help you build and reinforce your fitness habit. Conversely, any attempt to establish a habit that is not connected to your deepest passions and motivations is likely to fail.

For millennia, observers of habit formation have said that the best

---

Tyler on Cross-Training as a Response to an Injury

I broke my ankle while I was in college—a devastating turn of events for someone who was an intercollegiate track and cross-country competitor. But I knew I had to keep in shape if I wanted to return to the team after my injury healed, so I tried swimming.

I had never included swimming in my conditioning program before, but I began to train in the pool as though I were a competitive swimmer. As a result, I was in good overall shape when my ankle finally healed, and I was able to return to the track team with minimal loss of aerobic capacity.

But as important as this experience was for me as a track competitor, it's taught me an even more important lesson now that my college days are well behind me: namely, that cross-training can be a valuable strategy for maintaining a fitness program as we grow older. As a result of my swimming experience in college, I now have an alternative if I just don't feel like running on a particular day: I can jump in the pool at the Cooper Aerobics Center and swim a mile or so.

Cross-training certainly doesn't have to be limited to one alternate sport, such as swimming. I have friends who alternate their normal workout with use of various exercise machines, such as a stair-stepper or circuit weight training. In any case, the older I get, the more I become convinced that cross-training is a major secret to fitness motivation.

---

and strongest habits are those that have become a part of the individual's basic nature. The first-century Greek author Plutarch said, "Custom is second nature,"[23] and Montaigne, the sixteenth-century French writer, echoed the same sentiment in his *Essays:* "Habit is second nature."[24]

In the tradition of these two sages, you are now on the road to developing fitness and health habits that will soon become second nature. You have absorbed some valuable information that will enable you to get started on a Start Strong, Finish Strong program. In particular, you now know your hot button or buttons—the inner switches that can motivate you to make significant changes. You know how to use hot buttons to form lasting fitness habits. And you also know the probable consequences if you fail to square off the curve of your life.

Now, all you need is a practical program to make it all happen. And that brings us to Part Two and the seven simple Cooper start-ups that will revolutionize your body, your mind, and your life.

Part Two

The Seven Simple Cooper Start-ups

Five

Start-up #1—Don't Put Off Your Gold-Standard Physical Exam

A *complete* preventive-medicine exam is the absolutely essential first step in your Start Strong program—for at least three reasons:

- To alert you and your physician to any *hidden health problems* that could now threaten your health or your life.
- To establish *baseline measurements* that could identify a danger to your health in the future.
- To provide *motivation* for you to improve your health and fitness— beginning right now.

Why should you take these reasons to heart? Here are just a few considerations, which we hope will encourage you to make an appointment today:

REASON #1: HIDDEN HEALTH PROBLEMS

Perhaps the most important function of a complete physical examination is that the evaluation gives your doctor a great opportunity to identify hidden health problems that may have the potential to kill you. Many times at the Cooper Clinic we have identified serious heart problems during stress tests; tumors and other heart problems during fast computerized tomography (CT) exams; diabetes as a result of blood tests; osteoporosis during bone scans; and countless other conditions. Yet without a complete exam, sudden death may be the first symptom that reveals you have a serious problem.

These points come alive in the context of a couple of actual experiences involving some friends of ours:

The inconsistent couple: A woman in her midfifties, who had experienced heart arrhythmias (irregular heartbeats), came to us for an exam. But her husband—who also had serious health concerns—refused to join her.

What was so bad about the husband's situation? First of all, he was a heavy smoker. Second, he was the son of a father who had undergone a bypass operation after having a heart attack at age sixty, and the brother of a man with very high cholesterol. Both the smoking and the bad family history constituted serious risk factors, greatly raising his chances for a heart attack, stroke, or other cardiovascular catastrophe.

When Ken asked what he was doing to counteract his risk factors and improve his fitness, he answered, "Not much."

He said he was playing a lot of golf, though he was using a golf cart. On the positive side, he had managed to quit smoking.

At one point, Ken told him, "I'm not going to give up!"

But unfortunately, this husband ran out of time. His car stopped on him while he was out for a drive, and he made the mistake of pushing the car onto the side of the road when the temperature was close to 100 degrees. Immediately he began to feel nauseated. He called his wife, and she told him to get into the shade and find something to drink. So he entered a nearby building, managed to find a glass of water, and sat down in a chair. A few minutes later, however, he had slumped to the floor.

After a call to 911 by his wife, an emergency medical crew arrived and began to administer first aid, including defibrillation (shocking his heart). He was finally resuscitated, but he had been without oxygen too long, and the brain damage was too great. He never regained consciousness. The cause of death was determined to be an acute MI (myocardial infarction, or heart attack), with multiple vessels 80 to 90 percent occluded (blocked).

What had been this man's biggest mistake?

It wasn't that he had "chosen" the wrong family history or even that he had been a heavy smoker—though both these risk factors contributed significantly to his condition. No, his biggest mistake was that he had failed to come in for a complete physical exam, which would have included a stress test and a fast CT scan. With those evaluations, we most likely would have picked up his occluded (blocked) coronary arteries, and medication and surgery might have given him a new lease on life.

The wise executive: Another patient, a retired airline pilot and multiyear jogger, came to us when he was in his early seventies. With our usual battery of tests, including a state-of-the-art stress test, we identified a coronary artery blockage, which eventually required a five-vessel bypass operation. After the surgery and rehabilitation, this man went back to his jogging program and in October 2005, he participated in a two-mile competitive event, running the distance in under 21 minutes—even though he was eighty-seven years of age.

This pilot is also representative of our average male patient, who, through wise Start Strong, Finish Strong principles, adds about ten years to his life span and also significantly improves his quality of life. In fact, the average life expectancy of all patients at the Cooper Clinic is well above the national average of less than seventy-seven years.

Without such a *complete* exam, however, dangerous or even lethal health problems may go undetected (see also the accompanying account, "Ken on the Jim Fixx Syndrome").

Ken on the Jim Fixx Syndrome

More than twenty years ago, I authored a book entitled *Running Without Fear: How to Reduce the Risk of Heart Attack and Sudden Death During Aerobic Exercise,*[1] which was written in response to the tragic demise of my friend Jim Fixx, the running guru who wrote a major best seller in 1977, *The Complete Book of Running.*[2] Although Jim inspired millions to don their running shoes, his death during that ill-fated workout on a Vermont highway in 1984 might have been avoided if only he had added a regular, complete preventive-medicine exam to his fitness program.

In a nutshell, his story unfolded this way:

Jim had a horrendous family history of heart trouble. His father, Calvin, had suffered a heart attack when he was only thirty-six years old, and he had died of a heart attack when he was just forty-three. It may not have been a coincidence that Jim began to run regularly when he was about thirty-six—or the age at which his father had suffered his first heart attack.

But running by itself isn't enough. Like many people, Jim avoided the doctor's office like the plague—and that proved his undoing. In 1973, at age forty-one, he did undergo a stress test because he was writing an article on the subject. But the test was conducted at a "submaximal" exercise level, or well below both his predicted maximum heart rate and the level that would have been necessary to detect any cardiovascular disease.

Much later, just six months before his death in 1984, I invited Jim to undergo a stress test at the Cooper Clinic. He was working on an article on Johnny Kelley, the renowned Boston marathoner who, at the time, was pushing eighty years of age. Jim declined my offer, giving no reason. But I later learned from his sister that he had a respiratory ailment and was probably worried that he might not perform well on the test.

That decision may have sealed his fate. If Jim had undergone the stress test, there was a very good chance that we would have identified his coronary artery disease, including the fact that he had three severely blocked coronary arteries leading to his heart. We then would have pre-scribed proper medication or surgery.

His autopsy revealed the consequences of his failure to undergo an exam: scar tissue on his heart indicated that he had suffered at least two heart attacks prior to the one that killed him on that highway in New England. One or both of the "silent" heart attacks might have produced only mild chest discomfort or might have escaped his notice entirely. But as far as we know, he never had any signs or symptoms of heart dis-ease before his fatal run.

Even though the memory of Fixx and his tragic experience may have faded somewhat over time, a crucial lesson remains for us: don't delay scheduling your first gold-standard exam, and don't neglect regular follow-up exams. Your life depends on it.

REASON #2: BASELINE MEASUREMENTS

When you go in to see your doctor with a particular complaint, he or she will be in a much stronger position to prescribe the right drugs or recommend the appropriate medical procedure if you have provided a complete set of medical measurements and evaluations. Physicians are quite interested in *changes* that occur in your body and blood as you grow older. But without a set of baseline readings, it's difficult or impos-sible to determine whether any changes have occurred.

One of our patients, Will, who has undergone several of our gold-standard exams, represents the experience of countless others with this baseline-measurement issue. In 1997, when he was in his midfifties, he had a complete exam, including a CT scan, which provides a picture of a patient's heart, lungs, other organs, and blood vessels. The scan report also gives a coronary artery calcification score, which shows any calcified plaque buildup in the arteries supplying blood to the heart—an important read-ing because clogged coronary arteries are the main cause of heart attacks.

Will's very low calcification score in 1997—which was far below the average scores for others in his age group—showed that at the time he had absolutely nothing to worry about as far as his coronary arteries were concerned. Will grew even more confident about his health outlook because he had been on a reasonably low-fat diet and a regular aerobic exercise program for years. His marginally high total cholesterol, which typically ranged from about 190 to 220 mg/dl didn't seem of particular concern to him, either. But then, he made an almost fatal mistake: for several years, he neglected to go in for another exam.

Fortunately for Will, he did finally return for another complete physical in 2004. This time, the CT scan revealed some disturbing developments in his coronary arteries. During the seven-year period during which he had missed his exams, his calcification score increased to put him in the "average" category for his age. (For an explanation of the calcification scores taken from a large population of patients who have undergone CT scans over a number of years, see the charts on pages 370 to 371 of the Appendix.)

Now, *without* the prior baseline score determined in 1997, this reading would probably have been tabbed as worth monitoring in the future, but not necessarily as something to act upon immediately. But *with* the prior baseline score, our Cooper Clinic physician who conducted the exam immediately determined that the increase in calcification had been occurring at a significant, if not alarming, rate of over 40 percent per year!

Also, another component of Will's gold-standard physicals over the years helped provide a possible explanation for the rather dramatic increase in calcification: his family medical history showed that several of the male members of his family had begun to run into cardiovascular problems when they reached their fifties and sixties. For example, one of his grandfathers had died of a heart attack in his midfifties, and another grandfather had succumbed to a stroke in his late sixties. Even more ominous, his father had died of a heart attack in his early sixties.

In other words, what may have been happening with Will was that his low-fat diet and regular exercise regimen had carried him into his fifties in fine health. But then, as he moved toward sixty, his genetic history kicked in. Without medical intervention, he couldn't escape the inherited tendency of males in his family to develop serious cardiovascular problems in the fifty-five to seventy age range.

But that gold-standard medical exam in 2004, and especially the CT scan, alerted Will's doctor to the need for extra help to counter Will's genetic predisposition. As a result, Will went on low doses of a statin drug, which lowered his total cholesterol to 170 mg/dl and took his "bad" LDL cholesterol down to about 90 mg/dl—ordinarily considered an acceptable score.

But we now believe that even more may be required. With a history of heart disease in the family and one or more coronary risk factors, a patient should have LDL levels close to 70 mg/dl. Some studies conducted at the Cleveland Clinic have shown that lowering LDL cholesterol to 60 mg/dl using the drug Crestor in doses of 40 mg per day—and keeping the LDL at that level for two years—can actually cause a 10 percent reversal of plaque in the coronary arteries.

In any event, with Will, as with many of our other patients, the baseline numbers in the physical exam were critical in helping us monitor changes in those numbers and treat him most effectively in light of the changes.

REASON #3: MOTIVATION

A complete preventive-medicine exam can be decisive in motivating patients to change their ways—especially when the exam includes hard visual or numerical evidence of a particular health problem. For example, we've seen countless patients literally *rush* to comply with health and fitness recommendations when they were confronted with very high cholesterol or blood pressure numbers, or, better yet, with a picture of their calcified coronary arteries.

In an April 2006 report in the journal *Atherosclerosis,* for instance, when patients saw a scan showing plaque accumulation in their own arteries, their adherence to a lipid-lowering drug program increased significantly.[3]

In this study—which was conducted by N. K. Kalia and colleagues at the Division of Cardiology, Harbor-UCLA Medical Center, Research and Education Institute, in Torrance, California—the researchers evaluated more than 500 heart patients with electron beam tomography (EBT).

The patients were all placed on statin therapy to reduce their elevated blood fats (lipids), which had raised their risk for a coronary problem. The EBT, which produced pictures of their arteries that the patients could study, showed their levels of coronary calcium accumulation (i.e., the amount of calcified plaque in their arteries that could block blood flow to the heart and trigger a heart attack). Then the patients were monitored as to their compliance with cholesterol statin drug therapy over the next two to three years.

Kalia and his colleagues found that the statin compliance was lowest (44 percent) among those with the lowest calcified artery score—that is, those who had the least amount of blockage in their coronary arteries. But 91 percent of the individuals with the highest scores stuck consistently to their statin therapy program.

The researchers concluded that "patients visualizing coronary artery calcium may improve . . . adherence to lipid-lowering therapy."

A senior member of the research team, Dr. Matthew Budoff, stated his conclusions about the study this way: "This is one of the best and easiest methods to improve patients' compliance, not only with cholesterol medications, but with diet and exercise as well. Patients' seeing the calcified plaque in their own coronary arteries was a powerful motivator of good behavior [for] over three years."[4]

In other words, if you actually *see* those coronary arteries getting clogged up, you're *very* likely to take steps to do something about it. But despite such compelling reasons to undergo a gold-standard exam, we often resist the idea. So what's the problem? What's holding us back?

Why Do We Resist Getting the Exam?

We have probably heard just about every excuse known to man or woman for not getting a complete preventive-medicine physical. But here are some of the most common:

Objection #1: *This kind of exam takes too much time—*
I'm a busy person!

Although this objection often goes unstated, it's probably the most common reason of all. Too many people imagine that they are the busiest individuals on earth and conclude that they just can't spring free. Yet this objection is somewhat illogical because it takes almost no time at all to undergo a complete annual physical at an efficiently run preventive-medicine facility.

At the Cooper Clinic in Dallas, for instance, if you plan on coming in from out of town, you'll probably devote part of one day to travel, and then most of one full day to the actual examination. Those who need to get back home quickly can usually fly out the same day that they've had the exam. So for most people, it takes less than two days, including travel time, to finish the whole checkup.

Furthermore, the very small amount of time you spend on a gold-standard physical may very well save you days, weeks, or even years of being consumed by an illness or by recuperation.

Objection #2: *It costs too much money.*

At a center like the Cooper Clinic, a complete physical would cost you in the range of about $1,500 to $3,500, depending on whether you undergo only the basic, standard tests—such as a complete blood workup and stress test—or whether you undergo additional prescribed tests, such as an echocardiogram, nuclear scan of the heart, CT angiogram, or a colonoscopy.

Now, this outlay of funds may at first glance seem rather exorbitant, especially if you're used to spending only a few hundred dollars at the most for a less extensive physical. Also, our health-care system is still rooted in the old-fashioned notion that medical care is meant for those who are sick, not those who are well. Unfortunately, many of our medical insurance programs buy into the false assumption that the only care worth paying for is "sick care," not preventive care. As a result, you may find that you have to pay for much if not all of your preventive-medicine exam out of your pocket—unless, of course, you are a participant in a forward-looking insurance program that encompasses such exams.

But reflect for a moment: if you could prevent the loss of tens or hundreds of thousands of dollars—and the loss of weeks or months out of your life—in the near future, would you spend $1,500 to $3,500 right now to do so? Most of the people we know would answer yes to that question and never look back.

Of course, you may really not be able to afford the cost of a complete gold-standard exam every year. But that shouldn't deter you from going in every two or three years for such a checkup, or undergoing more limited annual exams that come as close to the gold standard as possible. A regular medical checkup in your family doctor's office with some of the basic components of the complete preventive exam is certainly better than not being checked at all—and may very well alert your doctor to possible problems that will require further tests. This basic evaluation should include laboratory tests such as a blood workup; resting ECG; investigation of your blood pressure and heart rate; evaluation of unusual physical formations or lumps, and basic bodily functions; and a frank discussion with your doctor about symptoms or abnormalities you may have noticed. Such a physical should cost no more than a few hundred dollars, much of which may be covered by your health insurance if you have some medical condition that the physician is monitoring, such as elevated cholesterol or blood pressure.

Objection #3: *The exam covers too many unnecessary items—chances are I'll never have a problem with 99 percent of the things I'm being tested for.*

Ken on Cost-Effective Personal Health

When patients question me about the cost of an exam, I like to ask, "What did you pay last year for the insurance on your car, or your home?"

After they respond, I usually say, "You can buy a new car or build a new house. But you have only one body. And the body is masterful in disguising its problems—until it's too late. That's why the most common first symptom of severe heart disease is sudden death."

In fact, 40 percent of the people who die from heart disease have no history of heart problems. So what's the best health strategy to help you guard against this danger? A complete preventive-medical exam.

My final words to them typically go like this: "What you pay for such an exam is the best health and life insurance you can buy."

It would be great if you could know exactly what illness or condition you're likely to suffer or die from, because then you could order and pay for a limited round of tests that would focus only on your special problem. But, unfortunately, such medical crystal balls just aren't available—and probably never will be.

To be sure, we can evaluate risk for different health problems—that's a large part of what a preventive exam is all about. For example, we may determine from your family history, blood lipids, blood pressure, and other factors that you are at a great risk of experiencing heart problems or cardiovascular challenges in the near future. Then, after we have outlined your particular risk, we can be sure to check those components of your exam especially closely to see if your risk is increasing, or if your lifestyle adjustments and medical interventions are lowering your risk.

But even if you seem at greatest risk for one condition, we know from experience that we can't overlook other possibilities. Too often, for example, a CT scan administered during a regular annual physical at the clinic will reveal that a heart patient has developed a tumor or some other condition that has nothing to do with his or her heart.

In short, there are virtually no tests in a well-designed preventive-medicine examination that are "unnecessary." All are essential for you and your examining physicians so that you can be as sure as possible that *all* your health risks are being properly managed.

Now, let's get to the heart of the matter—the details about what tests should be included in your exam.

Checklist for the Gold-Standard Physical Exam

Although exams vary from clinic to clinic, you should expect the following tests when you go in for a gold-standard preventive-medicine exam. We've kept this description of the twenty-five key tests relatively short so that you can use it as a kind of checklist to be sure you're getting everything you need when you go in for your exam.* Many clinics will regard some of these items as optional or will outsource certain exams to specialty clinics or hospitals in their area. If you're given the option to have a particular test but find you have to go to another location in the city to get it, don't be put off by the inconvenience. Be sure to take advantage of the opportunity.

How often should you go in for one of these complete, gold-standard exams?

In general, we recommend that everyone have a complete baseline

---

*A somewhat similar list was included more than twenty years ago in Ken's *Aerobics Program for Total Well-Being* (New York: M. Evans and Co., Inc., 1982, 221ff.). But even though much has stayed the same in preventive-medicine testing during the intervening years, much has also changed—especially with such new diagnostic devices as the fast computerized tomography (CT), also known as the EBT (electron beam tomography) scan. Also, the latest gold-standard exam includes more precise blood tests for blood components that may signal newly recognized cardiovascular risk factors.

physical with all of the tests listed below as early as possible—and at least by age thirty-five. At age forty, you should begin to undergo a complete exam every two to three years. When you reach fifty years of age, you should increase the frequency of the gold-standard physical to once every year to eighteen months. For everyone over sixty, a modified, if not a complete, exam should be done annually.

But of course, if you have a particular health condition your doctor is monitoring, you should go in more often for special tests and checkups as they are needed. Also, certain tests, such as the pelvic exam and Pap test for women (described on page 97), should be done at least annually.

Beyond the "Quick Cure"

For the complete physical at the Cooper Clinic, we have pioneered what we believe is the best way to obtain optimum results, not just a "quick cure"—a preventive-medicine exam, which involves a four-step approach:

First, we conduct a thorough, comprehensive preventive-medicine-type examination.

Second, we make the exam an educational and motivational experience. To this end, our physicians see only four patients per day, and spend at least one and a half hours with each patient.

Third, we provide the patients with implementation programs that are safe, effective, and realistic. In other words, we don't set goals that are too high or unrealistic or mandatory.

Fourth, we urge the patients to come back to us at variable intervals, depending on their wishes and response, for follow-up evaluations.

In general, most physicians do a good or reasonably good job in evaluating a patient (the first step). But they often do a less than optimum job in the other three steps because of insufficient time. The need for those last three steps is a major reason preventive medicine is a specialty of its own, unable to be combined with acute care specialties. So do your best to find a preventive-medicine specialist to conduct this gold-standard exam for you.

TEST #1: COMPREHENSIVE HEALTH HISTORY

Typically, the clinic will supply a questionnaire that will include such information as your personal history of disease, prescription medications, dietary supplements, and surgery; your family's history of disease; your eating habits; your drinking habits (i.e., number of alcoholic drinks per week, number of glasses of water per day); your substance use (smoking, etc.); and your exercise routine.

TEST #2: BASIC PHYSICAL MEASUREMENTS

The physician's assistant should record your height, weight, percentage of body fat (using calipers to measure skinfolds, or another measuring device), blood pressure, pulse rate, measurements of your waist and chest, and an evaluation of your bone size.

Also, we now recommend determining the ankle/brachial index, which measures the systolic blood pressure in both arms and both ankles. The ratio should be greater than 1.0. A lower reading indicates a decreased blood flow to the lower extremities, a condition that may need to be corrected. Because this index is a good predictor of future coronary problems, physicians are increasingly regarding a low measurement as a new coronary risk factor.

TEST #3: EXAMINATION OF HEAD AND NECK

This exam, which includes both visual inspection and palpation with the hands, will alert the physician to any unusual size of the head or neck or the presence of swollen lymph nodes, nodules on the thyroid gland, and quality of pulse in the neck (at the carotid artery). At times, listening with a stethoscope over the carotid arteries will reveal a bruit, or "whistling" sound, which is indicative of significant obstruction that may require surgical correction.

More than once, we've picked up nodules or tissue masses on the thyroid gland, which have turned out to be malignant. Catching such an abnormality early can enable your physician to take preventive measures to correct conditions that could be very serious or even fatal if they are allowed to continue untreated.

TEST #4: PHYSICAL INSPECTION OF EYES

Just looking closely into the eyes using a beam of light can uncover a variety of diseases or serious health conditions. These include cataracts; "floaters" and other changes in the retina as a result of high blood pressure; brain tumors; or diabetes.

TEST #5: FEELING THE LYMPH NODES

We've already mentioned palpation of the neck, but the lymph nodes of the underarms and groin should also be checked. This exam is especially effective in picking up various types of infections and early malignancies.

TEST #6: CHEST EXAM WITH A STETHOSCOPE

This exam will often provide the first indication of emphysema, asthma, tuberculosis, or a variety of heart problems.

For example, a murmuring sound made by the heart during this phase of the checkup may signal the presence of a heart valve problem, which will require patients to take a round of antibiotics before they go in for a dental exam. Those with this condition who fail to take antibiotics may suffer a fatal infection called bacterial endocarditis. Also, during this part of the exam, irregular heartbeats may indicate the need to take medications or other measures to correct an underlying problem with the rhythm of the heart.

TEST #7: PHYSICAL MANIPULATION OF
THE ABDOMINAL AREA

Just feeling for abnormalities in the abdominal cavity can reveal an enlargement of the liver, which may indicate cirrhosis of the liver; congestive heart failure; or an abdominal aneurysm. Also, palpation of this area may alert your doctor to various lumps that could indicate the presence of an abnormal mass or malignancy.

If your examining physician finds a suspicious mass, he or she may order an X-ray CT scan or abdominal sonogram to provide a picture of exactly what's going on inside. With a sonogram, the specialist conducting the test will have a chance to pick up other problems with the gallbladder, spleen, kidneys, or pancreas. We have identified a number of malignancies this way and have also identified aneurysms (weak points on arteries), which surgeons have been able to correct before a potentially fatal rupture occurred.

TEST #8: RECTAL EXAM—INCLUDING PROSTATE
EXAM FOR MEN

Many patients—and even physicians—like to skip this exam because of its location and discomfort. But the test is important in helping physicians identify malignancies in this part of the body, and is absolutely essential for men in detecting prostate problems.

The physician must insert his finger into the male rectum in order to feel the condition of the prostate gland. A hard or enlarged prostate, or one with a nodule, may indicate a malignancy. In such cases, the physician will usually refer the patient to a urologist, who will perform a needle biopsy. Prostate cancer that is identified and treated early tends not to be fatal, unlike prostate cancer that has gone untreated for a lengthy period.

TEST #9: PELVIC EXAM AND PAP TEST FOR WOMEN

The frequency of cancer of the cervix in women has declined significantly since the 1930s, mainly because of the effectiveness of the annual Pap test and pelvic exam. Unlike the general recommendations mentioned above, this test should be conducted annually after a woman reaches childbearing years.

TEST #10: RANGE OF MOTION AND STRENGTH OF BONES AND MUSCLES

In this visual and physical check, the physician will see if you have a normal range of motion and strength in your arms and legs. The doctor may ask you to hold an arm or leg out and then may press or pull on it to evaluate your strength in different muscles.

TEST #11: SKIN EXAM

In this visual check, the doctor will scan your entire body to be sure that you don't have suspicious lesions or blemishes that may suggest a malignancy. If he or she finds something suspicious, your doctor will send you for additional consultations with a dermatologist or other specialist. Remember that skin cancer is often easily cured if diagnosed at an early stage. Don't die of something stupid.

TEST #12: NEUROLOGICAL EXAM

The well-known reflex response, involving tapping the knee or tickling the bottom of the foot, could point to a disc problem in the back or perhaps a neurological problem. Reflex tests are also often the first step in identifying brain tumors. Other tests may be employed to evaluate the cranial nerves and cerebellar function in the brain.

TEST #13: BLOOD, URINE, AND OTHER LABORATORY ANALYSES

As we have identified additional risk factors in recent years, the number of elements in blood tests has increased significantly. For example, at the Cooper Clinic we now regularly test for homocysteine and C-reactive protein, which have been recognized as important new risk factors for cardiovascular disease. We also routinely do a PSA test for men to check for possible prostate cancer. If the result of this test is elevated, you may be given a percent-free PSA, which is more accurate. These tests weren't a part of regular, comprehensive blood testing a couple of decades ago.

A complete set of lab tests can be divided into the three categories listed below. Because many of the items tested are usually written in medical shorthand, we've tried to take some of the mystery out of your report by highlighting a few of the specific tests that are of special interest to many patients. But these explanations are not the whole story. You can assume that many other tests will be included in your analysis, and so you should be ready to ask your physician for further explanations.

Each of these laboratory test results, which should be reported to you as a list on two or more printout sheets, will have a column with the normal range of results, or with a "negative-positive" indication. If you are within the normal range of readings, there will be no special indicators on an item. But if an item is high or low in relation to the normal range, the lab will include (H) or (L) next to the measurement.

Blood and Other Chemistries (30 or more tests)

- *Cholesterol* readings, including "bad" LDL cholesterol, "good" HDL cholesterol, and a total cholesterol/HDL ratio. Abnormal cholesterol is a risk factor for cardiovascular disease.
- *Triglycerides,* another important blood lipid. When elevated, triglycerides are both a cardiovascular risk factor and a component of the "metabolic syndrome," described on page 111.

- *Glucose,* or blood sugar. High levels of blood glucose may indicate a diabetic tendency or actual diabetes.
- *Uric acid* is a breakdown product of protein. Significant elevations may be associated with gout or kidney stones.
- *Calcium, phosphorus, potassium,* and *sodium* are minerals important for various chemical processes in the body.
- *Bilirubin,* which is metabolized by the liver, is a pigment produced from the normal breakdown of old red blood cells. High levels, especially when associated with other abnormal liver functions, may require further medical evaluation.

   At times we see an elevation of the bilirubin in highly conditioned athletes, but this is of no special significance.

- *ALT, AST, LDH,* and *alkaline phosphatase* are enzymes related to your liver function, though they may also come from other tissues, such as muscle or bone. These tests may be abnormal as a result of alcohol or prescription drug use (particular statin drugs used to control cholesterol) or of liver or gallbladder abnormalities.
- *BUN* (Blood Urea Nitrogen), GFR, and *creatinine* are tested to measure your kidney functions. Mild elevations of BUN may result from too little fluid intake.
- *Total protein* and *albumin* (a type of protein) indicate liver function, and minor changes (slightly above or below normal) are usually not significant.
- *CPK* is an enzyme found in skeletal and heart muscles, as well as in the brain. Slight elevations are relatively common following vigorous physical activity or mild muscular trauma. *Caution:* Excessive muscle activity can at times cause a marked, serious elevation, leading to a shutdown of kidney function (i.e., renal failure requiring dialysis).
- *Hemoccult* (or Seracult) is a test for blood in the stool. A clinic or physician will typically ask you to perform this procedure at home and bring the specimen with you for the exam. This is part of a

screening procedure for the early detection of bowel cancer. But an abnormal ("positive") stool test for blood may result from mild bleeding due to a variety of sources in the gastrointestinal system.

- *TSH* (thyroid-stimulating hormone) is a sensitive measure of your thyroid function. Thyroid hormones serve as a kind of metabolic "thermostat" to regulate levels of biochemical activity in most of your tissues. But the TSH may become significantly elevated when your thyroid gland isn't producing enough thyroid hormone.

  The TSH measurement is also helpful in monitoring the effectiveness of thyroid-replacement therapy. *Caution:* Oral contraceptives, hormones, steroids, aspirin, and other medications can cause false increases or decreases in your TSH reading.

- *Sed Rate,* or *ESR,* is a nonspecific test for infection or inflammation in the body.

- *RPR* is a screening test for one type of venereal disease.

- *Fibrinogen* is a clotting factor in the blood. High fibrinogen levels have been associated with an increased risk of heart disease. A fibrinogen in the range of 20 to 400 or less is considered to be an advantage.

- *Ferritin* is an indicator of the amount of iron that the body is storing. It's helpful in differentiating iron-deficiency anemia from other types of anemia and identifying possible hemochromatosis, a serious disease involving cirrhosis of the liver, diabetes, and other problems.

- *Pap smears* are examined microscopically for any evidence of cancer or precancerous changes of the female genital tract.

- *PSA* (prostate specific antigen) is a blood test used in male patients to detect cancer of the prostate. Elevations may occur with prostate infections, benign enlargement of the prostate gland, or prostate cancer. If your level is high on a single exam or is increasing significantly on a series of exams, further evaluation is indicated.

- *Homocysteine* is an amino acid that has been associated with vascular disease (heart attacks and strokes), Alzheimer's disease, colon cancer, and osteoporosis. Elevations can be treated with certain supplements (folic acid, and vitamins B_6 and B_{12}—see Chapter 10).

- *hsCRP,* C-reactive protein, is a protein in the blood that's related to inflammation. Research has identified this inflammation as an important new, independent risk factor for coronary heart disease, as well as an indicator of an infectious process anywhere in the body.

Complete Blood Count (15 tests)

- *WBC* refers to white blood cell count. This number may be elevated when there is infection in the body. The "differential" measurement reports the percentage of different types of white cells in the blood and is useful in screening for infection or blood disorders.
- *Hemotocrit (HCT)* and *hemoglobin (HGB)* are measures of red blood cell volume. Low values may indicate anemia.

Urinalysis (10 tests)

- *pH* is a measure of urine acidity.
- *Specific gravity* refers to the ability of the kidneys to concentrate the urine.
- *Protein, glucose,* and *red blood cells (RBC)* should not normally be found in the urine.
- A few *white blood cells (WBC)* and *casts* (debris from old cells) may be present in normal urine, but shouldn't be present in large numbers.

As mentioned above, the above summary includes only some of the most important tests we use at the Cooper Clinic, which have helped us identify and treat hidden diseases and conditions that are often life-threatening. You can expect a complete workup to include many other lab tests, and if you find that your results are too high or too low in any of these, your physician will explain the implications to you.

TEST #14: VISION TEST

This test, which should be done in addition to a physical inspection of your eyes, will show whether your vision needs to be corrected by lenses or laser surgery. The exam should include your distant and near vision capabilities, both corrected and uncorrected by lenses, and your ability to discriminate colors. Also, the exam should include tests for glaucoma and macular degeneration.

TEST #15: HEARING TEST

Both ears should be tested in a soundproof audiometry booth. Technicians will typically check eight different levels or frequencies of sound.

TEST #16: SPIROMETRY TEST FOR LUNG FUNCTION

This pulmonary-function test is useful in helping your doctor detect whether you have a lung disease. When you blow all the air in your lungs out into a special canister, the technician checks for both your "vital capacity" (total amount of air you expelled) and your "timed vital capacity" (the speed with which you blew the air out). By measuring the amount and flow of air in your respiratory system, your doctor is in a position to make an early diagnosis of asthma, bronchitis, or emphysema. This test is especially helpful in monitoring the lung health of smokers.

TEST #17: COLONOSCOPY

Colon cancer, which is one of the most common of all cancers and responsible for tens of thousands of deaths each year, represents one of the greatest threats to health, especially as patients move into middle age. For patients who don't undergo a complete colonoscopy (examination of the entire colon), we still offer testing by the flexible proctosigmoidoscope (or just "sigmoidoscope"). This device, which is inserted into the colon through the rectum, allows the physician to examine about one-third of the colon for polyps, tumors, or other abnormalities. Preparation involves fasting beginning the day before the test and undergoing a self-administered enema to clear the bowel area.

But the gold standard for colon inspection is the regular optical colonoscopy, with the "virtual colonoscopy" close on its heels. Both of these tests, which are offered at the Cooper Clinic, provide a high degree of accuracy in detecting abnormalities in the entire length of the colon. Also, both require the patient to take certain steps a couple of days prior to the exam. These include observing a strict diet and ingesting medications that clear the bowel area and make observation by the physician easier.

There is a definite difference in time, technique, and expense for each procedure. The regular colonoscopy requires the patient to be given a mild anesthetic and to undergo about three hours of close monitoring following the procedure. The virtual colonoscopy, in contrast, is done without an anesthetic and typically takes about a half hour to forty-five minutes to complete. During this time, the patient is placed in a non-claustrophobic computerized tomography tube, where pictures are taken of the inside wall of the colon. Then, the pictures are downloaded into a computer and examined by a specialist to determine if there are any abnormalities that must be corrected.

What are the advantages and disadvantages of each procedure? Obviously, the regular colonoscopy takes longer and is more invasive in that it requires anesthesia. There is also the risk—though slight, if the specialist is experienced in the procedure—that the colonoscope inserted into the colon may puncture or damage the colon wall. In addition, a regular colonoscopy is typically considerably more expensive than a virtual colonoscopy, costing two to three times what you would have to pay for the virtual.

But an advantage of a regular colonoscopy is that it is more established in most hospitals and clinics, and can involve an all-in-one experience. In other words, if the specialist finds suspicious growths, they can be removed on the spot, or specimens can be taken for biopsy. In contrast, if such problems are discovered during the virtual colonoscopy, a separate procedure has to be scheduled for removal or biopsy. Also, according to studies comparing the procedures, the optical colonoscopy continues to be regarded as somewhat more accurate in identifying colon problems, though as computer programs and technology improve, that gap is closing fast.[5]

Key factors in conducting a colonoscopy of any type are the competence and experience of the physician conducting the exam. For example, a 2006 study in the *New England Journal of Medicine* showed that the sensitivity in finding polyps of early cancers in a regular "optical" colonoscopy was directly related to the time the physician took to do the exam.[6]

If physicians spent less than six minutes in withdrawing the colonoscope from a patient's appendix area to the rectum, the researchers found that the examiner missed a significant number of polyps. Specifically, those who spent six minutes or more withdrawing the instrument—considered by experts to be the minimum time for the procedure—had a detection rate of more than 28 percent for polyps, as compared with a rate of less than 12 percent for those who spent less than six minutes.

A helpful strategy for the patient is to ask the physician about his or her detection rate. For male patients over fifty, the examiners should be finding 25 percent of cases with polyps, and for women over fifty, 15 percent. If the doctor can't tell you the detection rate when you ask the question, you should probably look elsewhere for your colonoscopy.

To sum up, then, if you have a personal history of colon cancer or a very strong family history, you should probably plan on having regular colonoscopies as part of your physical exam at least every five years after age fifty. But if you have no personal history and a weak family history of such problems, the virtual colonoscopy may be the right test for you. In the end, this is a decision that you and your physician must make in light of your particular circumstances and health profile.

TEST #18: CHEST X-RAY

Chest X-rays help your physician determine whether your heart, lungs, and other organs are within normal size limits and are otherwise healthy. For the diagnosing of early lung cancers, however, the chest X-ray is not effective.

TEST #19: ELECTRON BEAM TOMOGRAPHY (EBT)—OR "FAST CT SCAN"

This device, which has been growing in popularity in recent years, is proving to be an extremely useful tool for alerting physicians to the calcification of the coronary arteries (i.e., the buildup of calcified plaque in heart arteries), which is the greatest cause of heart attacks. Also, the procedure provides pictures of all internal organs in the trunk, including abnormalities such as tumors. At the Cooper Clinic, we routinely give this exam to patients who come in for a comprehensive evaluation after age forty. We've picked up numerous abnormalities, cysts, and tumors of the liver, spleen, pancreas, adrenal glands, and kidneys.

The procedure works this way:

There are no special preparations, such as dietary restrictions, before you have the test. You'll remove any metallic objects in your clothing and then have three ECG electrodes placed on your chest to signal to the EBT scanner when to obtain each image. Otherwise, you can remain fully clothed.

You then lie down on your back on the scanning table and are instructed to take a deep breath periodically and hold it for several seconds as the scanner is operating. You're then moved slowly back and forth in an open tubular structure that houses an electron beam generator. The beam is used to "take pictures" of the insides of your upper body, and the results are then transferred to a computer for further processing. The entire scanning procedure takes only about ten to fifteen minutes.

We've found the fast CT scan to be especially effective when it's coupled with the next exam, the stress test. (See the Appendix, pages 370 to

371, for age- and sex-adjusted coronary artery calcification [CAC] scores for people without a history of coronary heart disease.)

TEST #20: STRESS TEST

The stress test, or exercise electrocardiogram (ECG), is usually conducted by having the patient walk on a treadmill, but may be done with a cycle or other device that will raise the heart rate to the maximum. For patients who can't walk or cycle, a pharmacological stress test is performed. This procedure involves injecting a medicine into the body to simulate exercise (i.e., elevation of the heart rate and blood pressure).

The purpose of the stress test is to test the health of the heart when the person's endurance level is pushed to exhaustion. Although a resting ECG can be helpful, an exercise ECG under maximal conditions is essential to evaluate a person's true heart health and true risk for cardiovascular disease.

In brief, the Cooper Clinic Protocol we use for stress tests includes these elements:

- You undergo a complete screening before the stress test, with a check of such functions as your blood pressure and heart rate, and also at least four resting ECGs. The ECGs should be done with at least twelve "leads," or electrical lines connected to electrode pads attached to your upper body.
- For the actual stress test, you should have at least ten leads attached to electrodes on your chest and upper body. This approach gives you a standard twelve-lead ECG at rest and during exercise. A good rule of thumb is the more leads and electrodes, the more accurate the test.
- Walk a minute or two on the treadmill to get your bearings and balance. At this stage, it's okay to hold on to the treadmill bar.
- When the actual stress test begins, don't hold on to the bar. If you do, an accurate measure of your fitness won't be possible because

The Stress Test Under a Microscope

The Balke protocol consists of walking at a constant speed (3.3 mph, or 90 meters per minute) with the treadmill flat for the first minute. At the conclusion of the first minute, the incline is increased by 2 percent. At the end of each subsequent minute, the incline is increased by 1 percent until the twenty-fifth minute. After that, the speed is increased 0.2 mph per minute until the patient reaches exhaustion or "predicted maximum heart rate" (PMHR).

PMHR is usually calculated by using this formula: 220 minus the age of the patient = PMHR. But for conditioned people, this formula is more accurate: 205 minus ½ the age of the patient = PMHR.

In addition, the technician monitoring the test will ask the patient how hard he or she is working according to the Borg scale of perceived exertion, with 6 being the lowest level of perceived exertion and 20 being the highest level. A rating of 6 means the person is totally at rest, whereas a 20 is very, very hard. Ordinarily, the technicians will stop the test either when PMHR is reached or when the Borg measure of work is a 19 or 20.

When exhaustion is achieved, the incline of the treadmill is reduced rapidly to 0 percent, and the speed is dropped to 2.2 mph. The cool-down period lasts for five minutes on the treadmill, followed by five more minutes of ECG monitoring in the supine (lying on the back) position.

To compare performances on the Bruce and Balke protocols, multiply the minutes on the Bruce test by 1.7 to predict what the time would have been using the Balke test. For example, a maximal performance of nine minutes on the Bruce protocol is equal to fifteen minutes on the Balke test.

For levels of fitness as determined by time on the Balke test, age and sex adjusted, go to pages 373–374 in the Appendix.

holding on to the bar will reduce the emergency expenditures by at least 30 percent.

- We use a version of the Balke method as part of the Cooper Protocol. The Balke approach requires the patient to walk a longer period, with a more gradual increase in treadmill rate and incline, than do other techniques, such as the Bruce method. (For a more detailed description of the two methods, see the accompanying box.)

- You should walk on the treadmill until you *have* to stop, either because you're totally out of breath or your legs won't keep going. By "exercising to exhaustion" in this way, you'll cause your heart rate to rise to its maximum rate (or very close to it). It's at this point of maximum heart rate that latent heart problems tend to become obvious on the ECG.

- After you've reached your maximum heart rate, cool down on the treadmill with five minutes of slow walking.

- Lie down on your back for a few minutes after the test. During this final phase, your physician or a qualified technician will continue to monitor your blood pressure, ECG, and other vital signs.

As indicated above, combining a good treadmill stress test with a fast CT scan can provide you with the best possible evaluation of your heart function. And now, with the new "64 slice spiral CT," it is possible to perform a coronary angiogram (arteriogram) as a part of a routine physical. This procedure is noninvasive, less expensive, and less traumatic than a regular angiogram. All that is required is the injection of a contrast medium into a vein in the arm, and, immediately afterward, the administration of the CT scan. The accuracy of this approach is remarkable when it is compared with the routine coronary angiogram that is performed in hospitals. In the future, the 64 slice spiral CT may replace the ultrafast CT because of its greater sensitivity.

TEST #21: BONE-DENSITY SCAN

Women past fifty and men past sixty should undergo a bone-density scan to determine whether there is any bone loss, i.e., osteopenia or osteoporosis. Typically, a bone-density test will focus on the spine and the hips.

TEST #22: MAMMOGRAPHY

Because breast cancer is such a threat to women of all ages, we recommend that you have a mammogram at least by age thirty-five (earlier if you have a family or personal history of breast cancer or breast abnormalities). Then—if there is no personal or family history of this cancer— you should have a mammogram every other year between the ages of forty and forty-nine, and annually beginning at age fifty. We now use digital mammography, which is more sensitive and more accurate in diagnosing early breast cancers, and in the future we'll be offering MRI (magnetic resonance imaging) mammography as the gold standard.

TEST #23: STRENGTH AND FLEXIBILITY TESTS

Different clinics will use varying equipment or protocols to test strength and flexibility. But in general, you should expect tests that check the flexibility of your lower back, hamstrings (back of thigh), and arms and shoulders. Strength tests will focus on the muscles of your quadriceps (front of your thighs), hamstrings, abdomen, chest, upper arms (front and back, or biceps and triceps), and shoulders.

Strength and flexibility become increasingly important as you grow older—and especially when you pass age fifty. To get an idea about how you can design a program to improve your strength and flexibility as you age, see Chapter 7 ("Launch a Personal Plan").

TEST #24: DENTAL EXAM

Too often, patients who pay close attention to the rest of their body fail to pay enough attention to their teeth. Yet terrible, expensive health problems, including decaying teeth and gum disease, become the bane of many older people. Also, chronic headaches have often been traced at the Cooper Clinic to dental problems, including a bad bite. So don't neglect this important component of your exam.

As part of our exam, our dentist will visualize and photograph the posterior pharynx and vocal cords, looking primarily for polyps and the normal or abnormal function of both cords. This evaluation is particularly important for current or past cigarette smokers.

TEST #25: PSYCHOLOGICAL EXAM

Finally, most complete preventive-medicine exams will provide you with a questionnaire about your perception of your emotional condition and the stress in your life. An estimated 60 to 90 percent of all visits to the doctor are stress-related in some way,[7] and so if you can identify and relieve the stress in your life, you're much more likely to maximize your health—and stay out of the doctor's office. As part of the mental evaluation, we now use a simple questionnaire to find possible early signs of dementia.

Breaking News About Your Exam

When we conduct the above tests as part of your comprehensive physical, we are always looking for ways to exploit the latest scientific findings to your advantage. Here are just a few of the current trends that we expect to become well-established in the near future:

Maintaining Super-low "Bad" LDL Cholesterol Levels

Some of the latest recommendations from the National Cholesterol Education Program (NCEP)[8] say that for high-risk heart patients (i.e., those with diagnosed coronary heart disease), "bad" LDL levels should be below 70 mg/dl. A level of 60 for two years or longer has been shown to actually *reverse* coronary atherosclerosis in some people.

Patients at moderately high risk (i.e., with two or more risk factors, such as cigarette smoking; high blood pressure; low "good" HDL cholesterol; or an immediate family history of early coronary heart disease) should keep their LDL cholesterol below 100 mg/dl, with an ultimate goal of 70. Even if there is no history of heart disease or coronary risk factors, it's still advisable to keep the "bad" LDL cholesterol below 100 mg/dl.

Because cholesterol is increasingly seen as a major threat to heart health, your physician may recommend strict diet and exercise programs, plus a prescription medication if lifestyle attempts don't do the job.

Guarding Against the Metabolic Syndrome

The metabolic syndrome is increasingly being recognized as a major "combination risk factor" for cardiovascular disease.[9] The syndrome exists when *three* of the following five signs are present in a given individual:

1. *Abdominal obesity* (i.e., waist circumference equal to or greater than 40 inches for men or 35 inches for women)
2. *Elevated triglycerides* (equal to or greater than 150 mg/dl)
3. *Low "good" HDL cholesterol* (less than 40 mg/dl for men or less than 50 mg/dl for women)
4. *Elevated blood pressure* (equal to or higher than 130/85 mm/Hg). This level of blood pressure, which may strike you as quite normal, given standards of the past, is now considered elevated—and a significant risk factor for cardiovascular disease.
5. *Elevated fasting blood glucose* (equal to or greater than 110 mg/dl). This condition may signal the presence of diabetes or at least a propensity toward diabetes.

Monitoring ALL Risk Factors

For a long time, the common wisdom in medical circles was that more than 50 percent of heart patients lacked any of the conventional risk factors, such as cigarette smoking, diabetes, high cholesterol, or hypertension.

But the most recent research puts this misconception to rest. In fact, 80 to 90 percent of patients with coronary heart disease have at least one conventional risk factor.[10] And if you include the new "emerging" risk factors, such as C-reactive protein (one of the items we test in our blood workup) and the AB index, virtually all heart patients have at least one risk factor.

What does this new research finding mean for you? Simply this: you should pay close attention to every finding on your complete preventive-medicine exam and regard no cardiovascular risk factor abnormality as unimportant. When you have your health numbers in hand, you'll find that there is almost always something you can do to fine-tune your health and fitness profile—and ensure, as best you can, that you'll finish strong.

Your Best Insurance Policy

Clearly, the gold-standard physical exam we've described goes far beyond the garden-variety physical checkups most people get in a doctor's office. But getting one of these exams—which your insurance may not reimburse you for—will provide the best "insurance policy" you've ever taken out on yourself. Let's summarize a few of the reasons:

- A complete checkup will increase the odds that any hidden health problems you have will be found.
- The earlier such a health problem is found, the more likely it is that your doctor will be able to cure you at minimal cost.
- Conversely, the longer you wait, the more likely it is that you may die or be forced to undergo costly and debilitating medical procedures.

- By seeing clearly the exact flaws in your fitness and health, you'll be more motivated to do something about them.
- By developing baseline measurements for all the major areas of your health and fitness, you'll give your doctor a head start in treating you when you face some health challenge in the future.

If you question the value of this type of examination, you might consult the approximately 10,000 "healthy" patients who have been diagnosed with heart disease. Or check with the 1,300 "healthy" men in whom we have found prostate cancer, or the 650 "healthy" women in whom we have found early breast cancer. We have also discovered more than 350 colon cancers, along with nearly two hundred lung cancers and more than a hundred kidney cancers. And remember: these cancers were found in people who came to the Cooper Clinic thinking they were healthy. They are among the 90,000-plus men and women evaluated one or many times over the past thirty-six years, including more than one million person-years of follow-up. Our survival rate among patients is far above the average because we usually pick up cancers at the earliest stage when there is the best chance for a cure.

One man refused for many years to take a complete exam with this protective screening—even though his fellow corporate executives came in regularly for their checkups. His excuse: "I'm afraid you'll find something wrong."

Ken's response: "The problem with that reasoning is that if there's something wrong and we don't find it now, we will find it in the future. And then it may be too late."

Now, this man is a regular at the clinic, and various preventive measures have kept him in good health.

In short, a gold-standard physical exam is an absolutely essential first step in a Start Strong, Finish Strong program. Without it, you'll be flying blind as you begin to develop other parts of your program, such as the no-frills fitness plan that we are now ready to discuss in the next chapter.

Six

Start-up #2—The Active Mind-set: Focus on the Amazing Benefits of Fitness

Next to a complete preventive-medicine exam, physical fitness is the single most important factor in your Start Strong, Finish Strong program. But we don't want you to plunge into any unaccustomed physical activity just yet—especially not if you're a complete newcomer to this fitness business.

Instead, as a way of jump-starting your motivation and heating up the hot buttons that you identified in Chapter 3, we want you to focus for a few minutes on what you stand to gain by ratcheting up your fitness level. Believe us, when you know the facts, you'll be impressed, if not amazed. And when you finish this chapter, you should be more than ready to get off the couch and into a personal exercise program.

We've long known that the four most important things that accelerate aging are inactivity, obesity, cigarette smoking, and stress. But if we had to pick one of these four as the "first great health sin among equals," inactivity would be it. In fact, research that has emerged from the Cooper Institute and other research centers in recent years has confirmed this unexpected truth: *it's better to be fat and fit, rather than skinny and unfit.* It's also better to be a cigarette smoker and fit than a nonsmoker and unfit.

Of course, we don't advocate physical fitness to the exclusion of weight reduction or quitting tobacco use. Both weight loss and smoking cessation are extremely important for your health and longevity. But aerobic fitness still should be given a slight edge in your Start Strong program—and that's why we've given it the No. 2 spot in our list of health-and-fitness start-ups.

To understand a little better why the scientific findings we'll be discussing in this section may be true for you personally, let us introduce you to "Keith," who at age forty-seven epitomized many of the declining health issues that characterize "civilized" society.

Keith's Quick "Fitness Cure"

A mostly sedentary middle manager, Keith admitted that the most vigorous exercise he got during a typical week was walking from the parking lot to his office every day and strolling around the local mall on weekends. Fortunately, a complete preventive-medicine exam alerted Keith to the fact that his lack of physical activity was beginning to take its toll, with such results as these:

- Elevated blood pressure—a reading of 140/86 mm/Hg, which should have been 120/80 or lower.
- Unbalanced cholesterol—a "good" HDL cholesterol reading of 43 mg/dl (should have been at least in the 44 to 55 range, and preferably above 55) and a "bad" LDL cholesterol reading of 165 mg/dl (should have been closer to 100).
- A body fat percentage of 24 percent—which should have been no higher than 19 percent.

- A tendency to be mildly depressed several days each week.
- A sense of being overwhelmed by job stress.
- A decline of interest in sex.
- A tendency to have more aches, pains, and muscle injuries than when he was younger.

An important part of Keith's "prescription" when he left the office was to embark on an aerobic fitness program consisting of walking thirty minutes per day, five days per week. He was also instructed in techniques for gradually increasing the intensity of his exercise sessions and was introduced to some simple strength-training exercises, in accordance with the principles described in these pages. In addition, registered dieticians put him on a lower-fat, lower-calorie diet. As a result, at the end of two months of following this program, Keith showed these improvements:

- Blood pressure—a reading of 125/80 mm/Hg.
- Cholesterol—a "good" HDL cholesterol reading of 51 mg/dl, and a "bad" LDL cholesterol reading of 135 mg/dl.
- A body fat percentage of 22 percent.
- Rarely a tendency to be depressed.
- A sense of being able to handle job stress more effectively.
- A decided increase in his interest in sex.
- A tendency to experience few aches, pains, or muscle injuries.

Of course, these lifestyle improvements had not moved Keith into ideal health ranges, and he still had work to do. But remember where he had come from. In only two months, he had improved most of his important health numbers and had made significant progress toward his health goals—just by changing habits related to exercise and diet.

Yet these health and well-being improvements that Keith began to enjoy after only a few weeks of training represent merely the beginning of the many specific benefits of fitness. Here is a sampling of the wide array of advantages that leading scientists have discovered—and that can be yours as you move forward with the Start Strong, Finish Strong program.

The Remarkable Benefits of Fitness

Almost two decades ago, a landmark study at the Cooper Clinic in Dallas established beyond any doubt that you can increase your chances of living a much longer and healthier life with a simple but effective fitness program. This report, published in the *Journal of the American Medical Association,* showed that both men and women with the lowest levels of fitness suffered more than twice the death rate of those with just a moderate level of fitness.[1] Furthermore, being physically fit lowered the risk for all causes of death and serious disease, including heart problems, cancer, and diabetes.

In this study, we measured fitness in more than ten thousand men and three thousand women who were studied by determining their performance on a treadmill test—just like the one described in the previous chapter. How much exercise would it take you to reach this minimal level of fitness? The answer: not much.

For example, to reach this basic standard, you would have to walk two miles in less than thirty minutes three days a week. Or if you want to lower the intensity of your exercise to an even less demanding level, you could choose this approach: walk two miles in thirty-five minutes, four days per week; or walk two miles in forty minutes, five times per week. Also, if you choose to *increase* the intensity of your exercise further, your risk of death and disease will go down even more.

Now just think about this for a moment: if you're currently completely sedentary, all you have to do to increase your longevity and improve your heath *dramatically* is to amble along at a twenty-minutes-per-mile pace for a couple of miles, at least five times a week. What insurance policy could you buy that would be more effective or cheaper—or more pleasant—than that?

Since our report was published, more evidence has been piling up in support of our earlier findings. Here are some of those specific, scientifically established health-and-longevity rewards that a regular exercise program will provide:

Exercise will lower your blood pressure.

To have the best chance of preventing a stroke, heart attack, and other cardiovascular problems, current recommendations are to reduce blood pressure lower than ever: below 120/80 mm/Hg. Anything above that is regarded as either prehypertension or hypertension, and puts you at significantly greater risk.

What's the best way to achieve such low blood pressure readings?

The American College of Sports Medicine makes its position quite clear: "Exercise is the cornerstone therapy for the primary prevention, treatment, and control of hypertension."[2] This recommendation applies both to those who have normal blood pressure and want to prevent future blood pressure problems, and also to those with elevated blood pressure who want to bring it down.[3]

"There is little doubt that increasing exercise can reduce blood pressure," declared Marvin Moser in the *Journal of Clinical Hypertension*.[4] In line with generally recognized medical recommendations, he also called for consuming no more than moderate amounts of alcohol (no more than two drinks a day), reducing salt intake, and reducing weight. When all these lifestyle strategies are followed with moderate exercise, it's possible that as many as 20 percent of patients with hypertension wouldn't have to be treated with medication, he wrote.

What exactly is the best *type* of exercise for lowering and managing blood pressure? It's generally recognized that the best exercise prescription and dosage involve low to moderate intensity aerobic exercise.[5] More specifically, this approach involves such exercises as walking, running, cycling, and swimming. Closely in line with our recommendations at the Cooper Clinic, a Cleveland Clinic consultant has suggested that hypertensive patients should perform endurance exercise at least three to five times per week for twenty to sixty minutes per session. The intensity of the activity should cause the patient to work out at a heart rate of 50 to 70 percent of maximum. This would usually translate into a walking pace of three to four miles per hour.[6]

Exercise will lower your risk of heart disease.

The beneficial impact of aerobic exercise on the heart cuts across all ages and both genders. A Finnish study, for instance, examined the impact of moderate physical activity on 1,340 men and 1,500 women, aged thirty-five to sixty-three. The researchers found a preventive effect of the leisure-time physical activity in reducing coronary heart disease, diabetes, and hypertension.[7]

Similarly, in a 2002 Harvard investigation, researchers found that total physical activity—including running, weight training, and walking—was associated with reduced risk of coronary heart disease.[8]

Why is exercise so good for your heart? There are many reasons, including simply the fact that regular physical activity strengthens the heart and builds better circulation. It's long been known that fit people who exercise regularly tend to develop "collateral" circulation, or more efficient secondary vessels that enable blood to bypass blocked or partially blocked main vessels.

Some other factors may include the tendency of exercise to increase the "good" HDL cholesterol in your blood, which is a marker of low cardiovascular risk.[9] Also, just one sixty-minute session of exercising on a stationary bike showed changes in heart functions associated with a more stable environment for the heart. This result appeared to provide evidence of the protective effects on the heart of just a "single bout of submaximal exercise."[10]

Finally, one of those "emerging risk factors" mentioned in the previous chapter—C-reactive protein, or CRP, which indicates levels of inflammation in the blood—appears to decrease as fitness increases. A study at the Cooper Institute conducted by Alexander N. Jordan, Timothy S. Church, and Steven N. Blair investigated the impact of fitness on 141 men age sixty and older. They found an inverse correlation between treadmill performance times (an excellent measure of aerobic fitness) and CRP levels. In other words, higher levels of fitness were associated with lower levels of CRP.[11]

Exercise will improve your mental and emotional health.

An important Harvard study published in the *Journal of the American Medical Association* in 2004 found that long-term, regular physical activity, including walking, was associated with "significantly better cognitive function and less cognitive decline in older women."[12] This investigation, which was part of the Nurses' Health Study involving nearly 19,000 women age seventy to eighty-one, tested general cognition, verbal memory, category fluency, and attention. The women who were in the top 20 percent range of fitness showed a 20 percent lower risk of mental impairment than those in the bottom 20 percent.

Also, in a study published in the November 2006 issue of the *Journal of Gerontology: Medical Sciences,* researchers reported that, beginning in your forties, you can increase the odds that you'll stop shrinkage of brain areas related to memory and higher cognition if you engage in at least three hours of brisk walking each week.[13] The investigation, conducted by scientists at the University of Illinois, Urbana, adds strong support to earlier studies showing that people age sixty to seventy-nine who walked three miles in one hour, three times a week for three months, displayed improved thinking capacity, including a better ability to switch between mental tasks and screen out distractions.

The University of Illinois researchers found that aerobic exercise can increase the physical volume of the brain in those areas associated with neurons and neuron connections. By "growing" and activating new neurons, those who exercised actually reversed the aging process. In fact, by the end of the study, their mental performance and brain volume were equal to those who were three years younger. In contrast, study groups that did no exercise, or only nonaerobic stretching and toning exercise, showed no such changes in their brains. Additional studies have shown that during exercise, the areas of the brain most filled with blood and oxygen are those responsible for memory and creativity.

Other studies have demonstrated that regular exercise can lower your risk of suffering from depression, anxiety, and a host of other emotional complaints. Although any amount of exercise will help, a 2005 Cooper Institute investigation published in the *American Journal of Preventive Medicine* found that in treating mild to moderate depression, the more calories you expend in exercising, the more you improve emotionally.[14]

Exercise helps heart patients with their stress management.

We have long said that those who pursue a regular Start Strong fitness program find that exercise is "nature's best tranquillizer."[15] In other words, neurotransmitters of well-being, such as endorphins and dopamine, which are produced by aerobic exercise, facilitate sleep by making it easier to relax.

The scientific evidence continues to accumulate that exercise should be a component in any medical strategy for stress management. Researchers at Duke, for instance, have reported that patients with stable ischemic heart disease enjoyed a reduction in their emotional distress and improved cardiovascular risk when they combined exercise with stress management. The exercise included aerobic exercise training for thirty-five minutes three times per week for sixteen weeks.[16]

Higher levels of physical activity may lower the risk of Parkinson's disease.

This Harvard study followed more than 48,000 men and more than 77,000 women for more than a decade to see if there was any relationship between their physical activity levels and their risk of Parkinson's disease. The researchers found that the exercise seemed to have had no effect on the women's propensity to get the disease. But the Parkinson's risk in men who participated in more than ten months of strenuous exercise each year had a 60 percent lower risk than did those who regularly exercised less than two months each year.[17]

Exercise can improve your sex life.

Increased physical activity plus weight loss improved the erectile function in a group of obese Italian men, according to a two-year study reported in *JAMA* in 2004.[18] About one-third of the fifty-five participating men, who averaged forty-four years of age, showed improvement in their erectile function as a result of increasing their physical activity from 48 minutes per week to 195 minutes per week.

Another Italian study, reported in the May 11 issue of the *International Journal of Cardiology*, showed that moderate exercise can even help boost sexual function in men with heart failure. In this relatively short, eight-week investigation of fifty-nine men with chronic heart failure, half of the participants were assigned to an exercise program that included riding on a stationary bike and stretching three times a week. The other half remained sedentary. Those who exercised improved their ability to process oxygen (a primary test of fitness) and at the same time experienced improvement in several facets of their sexual performance, including the quality of their erections.[19]

Exercise can extend the life of those with adult-onset diabetes.

Adult-onset (type 2) diabetes, a growing health concern in the developed nations, will affect an estimated 366 million people throughout the world by the year 2030, a tremendous increase over the 171 million afflicted in the year 2000. Yet physical activity can reduce the risk of this health threat significantly, according to a nineteen-year Finnish study of nearly four thousand men and women, twenty-five to seventy-four years old. The study, published in *Diabetes Care* in April 2005, found lower death rates among these participants:

- Those with an occupation that required them to stand, walk, or lift;
- Those whose daily commute involved walking or cycling; and

- Those who did light or heavy gardening, running, swimming, or other exercise for at least three to four hours during leisure time.[20]

Weight-bearing exercise will counteract bone loss that occurs with aging.

After about age thirty, natural bone growth ceases, and steady bone loss begins in various parts of the body. If you don't act to delay or stop this bone loss, you're likely to end up with a fragile bone structure by the time you reach your later years.

Fortunately, you can begin to act against this deterioration at any age, and one of the best strategies is to include weight-bearing exercise in your fitness program. What constitutes weight-bearing exercise? Answer: anything that causes your muscles and bones to push or pull against resistance or gravity.

One of the most obvious weight-bearing exercises is brisk walking or, even better, jogging. Each time your foot hits the ground, your body weight *plus* the downward force of your weight puts pressure on your hips, legs, and feet—and on the bones in those parts of your body. This activity stimulates cells that make extra bone, thus helping to protect you against natural bone loss.

In addition to these "foot-striking" aerobic exercises, using free weights or machines that utilize resistance can help you place similar pressure on bones in other parts of your body, such as your wrists, arms, and shoulders. The result is greater bone mass—and greater protection.

Note: When this type of exercise is combined with adequate calcium supplementation (see Chapter 10), 1,000 IUs of vitamin D, and at least 400 mg of magnesium daily, the bone buildup tends to proceed more efficiently.

A 2004 study done by researchers at the National Aeronautics and Space Administration confirmed these principles rather clearly. Twenty men and women in the NASA community were divided into an exercise group and a nonexercise group for twenty-two weeks. All were assigned to seventeen weeks of bed rest, but the exercise group did upper- and lower-body exercises six days a week, while the nonexercise group just rested. At the end of the study period, the resting "control" patients showed statistically significant decreases in bone-mineral density in all regions of their body except at the upper thigh (femoral neck), the outer forearm (radius), and the arms. Their calcium balance in their bodies also decreased. The exercisers, in contrast, had significantly more "bone formation markers" and calcium.[21]

Reviewers in *The Physician and Sportsmedicine* journal concluded from this study that exercise may enhance calcium absorption. They also suggested that an adequate intake of calcium may be required to reap the full bone-stimulating benefits of weight-bearing exercise.

Exercise, combined with weight loss, may relieve arthritis.

Researchers at Wake Forest University studied 316 men and women, age sixty and older, who were suffering from osteoarthritis (wear-and-tear arthritis) of the knee. They found that a weight-loss diet, combined with exercise (including moderate walking sessions), had a greater effect on pain than did diet alone. The exercisers also improved in overall body function, flexibility, and mobility.[22] As we have said for years, exercise, including jogging, doesn't cause osteoarthritis, but it will aggravate pre-existing conditions.

Exercise improves your balance.

As you age, it gets harder and harder to keep your balance. After you pass about age fifty—and certainly by the time you reach your sixties—you may find that it's harder to stand on one leg to pull on a sock or shoe. Also, there may be an increasing tendency to teeter a little when you abruptly stand up or take a sharp turn while walking fast.

Exercise—both aerobic and strength conditioning—is a major solution to this balance problem. Researchers from the University of Lethbridge in Canada studied men in their sixties and early seventies, half of whom used oversize air-filled exercise balls to work on their flexibility, strength, cardiovascular conditioning, and balance. The active group exercised three times a week, forty-five minutes each session, over a period of fourteen weeks—and showed significant improvement in their balancing ability. The Canadian researchers noted that a major side benefit of this balance work is the decreased likelihood of older people suffering debilitating injuries from falls.[23]

Walking—by itself—can increase your immune response.

Brisk walking for thirty minutes by women who were regular walkers caused a modest, short-term increase in immunity, according to a study published in 2005 in *Medicine & Science in Sports & Exercise*.[24] The ability of the body to process oxygen also increases with intensity and duration of exercise—and this increase is associated with an overall improvement in aerobic fitness or endurance and better health.

These researchers noted that other studies have shown that regular exercisers report fewer upper respiratory tract infections, such as colds. Also, regular walkers experience about half as many days of upper respiratory tract infections as sedentary groups. Furthermore, near-daily physical activities reduce the number of work days lost to sickness. In contrast, competitive athletes who engage in vigorous but irregular athletic events, such as marathons, tend to have an increased risk of those upper respiratory infections if they exercise to the point of chronic fatigue.

The keys to maximizing your immune response with exercise, then, appears to be moderation and regularity.

Hiking on hilly terrain has multiple benefits.

In a novel study on alpine hikers, which was reported at a 2004 American Heart Association meeting, researchers found that walking *up* mountains lowered the triglycerides in the blood of forty-five volunteers, while walking *down* mountains lowered blood sugars (glucose). And there's more: hiking *both* up *and* down mountains lowered levels of "bad" LDL cholesterol.[25]

To put this in terms of specific diseases, focusing on climbing upward might lower the risk for heart disease (triglycerides), while focusing on the descent might lower a major risk factor for diabetes (high blood glucose). Also, by going both up and down, you can lower your cardiovascular risk for heart attacks and stroke.

The lead investigator, Heinz Drexel, M.D., from the Vorarlberg Institute for Vascular Investigation and Treatment, in Feldkirch, Austria, suggested that those who want to benefit from both the up and down effects of hiking—but who lack access to mountainous terrain—might include walking up and down flights of stairs in their exercise routine.

Exercise can not only lower your risk of getting cancer, but may also help you recover from breast cancer.

A few hours of walking or other exercise each week may help breast cancer survivors live longer, according to Harvard Medical School research.[26] In a study of nearly three thousand women, those who exercised more than one hour per week were less likely to die of their breast cancer than women who got less than one hour of physical activity each week.

Specifically, women under treatment for breast cancer who walked more than one hour a week at a relatively slow two- to three-mile-per-hour pace had a lower risk of dying than the women who walked less than an hour a week. Those who exercised a little more—walking three to five hours per week—had the lowest risk of dying, a risk that was even lower than those who walked longer distances.

You can use exercise to prevent injuries and prepare for unusual physical exertion.

If you know you'll be skiing, playing tennis, or engaging in some other relatively demanding sport for the first time in months (or years), it's easy and wise to tailor your regular workout to prepare unused muscles for the challenge. This approach, known as "kinesis" training, concentrates on building the exact muscles used in a particular sport or other physical activity. Serving a tennis ball, batting a baseball, swinging a golf club, or doing unusual and demanding work around the house can all be duplicated in your workout routine with excellent results.

For example, to guard against shoulder pulls or rotator cuff tears when you're serving in tennis, you might condition your serving muscles by using light hand weights to mimic the serving motion. Typically, you'd want to begin with a weight that would allow you to perform 8 repetitions fairly easily, and then you'd work up to 15 repetitions. Also, you might start off with one set of 8 to 15 reps and work up to two or three sets with the same number of reps. You'll usually need at least a couple of weeks, and preferably a longer period, to prepare for the unusual exertion.

This approach to exercise—also known as "specificity training" in reference to the concentration on specific sports movements—will work with any physical activity, and has found solid support in scientific research. One such study involved the use of specificity or kinesis training to prevent injuries focused on ankle problems. It's been estimated from emergency room statistics that 23,000 people in the United States injure an ankle every day, whether engaging in some athletic effort, wearing a new pair of high heels, or just taking an awkward turn in some daily task.[27]

To guard against this danger, men should do balance training and engage in stretching exercises for the calves and Achilles tendons, according to a presentation by biomechanical engineer Dr. Bruce Beynnon at a 2006 meeting of the American Orthopaedic Society for Sports Medicine. In contrast, according to Beynnon, women should concentrate on exercises that isolate and strengthen the muscles around the ankles that roll the foot inward and outward.

Beynnon and his fellow researchers at the University of Vermont came to these conclusions after studying the athletic experiences and injuries of 901 members of men's and women's varsity teams in soccer, basketball, lacrosse, and field hockey. The athletes played their sports in several high schools and universities in New England.[28]

These are just a few of the many benefits of regular exercise that have been featured in some of the most recent scientific studies. But what can you expect about maintaining a high fitness level as you age? Many people ask us, "Will my fitness level decline as I pass age fifty, no matter

Ken & Tyler: Don't Be Fooled by Fitness Terminology

In an effort to describe new exercise techniques—and also to package those techniques effectively for the popular market—fitness promoters have swamped us with new, important-sounding terms.

For example, the terms "aerobic exercise" and "aerobics" entered popular parlance in 1968 with publication of the first Cooper book, *Aerobics*. More recently, the term "cardio" has sometimes been used to refer to aerobic exercise, but we prefer to stick with the "aerobic" term for several reasons.

For one thing, the scientific community overwhelmingly uses aerobic to refer to studies being done on endurance exercise. Just as important, cardio may suggest cardiovascular exercise that benefits only the heart (or perhaps the heart plus the lungs in "cardiopulmonary"). Yet numerous studies have demonstrated that aerobic exercise provides many health and longevity benefits beyond the heart and lungs, such as reducing the risk of cancer and death from all causes.[29]

The term "anaerobic" refers to exercise that creates an "oxygen debt," or causes you to be out of breath. Sprinting is an example of this type of activity. Anaerobic conditioning can definitely help improve an athlete's performance, such as by lowering the time it takes to run distances (see the boxes dealing with interval and intensity training). But this type of workout will not provide the many health and longevity benefits of aerobic training.

Other common terms, which may be attached to strength training, include *isotonic* or *isophasic* exercise (contracting muscles through a range of motion, as with weight training and calisthenics); *isometric* exercise (tensing your muscles without moving them); and *isokinetic* exercise (moving your muscles through a continuous resistance, as can be done with certain weight or resistance equipment).

These strength- and weight-training strategies are essential for both men and women to maintain adequate muscle and bone strength, especially as the body ages. Women in particular should not be frightened by the thought that using weights may make them look "unfeminine" or "muscle-bound." It's difficult for any women other than serious female bodybuilders to put on too much muscle.

But even though strength exercises are necessary for everyone, they do not provide the cardiovascular and other health and longevity benefits afforded by aerobic exercise. An exception is the "Super Circuit" training we have designed at the Cooper Aerobics Center (described in Chapter 8). With this approach, the exerciser goes through ten strength-building stations involving different types of machines. But instead of resting for thirty seconds between machines, as is usually the case, the person engages in some type of aerobic activity to increase the heart rate. Examples include running in place, stepping up and down on a step, or jumping rope. Our studies have shown that the Super Circuit not only increases musculoskeletal strength, but also improves aerobic capacity to some extent.

In any event, it's essential for everyone to find some way to include *both aerobic and strength-building activities* in a personal fitness program.

what I do to try to hold off the aging process? Also, what should I look for as I move past sixty or seventy?"

In many respects, such questions are just another way of asking, "Will I *really* be able to finish strong with your program, regardless of how long I live?" The answer may surprise and encourage you.

What's the Effect of Age on Fitness— and Fitness on Age?

There is no doubt that you can hold the ravages of aging at bay with a regular fitness regimen. A 2001 survey of participants in the Senior

Olympics by researchers from the University of Pittsburgh Medical Center revealed that "Senior Olympians are in better physical, mental and emotional health than their sedentary peers."[30]

"It is not uncommon for Senior Olympics athletes to run, swim, or throw faster than sedentary people twenty to thirty years their junior," noted Freddie Fu, M.D., professor and chair of the department of orthopaedic surgery at the University of Pittsburgh School of Medicine. "Research has shown that seniors can make significant improvements in their physical and mental health by increasing their activity at any age."

Dr. Fu noted that "one astonishing [finding] in the 2001 survey was that more than 50 percent of the oldest female competitors—even at age eighty—still had normal bone density, a dramatic contrast to the low-bone-density levels typically seen in older women."

We find that such research is constantly confirmed by practical experience—such as that of eighty-one-year-old Rose Steward, who, despite failing eyesight, finished a 111-mile bike tour and more than a dozen road races in 1999. Steward was styled as the "oldest woman triathlete in the world" by the Perimeter Bicycling Association's sponsors of the premier race, El Tour.

Of course, you may be saying, "I'm not eighty years old, and I may never reach eighty. So maybe I won't start worrying just yet."

Okay, so don't worry. But do be concerned enough to take a little action. There are 76 million baby boomers in the United States who will become senior citizens in the next decade—and a number of boomers will soon be pushing age seventy, not so far from Rose Steward's category. But unlike Rose, about one-third of our older adults have some form of immobility or loss of independence. There's no reason for you to be one of the sad statistics if you face the facts and make some wise decisions beginning now.

The basic fact about exercise and aging is this: no matter how hard and conscientiously you work out, your body will begin to decline after your peak years—usually in the late teens through the twenties in most sports. Skills in a sport may improve into the thirties or even later, but the physical capacity to execute those skills will go down.

As proof of this principle, we need look no further than the careers of top older athletes in tennis, baseball, basketball, football, track, or any other physically demanding sport. Outstanding older athletes like Arthur Ashe, Dave Winfield, Andre Agassi, Bill Russell, and Gordie Howe are the exceptions, rather than the rule. And even in those special cases, the effects of age always begin to show up in the thirties, even if athletic skills and the ability to play the "mental game" are still improving.

Still, the decline will be slower in those who stay fit than in those who neglect their bodies. Recent research has confirmed that older athletes who participated in the Senior Olympics in 2001 and 2005 experienced a slow decline in their power as they passed age fifty and headed on through their sixties and into their seventies.[31] It wasn't until they hit age seventy-five that the processes of physical decline for these athletes began in earnest.

According to the University of Pittsburgh study, the speed of one-mile runners fell about 2 percent per year from age fifty to seventy-five. But from age seventy-five to eighty-five, speeds dropped by about 7 percent per year.

"We believe that these declines [after age seventy-five] involve three major factors—loss of cognitive function, loss of lean muscle mass, and the loss of bone-mineral density," said Vonda Wright, M.D., coordinator of the study. "We hope our investigations will help reveal more about physical-decline issues in Senior Olympians and help determine what interventions might be effective for seniors at all levels."

Many experts—including our scientists at the Cooper Institute—are hard at work trying to find ways to solve some of the primary problems involving loss of bone density, muscle mass, and cognition. At least a partial answer to the bone and muscle challenge is to encourage those seniors doing only aerobic work to include plenty of weight-bearing exercises for other parts of their body.

As for cognition, engaging in regular mental challenges as you get older, such as memorization or studying new subjects in extended education programs, can go a long way toward keeping your mental powers in shape. And don't forget that important 2006 study from scientists at the University of Illinois, Urbana, which was published in the *Journal of Gerontology: Medical Sciences* and was just cited a few pages back: from your forties on, you can help prevent a decrease in parts of your brain related to memory and thinking functions if you engage in at least three hours of vigorous walking each week.[32] Those who exercised as instructed ended up with brain volumes that were three years younger than they would have been otherwise.

With such exercise strategies, there is every reason to expect the process of aging and the functioning of the older body to slow down—if you *start* a sensible, regular aerobic-strength fitness program right now, regardless of your age, and *continue* with that program to the finish line.

So what might an easy-to-follow fitness program look like for you? To find out how to launch your own basic exercise program—even if you're totally sedentary or you've never exercised before—just turn the page and keep reading.

Seven

▪ Start-up #2—Your Basic
▪ Exercise Program:
Launch a Personal Plan

Any beginning exercise program should start with *aerobic exercise*— or endurance-type exercise such as brisk walking, jogging, swimming, or cycling—which gets the heart pumping and provides all sorts of benefits, such as those discussed in the previous chapter. But that's just the beginning.

We also now know that building your muscles and bones with *strength and resistance training*—such as work with weight machines, free weights, or calisthenics—increases in importance as you grow older. A major reason is that as we age, our bodies inevitably lose mass and strength. But weight-bearing exercise of all types—even including the pounding that occurs with jogging and running—helps contain this process of muscle and bone deterioration.

But how do you put these two components together into a simple, workable start-up program? Here's our recommendation for achieving the best balance at different ages.

The Aerobic-Strength Balance

Both aerobic (endurance) and strength training should be a part of every person's fitness program—and aerobic exercise should constitute at least 50 percent of a weekly workout schedule, no matter what your age. In other words, you should include endurance training such as walking, jogging, cycling, and swimming, plus muscle-building exercises. The muscle-building component might involve calisthenics, such as push-ups, sit-ups, and pull-ups, or weight training of various types.

As we've seen already, the aerobic or cardiorespiratory endurance component of your exercise is extremely important because of scientifically proven health and longevity benefits, which may not be associated with other types of exercise. For example, studies in many scientific centers, including our own Cooper Institute, have demonstrated clearly that the more fit you are—as measured by treadmill stress-test times for fitness—the lower your risk will be for mortality from all causes.[1] In other words, the higher your level of aerobic fitness, the less likely you are to die prematurely from a heart attack, cancer, diabetes, or any other cause.*

But as you grow older, the proportion of strength work should increase. In other words, you should do more strength work and less aerobic work—but always keep in mind that by the time you turn sixty, your aerobic exercise should still constitute at least half of your routine.

A major reason for this shift is that as you age, your bone density naturally declines and may put you at risk for osteoporosis. All weight-bearing exercise, including different types of strength training, will help you ward off osteoporosis by building up your bone mass. This danger of

---

*In recent years, the term "cardio exercise" has sometimes been used interchangeably with "aerobic exercise." But the "cardio" term is something of a misnomer because it may suggest that endurance exercise has only cardiovascular (heart and blood vessels) benefits. In fact, our studies and those of other scientists show that aerobic (endurance) exercise provides health and longevity benefits that go well beyond the cardiovascular.

bone-thinning disease is especially serious for older women who are small-boned or have other risk factors, such as a fair complexion, northern European or Asian ethnic background, low percentage of body fat, and family history of bone disease. But the risk of a bone-loss disease is also very real for many men who are in their sixties or older.

In addition to helping ward off the osteoporosis threat, strength training is quite important to help older people maintain their ability to function well when confronted with tasks that require unusual muscle exertion. The better shape your muscles are in, the lower your risk of pulling or straining a muscle. Also, by keeping your muscles in shape, you'll be less likely to lose functioning ability as a result of the natural process of aging. Among other things, you'll maintain better balance and thus be less likely to take a dangerous fall.

When we speak to audiences packed with older people, we often say, "If, at sixty years of age, you're a person who concentrates almost exclusively on aerobic conditioning, you may be able to run five miles in forty minutes. But you may also find that you can't pick up a sack of groceries without straining your back. So it's essential to combine weight or resistance training with aerobic activity as you age."

To head off such health threats, we advocate the following aerobic-strength training balance:

- If you're forty years old or younger, devote 80 percent of your workout time to aerobic training and 20 percent to strength training.
- If you're forty-one to fifty years old, shift to 70 percent aerobic and 30 percent strength work.
- If you're fifty-one to sixty, do 60 percent aerobic exercise and 40 percent strength training.
- After you pass sixty, divide your workout time more evenly between the two strategies—while still giving an edge to aerobic exercise, which provides the most health benefits: 55 percent aerobic work and 45 percent strength work.

Your Start-up Fitness Plan in a Nutshell

When you finally settle on your personal fitness program, the end product should fit into this basic daily model—which you are certainly free to adjust as your endurance and strength increase:

- Five minutes of warming up with walking or running in place, continuous stretching, or light calisthenics, such as jumping jacks.
- Thirty to forty minutes of aerobic activity or strength work each day. (About three to five days per week should be devoted to aerobic exercise, two to three days to strength work. Alternatively, instead of devoting a separate day to strength work, the strength phase can be added after a particular day's aerobic phase.)
- Five minutes of cooling down, typically involving walking, continuous stretching, or light calisthenics.

Now, with this overview in mind, let's take a closer look at what your start-up program should actually include in the way of both aerobic exercise and strength training.

Now here are some specific thoughts about aerobic activity, strength training, and stretching for the beginner. Some of these exercises, such as the calisthenics and the stretching movements, can be used by beginners and by more advanced exercisers—and we'll be referring to them when we get into the discussion of advanced fitness in Chapter 8. But as you'll see, there is much more to be said about both aerobic and strength work as you get into better shape.

Going Aerobic

The starting point for any effective fitness program must be *aerobics,* or aerobic exercise—the term coined by Ken back in the 1960s and introduced to the general public by such succinct and authoritative definitions as the one employed a few years ago by the *Encyclopaedia Britannica.* Aerobic exercise is, in essence, endurance exercise—and the many medical benefits associated with this form of activity have already been mentioned in some detail.

Recent research has caused most experts to make an adjustment to the description in the *New Encyclopaedia Britannica.* The assumption in the encyclopedia description is that the twenty minutes of aerobic exercise would be vigorous. But later findings have shown that moderate-intensity activity is sufficient to produce significant health and longevity benefits. As a result, we now recommend that your goal for minimum aerobic activity be thirty to forty minutes per day of endurance activity, three to five days per week.

Aerobics: The *New Encyclopaedia Britannica* Speaks

"**aerobics,** system of physical conditioning developed to increase the efficiency of the body's intake of oxygen. Typical aerobic exercises (*e.g.,* walking, running, swimming, dancing, and cycling) stimulate heart and lung activity long enough to produce beneficial changes in the body. To be effective, aerobic training must include a minimum of three sessions per week. During each session, the exerciser's heart rate must be raised to his training level for at least twenty minutes. . . .

"The concept of aerobics was pioneered by physician Kenneth H. Cooper and popularized in his books *Aerobics* (1968) and *The Aerobics Way* (1977)."

—from *The New Encyclopaedia Britannica,* 15th edition, Chicago: 1989, vol. 1, p. 120.

At this moderate-intensity level, you'll get the "good enough" level of exercise that will increase your chances of better health and longevity.[2]

So how do you get started with an effective aerobic exercise program? A good approach for a beginner might proceed like this:

First, we would suggest that most beginners stick to walking as their basic activity. Walking is an excellent aerobic activity and will prepare your heart and muscles for other types of aerobic training—such as jogging, swimming, or cycling—if you decide to shift to those later. Now here's a chart describing your basic aerobic program:

THE BASIC COOPER AEROBIC TRAINING PROGRAM*
(Perform 3 to 5 times per week)

	Week 1	Week 2	Week 3	Week 4	Week 5
Warm-up (slow version of any aerobic exercise)	5:00 minutes	5:00 minutes	5:00 minutes	5:00 minutes	5:00 minutes
Aerobic training†	10:00 minutes	15:00 minutes	20:00 minutes	25:00 minutes	30:00 minutes
Cooldown (same as warm-up)	5:00 minutes	5:00 minutes	5:00 minutes	5:00 minutes	5:00 minutes
Stretching‡	5:00 minutes	5:00 minutes	5:00 minutes	5:00 minutes	5:00 minutes
Total Program Time	25:00 minutes	30:00 minutes	35:00 minutes	40:00 minutes	45:00 minutes

*This generic program can be used to get started with any aerobic exercise. For more specific programs tailored to specific types of aerobic exercise, see discussions in Chapter 8.
†We suggest you begin with walking. But remember that aerobic training also includes such endurance activities as jogging, swimming, bicycling, walking on a treadmill, stationary cycling, using an elliptical trainer, and walking on a stair exerciser.
‡See page 148 of this chapter for stretching exercises.

You'll note that this program starts you with only ten minutes of aerobic walking in the first week, but the entire exercise time for a session is twenty-five minutes. With this approach, you'll start your walking at a very easy level. But you'll also become accustomed to operating at a higher level of activity for a full twenty-five minutes more than the level to which you may have become accustomed—especially if you're a classic couch potato.

You'll note that this five-week approach will gradually increase the time and intensity of your daily activity. But at this point, don't worry about what your ultimate potential may be, and certainly don't even think about turning yourself into a great athlete. There will be plenty of opportunity to consider such topics in the next chapter. To start out, just focus on developing a fitness habit.

For the second phase of your exercise program—on those days when you're not doing aerobic activity—you should focus on those activities that will increase your physical strength.

Building Strength

Your "strength days"—typically two to three days per week—will provide the aerobic-strength balance you need to maintain full physical functionality as you age.

As you begin this second phase, keep in mind the many benefits that we've already discussed for strength work, including building bone density to protect yourself against osteoporosis, and increasing muscle strength to ensure maximum physical functionality as you age. Also, your main concern in this early phase should continue to be *developing your fitness habit*—in a way consistent with the principles outlined in Chapters 3 and 4. That means being physically active on a regular basis. Remember that to establish an ingrained habit you need to do some sort of moderate to vigorous activity, no matter how small, *every single day.**

During the strength phase of your fitness workout, which may involve

---

*You can also devote one or two of those alternate days to some physical activity like yard work or vigorous housework (e.g., walking behind a hand lawn mower or scrubbing the bathroom floor).

roughly thirty minutes when you start out, you might even want to try a light, introductory circuit training of the type described in the following chapter. But if you choose this option, be sure you proceed under the eye of a seasoned trainer or other exercise expert. Otherwise, you could be putting yourself at risk for serious injury. As an alternative, you might want to begin with a simple calisthenics program, such as the one described below.

Calisthenics Made Simple

If you don't have access to a fitness center or a professional trainer, you might try these simple strength exercises and stretches. This entire program will probably take you no more than twenty minutes per session, depending on how many seconds you rest between exercises or sets.*

BEGIN WITH THREE TO FIVE MINUTES OF RUNNING IN PLACE OR JUMPING JACKS.

This start-up will provide a short aerobic benefit and will also serve as a muscle warm-up for the rest of the program.

Running in Place: A self-explanatory movement, running in place is where you simply jog easily without moving from the same spot on the floor or ground, allowing your feet to return to the positions from which they started. Keep your arms bent and pump them naturally, as you would do in an ordinary jog or run. Try to run on a soft or cushioned surface, wearing the appropriate athletic shoe.

Jumping Jacks: Do one jumping jack by starting off standing at attention, with arms down at your sides. Then jump with both feet off the

---

*A "repetition" is one complete exercise movement and a "set" is one group of continuously executed repetitions. Try to limit your rest between exercises or sets to thirty seconds.

floor and raise your hands to a clapping position above your head. At the same time, separate your legs and allow your feet to return to the floor at a position about shoulder width apart.

Finally, complete the movement by jumping again and returning your feet and hands to the starting position. One cycle of these movements constitutes one jumping jack. Execute the movements continuously for the three- to five-minute warm-up at a repetition rate that is not excessively fatiguing.

CONTINUE WITH THREE MINUTES OF ABDOMINAL CRUNCHES.

These crunches—which can be performed continuously or in sets, depending on your stamina—should be performed this way:

Lie flat on your back, with your knees bent at a 45-degree angle and your feet flat on the floor. Cross your arms across your chest, with right palm grasping left shoulder, and left palm grasping right shoulder.

Curl your upper body off the floor toward your knees. Your shoulders and head should be off the ground. Hold this position for one count and then lower your head and shoulders slowly to the starting position. This entire movement constitutes one repetition.

During the three-minute abdominal exercise period, do as many repetitions as you can before you experience mild fatigue. Then rest twenty to thirty seconds and begin again. Repeat until the three minutes are up. (Each group of crunches constitutes one set.)

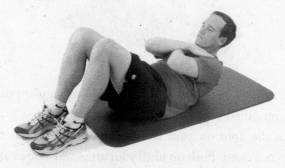

WORK YOUR UPPER BODY—INCLUDING ARMS, SHOULDERS, AND CHEST—FOR FIVE MINUTES.

Two exercises you might include in this phase are push-ups and pull-ups. Here's the drill:

Push-ups: For standard push-ups, lie flat on your stomach on the floor, with each hand placed flat on the floor next to your chest. Push your entire body up until your arms and elbows are in a straight position. Your body should be supported only by your hands and toes, and your back should be straight.

Then lower your body back to the starting position. This entire movement constitutes one repetition. Spend approximately three minutes doing these push-ups, employing as many sets as you need. Rest twenty to thirty seconds between sets.

For variety, you can alter the speed with which you do the exercise, such as doing them quickly in one set and then slowly in the following set. Varying the speed will condition different muscles and will also help prevent the tedium that may arise from doing each exercise the same way every time.

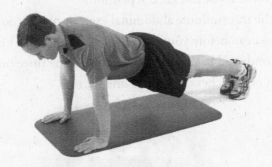

Modified Push-ups: If you have trouble doing regular push-ups, begin with this modified version:

Lie flat on the floor on your stomach, with your hands flat on the floor next to your chest. Push up until your arms and elbows are straight, but keep your knees and toes on the ground. Then lower your body back to the starting position.

Devote about three minutes to repeating this movement, using as many sets as you need. You should rest twenty to thirty seconds between sets.

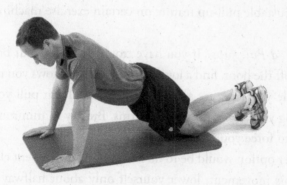

Pull-ups: Grasp a horizontal chin-up bar, using an overhand grip. The bar should be firmly secured, but otherwise can be located anywhere, such as on a child's jungle gym in the backyard or on a public playground. Also, there's nothing wrong with using a tree limb in your backyard; but be sure the limb is strong and secure.

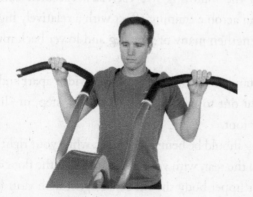

Begin with your arms supporting your body in a hanging position, with elbows straight. Pull your body up until your chin touches the bar, and then return to the starting position. This movement constitutes one repetition. Continue doing this exercise for two minutes, using as many sets as you need, with twenty- to thirty-second rest intervals between sets.

(The split bar Tyler is using to demonstrate the pull-ups may be available as an independent device for regular pull-ups or may be part of a weight-adjustable pull-up feature on certain exercise machines.)

Modified Pull-ups: If you have trouble pulling your body up with your feet off the floor, find a low bar or limb that allows you to bend your knees while your feet are still on the ground. Then pull your body up while using your legs to assist your arms. But try to minimize the use of your legs to force your arms to do most of the work.

Another option would be to do half pull-ups with bent elbows. In executing this movement, lower yourself only about halfway down from the bar and then pull yourself back up. One such movement constitutes one repetition.

STRENGTHEN YOUR LEGS AND LOWER BACK FOR FIVE MINUTES.

A series of the following five exercises, executed continuously, will help you get an aerobic training effect with a relatively high heart rate—while you strengthen many of your leg and lower back muscles.

Lunges: Stand with your feet shoulder width apart and your arms extended straight out to your sides. Take a long step, or "lunge," forward with your left foot.

Your left leg should be bent at the knee, while your right leg is extended straight out to the rear, with your toe planted on the floor at your starting position. Your upper body should be straight, with your hips dipping as far as possible toward the floor. The knee of your left, "lunging" leg should not move beyond the perpendicular plane traced by your left foot.

Return to the starting position to complete the first repetition. Now

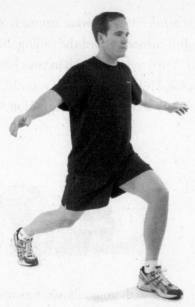

repeat the movements with your right leg for the second repetition. Continue for one minute.

Half squats: Stand straight while holding on to a bench, the back of a chair, or some other sturdy structure. Bend your knees until your thighs are almost at right angles to your lower legs. Hold this position for one second, and then return to the standing position. These movements constitute one repetition. Continue for one minute. (These are called "half squats" because knees are not bent beyond a 90-degree angle. Full squats would involve greater bending of the knee and are dangerous. See the accompanying box on leg strength training on page 148.)

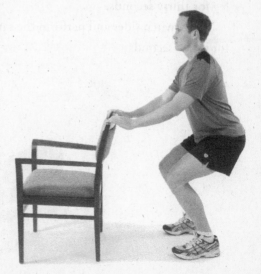

Lying Back Extension: Lie on your stomach with arms extended along your sides, palms turned toward the ceiling. Raise your feet, arms, and head off the mat. You'll feel the stretch in your lower back, hamstrings, and "glutes" (buttocks). Hold for as long as you can, without feeling undue strain. Eventually try to work up to a duration that may run as long as thirty seconds.

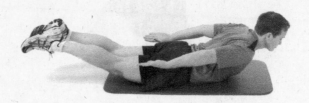

Rear Leg Lifts: Kneel with your elbows, forearms, knees, and lower legs on the floor. You should be in a "high crawl" position.

Keeping your left leg bent and planted on the floor, slowly extend your right leg straight up and back. You should "push" your right foot as much toward the ceiling as you can.

Return your right leg to the starting position. This series of movements constitutes one repetition. Continue the repetitions with the right leg for thirty seconds.

Now switch sides and perform the same movements with your left leg for thirty seconds.

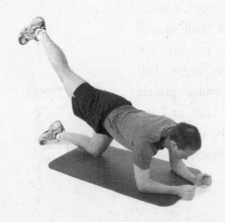

High Kicks: Begin by standing straight with your feet about a foot apart. Keeping your right knee as straight as possible, kick your right leg up in front of you as far as you can, and then return it to the starting position. Perform the same kicking movement with your left leg. The double kick counts as one repetition. Continue for one minute.

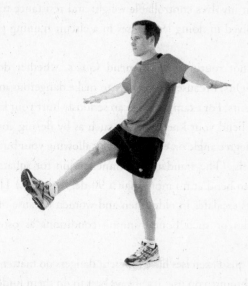

Caution: Older people or those unused to such activity will need to hold on to a chair while performing these movements.

END WITH FIVE MINUTES OF STRETCHING.

To fill up the five minutes with effective stretching, you can choose among these stretching movements, which our members and patients use with great success at the Cooper Aerobic Center. These can be incorporated as part of the above calisthenics routine, or as the final part of an aerobic or strength workout. We'll be referring to this routine as we introduce you to various programs, both in this chapter and in Chapter 8.

Ken and Tyler on Leg Strength Training

Using the wrong technique in certain types of strength training for the legs—especially building up the quadriceps ("quads") on the front of the thighs—can lead to serious injuries. For this reason, we prefer quad training that involves controllable weight and resistance training, such as that involved in doing leg presses in a circuit training program (see Chapter 8).

We do not routinely recommend squats, whether done with or without weights, because it's too easy to make dangerous mistakes with the movements. For example, you can seriously hurt your knees or your back if you bend your knees too far, such as by flexing your knees beyond a 90-degree angle or, even worse, by allowing your buttocks to rest on your heels. (The standard recommendation for squats is to allow your knees to bend at no more than a 90-degree angle.) The danger in doing squats escalates in older men and women because of underlying weak muscles or such bone-thinning conditions as osteopenia and osteoporosis.

Because quad exercises have inherent dangers no matter what equipment or technique you use, it's always best to do them under the supervision of a qualified trainer.

The Standard Cooper Stretching Routine

These stretching exercises should be inserted into your aerobic, circuit training, calisthenics, or other program as indicated in the explanation of those programs. Or just include them at the end of each exercise session. You should select only five to use as part of the five-minute cooldown phase of a regular aerobic or strength session. But try to include all ten stretching exercises at least once during your weekly workouts.

1. Seated Back Stretch

- While seated on a FitBALL, chair, bench, or floor, keep your posture tall and straight.
- Extend right arm over head.
- Lean to the left until you feel mild discomfort (a sense of stretching out) along your right side. Hold the position for 15 seconds.
- Repeat the movement with the opposite arm.

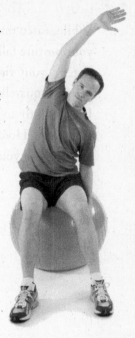

2. FitBALL Chest Stretch

- Lie with your upper back on a FitBALL, bench, chair, or other sturdy, raised surface. You should be facing the ceiling with your head inclined backward. (If you don't have a raised surface available, just lie with your back flat on the floor.)
- Extend your arms straight out to your sides until you feel a mild discomfort (sense of stretching). Hold this position for 15 seconds.

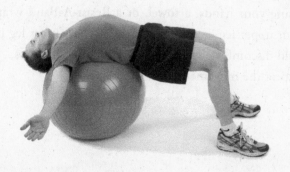

3. Seated Groin Stretch

- While seated on the front part of a FitBALL, chair, or bench, keep your posture tall and straight.
- Extend your right leg out to the side and keep your right foot planted squarely on the floor (both toes and heel).
- Lean slightly to the left until you feel mild discomfort (stretching sensation). Hold this position for 15 seconds.
- Repeat with your left leg.

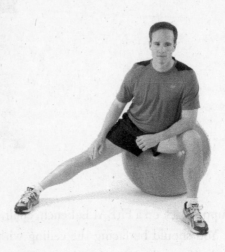

4. Lying Hamstring Stretch

- While lying on your back on a mat or soft floor, extend your left leg upward, keeping both legs as straight as possible.
- Using your hands, a towel, or a Resist-A-Band wrapped around your upper leg, gently pull back on your upper leg until you feel mild discomfort. Hold the position for 15 seconds.
- Repeat the movement with your right leg.

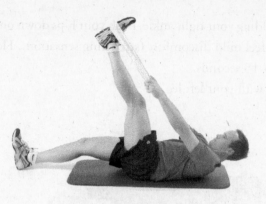

5. Lying Hip Stretch

- While lying on your back on a mat, cross your right foot over your left knee. Your left knee should be bent and raised off the floor, and your right ankle should be resting on your left knee.
- Using your hands or a towel, reach behind your left knee and gently pull back until you feel mild discomfort (a stretching sensation). Hold the position for 15 seconds.
- Repeat with your right leg.

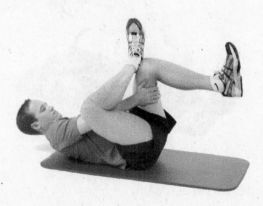

6. Lying Quadriceps Stretch

- While lying facedown on a mat, reach back with your right hand and grasp your right ankle.

- Still holding your right ankle, push your hips down on the mat until you feel mild discomfort (stretching sensation). Hold the position for 15 seconds.
- Repeat with your left leg.

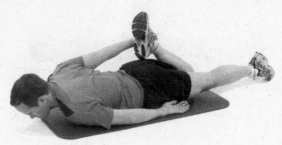

7. Lying Glute/Low-Back Stretch

- While lying with your back on the mat, gently pull your knees up to your chest until you feel mild discomfort (stretching sensation).
- Hold the position for 15 seconds.

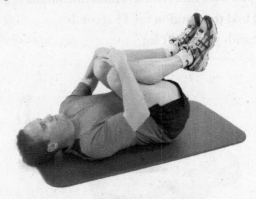

8. Lying Abdominal Stretch

- While lying on the mat facedown, push up on your elbows (supporting your upper body with your elbows), arching your lower back until you feel mild discomfort (stretching sensation). Hold the position for 15 seconds.

- As you're pushing up and supporting your upper body on your elbows, you should be facing directly forward.

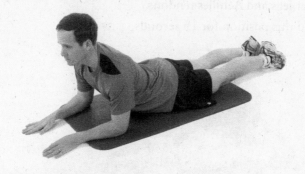

9. Seated Triceps Stretch

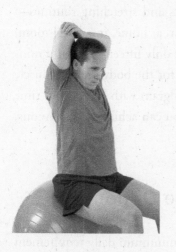

- While seated on a FitBALL, chair, or bench—or while standing—place your right arm behind your head, with your right hand extended down along your upper back in a "back-scratching" movement.
- Grasp your right elbow with your left hand and gently pull backward and downward until you feel mild discomfort (stretching sensation). Hold the position for 15 seconds.
- Repeat the movements with your opposite arms.

10. Kneeling Back Stretch

- Kneel on a mat with knees, shins, and tops of feet on the floor.
- Lean forward so that hands and forearms touch the floor. Elbows should remain straight with palms facing inward.

- Lower head and hips toward the floor so that you feel tension throughout your back, your thigh muscles, and the backs of your lower legs and Achilles tendons.
- Hold this position for 15 seconds.

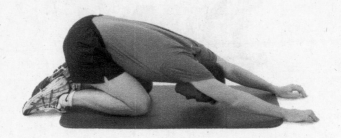

As you can see, these simple calisthenics and stretching routines—which can be performed without equipment, at home, in a hotel room, or in practically any other venue—will take only fifteen to twenty minutes. Yet they will provide a good workout for the body's major muscle groups. Furthermore, if you execute the program with little or no time between exercises or sets, you'll find that you can achieve a continuous, if moderate, aerobic effect.

The Intermittent Exercise Option

Some recent research indicates that the minimum daily requirement of thirty to forty minutes of moderate-intensity aerobic exercise can be broken up into segments during different parts of the day. The usual suggestion is to divide your routine into three segments of ten to fifteen minutes each. So you might jog ten to fifteen minutes early in the morning, then walk briskly ten to fifteen minutes at lunchtime, and finally, jog or walk briskly again ten to fifteen minutes before you sit down for supper in the evening.

This approach has gained approval from former U.S. Surgeon General David Stacher, who has recommended that to get some health and longevity benefits, all Americans engage in thirty minutes of exercise *collectively* most days of the week. In other words, you can split up your activity as you like so long as it totals thirty minutes per day. While we agree that getting some exercise, even in bits and pieces, is preferable to no exercise at all, we have a somewhat different take on the issue.

Our Preference: Continuous Exercise: Although the piecemeal approach to exercise is acceptable if you can stick with it on a regular basis, we prefer doing thirty to forty-five minutes of aerobic activity in one continuous session—for at least three reasons:

- First, most people are likely to miss one or two of those short sessions, as daily demands intrude at lunchtime or at the end of the day—and they'll fail to accumulate their necessary thirty minutes per day of activity.
- Second, the aerobic training effect will be greater if you do the exercise without any breaks.
- Third, if you do a complete aerobic session in the morning, you just might decide to do other physical activity at lunch or at the end of the day—and thus benefit from an even higher level of aerobic exercise than the minimum.

In any case, the more activity you can find time for, the better it's likely to be for your health and longevity—and weight loss.

The Basic Cooper Start-up Fitness Model

By now, you have a fairly good idea about what your start-up program should look like. But for more specific guidance, consider this model, especially if you're about to bridge that intimidating gap from sedentary couch potato to regular physical activity. *Caution:* Before you start, be sure that you undergo a complete gold-standard physical exam and get the go-ahead from your physician.

WEEK #1

Walk a minimum of twenty minutes, three to four days a week, either before or after work or during lunchtime. The distance you cover doesn't matter. The key thing is just to start moving and keep moving.

On alternate days, do some physical strength activity, no matter how light. For example, you might try the calisthenics routine described above one day, then do the entire stretching routine another day. On still another day, you might do some physical housework (e.g., cleaning a bathroom), or some yard work (pushing a power mower). On the seventh day, you might build in some extra walking, such as by parking a longer distance from your supermarket or house of worship.

WEEK #2

Walk continuously for twenty-five minutes three to four days a week, either before or after work, or during lunchtime. Again, the distance you cover doesn't matter. Fill the remaining days with physical strength activity, as described above in Week One.

WEEK #3

Walk continuously for thirty minutes, three to four days either before or after work, or during lunchtime. The distance doesn't matter. And don't forget to do some physical activity on the other days, as suggested in Week One.

WEEK #4

Walk continuously for thirty minutes, three to four days a week, either before or after work, or during lunchtime. This time, try to cover 1.25 to 1.50 miles during your outing. You can figure this out by walking on a track or measuring the distance with your auto odometer. Include physical strength activity on alternate days, as indicated above.

WEEK #5

Walk continuously for thirty minutes, three to four days a week, either before or after work, or during lunchtime. Now, try to cover 1.5 to 1.75 miles. Again, engage in strength activity on alternate days.

WEEK #6

Walk continuously for thirty minutes, three to four days a week, either before or after work, or during lunchtime. Try to increase your speed by covering 1.75 to 2 miles during your outing. And remember to do strength activity on the remaining days.

Now, let's explore a related question that fascinates everyone carrying some extra pounds around the middle: how, if at all, might these simple exercise programs—or the more advanced models described in the next chapter—help you with weight loss?

Using Exercise to Control Your Weight

The Classic Combination Approach: Generally speaking, to lose weight and keep it off, we recommend that you not rely on exercise alone. Instead, it's best to employ a complete exercise program, including aerobic and strength components, with a reduced-calorie, low-fat diet. Various studies have shown that your exercise should be combined with calorie reduction in order to maintain a lower weight—and these findings have consistently been borne out in practice.

Take the well-publicized case of my friend Mike Huckabee, former governor of Arkansas. In 2003, he launched a diet-and-exercise program to lose 110 pounds. And two years later, he had indeed lost a hundred pounds. In that same year, he also finished the Little Rock Marathon in a sprint. In Huckabee's case, as in most others, the secret to weight loss was the *combination* of aerobic exercise and diet, not just diet or exercise alone.

This principle means that as long as you're cutting calories, even the minimum three to five days per week, thirty minutes per day regimen of moderate exercise will help you with your weight control. This minimum level of activity will certainly contribute to the calorie burning that helps you get rid of extra pounds. But even more important, exercise appears to "rev up" your body's metabolism to make it easier for you to break through various weight barriers that may challenge you as your weight goes down.

Ken on Exercise and Weight Loss

You can't lose weight rapidly only through exercise—an effective weight-loss plan must combine *both* cutting calories *and* exercise. But even though exercise alone won't eliminate all those pounds, exercise can help you burn calories in at least two ways: by increasing your body's aerobic activity level and by increasing your muscle mass.

First, whenever you do aerobic exercise, you expend calories. And the more you exercise, the more calories you burn. Furthermore, your body will continue to burn calories after you finish your aerobic workout.

For example, assume you have a resting heart rate of 55 beats per minute (bpm) and you finish your aerobic workout with a maximum heart rate of 150. If you're in good aerobic shape, your heart rate should drop at least 12 bpm during the first minute, and at least 30 beats in the first five minutes, say to 120 bpm. Usually, it will then take up to two hours for your heart rate to return to your preexercise heart rate of 55 beats per minute. During those two hours, your body is still burning calories—at a higher rate than if you had never exercised at all.

A related strategy that we recommend is to exercise just before your heaviest meal of the day. That way, you'll "stoke the furnace" of your body through exercise, and tend to metabolize the food you consume more effectively. Also, our experience and a number of studies have shown that vigorous exercise just before a meal tends to suppress the appetite.

The second way of using exercise to lose weight is to increase your muscle mass by doing strength work. The more muscle you have, the more calories you burn. But be aware that the actual strength exercise itself is not as effective as aerobic exercise in burning calories. The reason: aerobic exercise raises the heart rate—and the "heat" of the body's calorie-burning "furnace"—higher than does strength work.

Can exercise alone result in weight loss? If you want to use exercise *independently* to lose weight, you'll have to increase the time you devote to physical activity, as the 30-60-90-minute guidelines by the U.S. government suggest. (These are discussed in some depth on pages 161 to 162.) The reason is fairly obvious: it takes a lot of exercise to burn up enough calories to lose weight.

Here's the challenge: to get rid of one pound of fat, you have to burn up 3,500 calories. To achieve this goal, here are some weight-loss possibilities for an exerciser who weighs 150 pounds:[3]

- Walking (brisk pace, outside or on a treadmill) at 4.5 mph—400 calories/hour
- Jogging (outside or on treadmill) at 5.5 mph—650 calories/hour
- Tennis singles—575 calories/hour
- Tennis doubles—430 calories/hour
- Bicycling (moderate pace, outside or on stationary bike) at 10 mph—400 calories/hour
- Handball or squash (vigorous)—860 calories/hour
- Swimming crawl (light effort, approximately 20–25 yards/min)— 300 calories/hour
- Swimming crawl (moderate effort, approximately 45 yards/ min)—550 calories/hour
- Swimming crawl (vigorous effort, approximately 55 yards/min)— 820 calories/hour
- Downhill skiing (constant activity)—422 calories/hour
- Roller-skating (moderate pace)—390 calories/hour
- Aerobic dancing (low impact)—430 calories/hour
- Ballroom dancing (fast or rock)—250–300 calories/hour
- Basketball (full court)—730 calories/hour
- Light to moderate snow-shoveling—600 calories/hour
- Calisthenics (continuous)—355 calories/hour
- Golf (walking with bag cart)—245 calories/hour
- Mowing lawn (walking behind power mower)—265 calories/hour

From this list, you can see that to lose one pound you would have to walk briskly for a total of nearly nine hours. Or you'll have to play six hours of singles tennis or four hours of handball to eliminate that pound. Also, if weight loss through exercise alone is your goal, you'll have to be sure that you don't start eating more as you exercise—a difficult task as you expend more energy through higher activity levels.

Another way of picturing this challenge is to think in terms of how much exercise it takes to work off different food servings.[4] Let's assume that you add an apple to your diet as you increase your exercise level. To get rid of the 101 calories in that piece of fruit, you'll have to walk nineteen minutes, or bicycle twelve minutes, or swim nine minutes, or run (not jog) five minutes.

And don't even consider adding one extra serving of spaghetti, at 396 calories. To eliminate that helping would require seventy-six minutes of moderate-paced walking, forty-eight minutes of brisk bicycling, thirty-five minutes of swimming, or twenty minutes of running (not just jogging).

A helpful reference point for weight loss through exercise might be to consider how you might apply some rather controversial—but potentially instructive—fitness guidelines recently put out by the U.S. government.

The 30-60-90 Debate

Howls of protest arose both from the general public and from the medical community when the U.S. government issued its Dietary Guidelines for 2005. The source of the dismay? There had been years of reports that great advantages could be gained from relatively modest amounts of exercise—such as a total of only about thirty minutes of non-continuous activity per day. But now the experts were suggesting that it would be necessary to exercise *up to ninety minutes per day* to benefit fully from physical activity. Many people were overwhelmed.

Specifically, the report recommended these rather formidable goals:

- 30 minutes of moderate-intensity physical activity most days of the week to reduce the risk of chronic disease in adulthood.
- 60 minutes of moderate- or vigorous-intensity activity to help manage body weight and prevent gradual weight gain in adulthood, assuming caloric intake remains the same.

- 60 to 90 minutes of daily moderate-intensity physical activity to maintain weight loss, independently of any dietary program that would diminish caloric intake.

In the category of "moderate-intensity exercise," the guidelines include any activity that would be the equivalent of walking fairly briskly, at about 3.5 miles per hour (a little over seventeen minutes per mile). Qualifying activities might include hiking at an easy pace, light gardening or yard work, dancing, golf, bicycling at a leisurely pace, stretching or other light calisthenics, or some light weight lifting.

The "vigorous-intensity" exercises might include running or jogging at 5 to 6 miles per hour (10 to 12 minutes per mile); walking at 4.5 miles per hour (13.5 minutes per mile); bicycling at 12 miles per hour; swimming, aerobics, heavy yard work such as chopping wood or shoveling snow, more vigorous weight lifting, or playing basketball.

Even with the variety of activities suggested, the new exercise recommendations may seem unrealistic. After all, 74 percent of American women and 66 percent of men currently fail to meet the thirty-minute guideline, and 41 percent of women and 35 percent of men engage in absolutely no leisure-time physical activity.[5] But in fact, you may find that some variations of the government recommendations will fit into your own program—if you integrate them creatively into the Start Strong, Finish Strong aerobics and strength guidelines outlined below.

The "Activity Add-on Principle" for Weight Loss

As the government's 30-60-90 minute recommendations for exercise indicate, thirty minutes per day of moderate-intensity exercise will certainly help give you protection from health- and life-threatening disease. Also, this amount of activity will at least *assist* you with weight loss if you cut calories in your diet. But thirty minutes alone isn't going to take those pounds off quickly, and won't take them off at all if you add an extra apple or two into the mix.

Sixty minutes per day of moderate-intensity exercise will help you hold off weight gain as you age. But again, you have to be careful not to add extra calories to replace those you're burning up.

Finally, ninety minutes per day of moderate-intensity exercise will help you keep off pounds you may already have lost—and can also result in independent weight loss (provided you don't add extra calories in your diet).

For some ideas about how to include some "activity add-ons" in your life—which can either provide you with extra calorie burners or just inject some significant physical activity on those days when you think you don't have time for exercise—see Tyler's add-on checklist in the accompanying box.

Tyler's Checklist for Activity Add-ons— at Home and Work

At work, at home, or during errands, try these fitness tricks to add health-enhancing, calorie-burning exercise to your life:

- Park farther away than you usually do from your office or from a particular store or supermarket. Set things up so that you have to walk briskly ten minutes each way to reach your destination. That will be an automatic twenty minutes of aerobic activity added to your schedule.
- Take the stairs instead of the elevator or escalator. And don't be cowed if you have to walk up several flights. If you can't make it all the way to the top at first, try only one or two flights for a couple of weeks. Then increase your stair-climbing by an extra flight or two.

(continued)

- Walk while you're talking on your cell phone. Just pace around your office or home, if that's your only choice. The size of the space doesn't really matter as long as you keep moving. Or if you have to use a landline phone, get an extra-long cord so that you can move around the full dimensions of your office or a particular room in your home.
- Determine what restaurants, shops, or parks are reasonably close to your home or job, and then walk to those places instead of driving. You'll be surprised how easy it is to put an extra fifteen-minute walk each way into your day.
- Always think in terms of *fitness multitasking*. In other words, you might lift light weights while talking on the phone, or build in a few crunches, stretches, or push-ups when a commercial comes on TV.
- Make creative use of *transition time* during the day. When you move from one room to the next at home, get into the habit of doing a few push-ups or modified push-ups, or a few repetitions with hand weights.
- Deliver your own reports or files around the workplace instead of using interoffice mail.
- Spend time with people who have the same health goals and habits that you do—and get them to participate with you in some activity add-ons.

Finally, don't worry if you don't want to follow the same routine every day. In fact, most people who maintain a high level of interest and yet avoid a rigid regimen have discovered it helps to vary the add-ons from day to day.

Finally, to keep focused on staying active rather than slipping back into a sedentary lifestyle, pose a pointed question to yourself each morning: "What physical activity can I add on to my life today?"

As you can see from the add-on checklist, it would be quite possible for most people to devote a basic thirty to forty-five minutes to a regular fitness routine three to five days a week *and also* to include some add-ons to further stoke the body's calorie-burning furnace. With just a little thought and alteration of your normal schedule, you should be able to do ninety minutes or more of moderate-intensity physical activity—and actually cause those extra pounds to melt away mainly from exercise.

But whatever strategy you choose, it's important to keep this principle in mind: *combining exercise—especially the calorie-burning aerobic kind—with a lower-calorie, low-fat diet is an essential part of any weight-loss regimen.* Finally, because relying on exercise alone for weight loss is such a formidable challenge, you'll need to get creative with your free time and work time if you want exercise to eliminate most of those unwanted pounds.

Get Creative!

It's essential to give your personal creativity free rein as you design a fitness program that you can live with now and into the future—for at least three reasons.

First of all, getting creative will help you find ways to make better *physical* use of your free time at home. The average person spends three to four hours per day in front of the TV set or computer screen.

Second, the process will help you inject more physical activity into your workday. You'd be amazed at how many hours you spend sitting at a desk when you could be doing the same tasks while walking or standing.

Third, the more creative you are in designing your physical activity program, the less likely it will be that you'll become bored and give up. Even though the two of us are professionals in the fitness field, we have to vary our routine regularly to keep our edge and interest level. Together, we get involved at one time or another with more sports and physical activities that we can keep track of: walking, jogging, running, interval training, skiing, swimming, calisthenics, treadmill training, resistance-machine workouts, basketball, mountain biking—you name it!

Creative Exercise Requires Breaking Some Rules

Too many exercise programs have fallen by the wayside during the first few months when important habits were being established because the programs became boring. To counter boredom, you might sometimes even have to resort to "breaking the rules."

In fact, there are no hard-and-fast rules about exercise for health and fitness—as long as you reach at least a moderate level of intensity. Furthermore, any physical activity can be modified to fit the ages and fitness levels of the players. So feel free to break the rules if that will promote more activity in your life or the lives of your friends.

For example, although you may be intrigued by volleyball, you may feel you're too old or lack the skill to play at the level of those hard-bodied men and women you watch on TV. But you don't have to play that way—so don't give up.

To make the game playable for you, you might try some "bounce volleyball": let the ball bounce on the court instead of requiring that players take it in the air. In effect, you'll convert ordinary volleyball into a kind of Ping-Pong volleyball—which is much easier to handle for older people or those who lack the special skills of the sport.

Another possibility would be a variation on slow-break basketball. First of all, as with the regular version, you would prohibit any fast breaks down the court. In other words, when the ball changes hands, the team in possession would have to walk-dribble the ball down the court, rather than running in an effort to beat the other team to the basket. In addition, you could allow double or triple dribbles, rather than the usual rule that you must pass or shoot after finishing a single sequence of dribbling.

For many years the Cooper Aerobics Center has sponsored a wheel-chair tennis league. Under the leadership of Bill Hammett, several out-standing players have developed significant skills, and in some cases have even achieved national recognition. In playing tennis these special ath-letes are allowed to let the ball bounce twice before they hit it. In other words, they have become very creative in adapting a traditional sport to their handicaps.

The options for this sort of rule-breaking are virtually endless, limited only by your own creativity. So allow your imagination to roam.

Whatever exercise variation you choose for your beginning program, you'll probably find after a few weeks or months that you want to ratchet up your intensity. As you see your endurance and strength increase—and your body becoming younger and younger—you'll become interested in seeing just how young and vigorous you can become. In other words, you'll want to explore your fitness potential, and that's what our final ex-ercise chapter is all about.

Eight

Start-up #2—Advanced Fitness: Explore Your Physical Potential

As you know from our previous discussions, the health and longevity benefits of simply going from a completely sedentary life to minimal activity are significant. But after you've enjoyed the advantages of becoming more active, why not take things a step further? Explore your potential to lift your body to higher levels of fitness. Here are some guidelines we use at the Cooper Aerobics Center.

First, we'll focus on the "Cooper Advanced Aerobic Training Program," including a description of the Cooper Aerobic Points System—which will enable you to evaluate the fitness value of practically any type of physical activity. Then, we'll launch into a discussion of strength work—or what we call the "Secret of Strength at Any Age." This strength section will introduce you to the finer points of resistance training with various types of exercise equipment.

The Cooper Advanced Aerobic Training Program

To improve your cardiovascular fitness—and protect yourself from heart disease, stroke, diabetes, and other life-threatening conditions—you should perform aerobic (endurance) activity several times each week *at increasingly higher levels of intensity.* This strategy will improve your fitness level (the ability of your body to process oxygen)—a major factor in reducing your risk for disease and death.

As we've mentioned before, exercises that qualify as the best aerobic or endurance activities include treadmill walking, treadmill jogging, outdoor walking, outdoor jogging, running, elliptical cross training, stationary cycling, outdoor bicycling, cross-country skiing, and swimming. But this list certainly isn't exhaustive: any activity that can keep your heart rate in the ranges and time periods indicated in the chart on page 170 will meet the aerobic criteria.

Guidelines for Advanced Aerobic Activity

Keep these guidelines in mind as you engage in more advanced aerobic activity:

- Consult your physician before beginning any exercise program—and especially demanding exercise programs.
- Do your aerobic exercise at least three to five times per week.
- Raise the intensity of your activity to a moderate to hard level, or to the level of your "target heart rate" (65 to 80 percent of your maximum heart rate).
- Exercise at your target heart rate for thirty to forty-five minutes or longer during each session.

General target heart-rate ranges for aerobic conditioning (in heartbeats per minute according to age) are as follows:

COOPER AEROBIC EXERCISE TARGET
HEART RATE RANGE TABLE

| Exercise Time | Age | | | | | | % Maximum Heart Rate |
	20 years	30 years	40 years	50 years	60 years	70 years	
20 minutes	160 heart-beats/ minute	150	145	135	130	120	80%
30 minutes	150 heart-beats/ minute	140	135	125	120	115	75%
45 minutes	130 heart-beats/ minute	125	115	110	105	100	65%

Generally speaking, to achieve a consistent training effect, the heart rate at which you exercise should decline as your exercise time increases, and vice versa. In other words, if you decide to work out only for twenty minutes, you should exercise more intensely (e.g., walk or jog at a faster pace) than you would if you work out for thirty or forty minutes. More specifically, if you exercise for twenty minutes, try to exercise at 80 percent of your maximum heart rate. But if you exercise for thirty minutes, keep your target heart rate at 75 percent of maximum. Finally, if you exercise for forty-five minutes, maintain a heart rate at 65 percent of your maximum.

You can determine your actual heart rate during exercise by using a variety of heart rate monitors (we recommend the Polar heart rate monitor). Some types of exercise machines have built-in monitors, but most of them are not that accurate. Or you can just stop exercising briefly and check your pulse, using your index or middle finger pressed against the inside of your wrist or a carotid artery (on each side of the neck). If you choose this check-your-own-pulse approach, the most accurate and convenient technique is to measure your heart rate for ten seconds, then multiply by six to get your heart rate per minutes.

So what should an advanced daily aerobic workout schedule look like?

The strategy for advanced training is basically the same as that for a beginning program. In other words, you begin by warming up for five minutes; next, do your chosen aerobic activity for a preselected period of time; then spend five minutes cooling down; and finally engage in some stretching.

Note: The latest thinking on this exercise sequence is that, instead of stretching, it's best to warm up using a low-level version of your regular aerobic activity, such as walking or slow jogging. In some cases, stretching at the beginning of a workout, before you're properly warmed up, may increase your risk of muscle pulls or other injury. But stretching should be done at the end of the workout to relax and extend muscle groups that have become contracted during the main part of the workout.

An effective way of thinking about a more advanced aerobic program is to focus on the *Aerobic Points System,* developed by Ken several decades ago and still used in many military, governmental, and corporate fitness programs. This system is based on the assignment of point values for different types of exercise in terms of the ability of the exercise to increase or maintain aerobic (cardiopulmonary endurance) fitness.

THE COOPER AEROBIC POINTS SYSTEM™

Ken originally developed the Aerobic Points System in the 1960s for the U.S. Air Force. This approach can be especially useful if you're looking for an easy way to keep track of the conditioning value of your level of aerobic physical activity, or if you want to steadily increase your fitness levels.

For example, if you want to maintain only a minimum level of activity for health and longevity fitness, you should acquire a minimum of 15 aerobic points per week. Remember that our research shows that health and longevity fitness translates to a 58 percent reduction in death from all causes, and up to a six-year increase in longevity.[1] You can accumulate 15 Aerobic Points per week in this fashion:

HEALTH AND LONGEVITY FITNESS

15 aerobic points/week

Walk 2.0 miles < 30:00 minutes 3x/week

Walk 2.0 miles < 35:00 minutes 4x/week

Walk 2.0 miles < 40:00 minutes 5x/week

Walk 3.0 miles < 45:00 minutes 2x/week

Aerobic dance 45:00 minutes 2x/week

If you want to maintain a higher level of aerobic fitness, you should perform a minimum of 35 points per week. This more advanced level of conditioning will translate to a 65 percent reduction in death from all causes, and up to a nine-year increase in longevity.[2] To increase your level of aerobic fitness, all you have to do is gradually increase the number of points you earn each week up to at least 35. This goal could be achieved in a number of ways, as illustrated on pages 173–85.

AEROBIC FITNESS

35 aerobic points/week

Run 2.0 miles < 20:00 minutes 4x/week

Walk 3.0 miles < 45:00 minutes 5x/week

Aerobic dance 45:00 minutes 4x/week

These 15- and 35-point charts provide just a suggestion about how you can employ the Aerobic Points concept.* To provide you with the

---

*For younger people, both men and women, points can be earned by means of exercise of greater intensity and shorter duration. For older men and women, points should be earned through lower-intensity and longer-duration activities. But the point requirement remains the same, regardless of sex or age.

full range of flexibility in choosing and evaluating your activities as you fine-tune your program, here are the aerobic point values for a number of common exercise choices. Feel free to substitute any of these exercises and activities for any other routines you may be following—provided that the new exercises have point values comparable to those of your old exercises.

AEROBIC POINTS VALUES—VARIOUS EXERCISES*

Walking/Running		
Distance	Time	Point Value
1.0 mile	Over 20:01	0
	20:00–15:01	1.0
	15:00–12:01	2.0
	12:00–10:01	3.0
	10:00–8:01	4.0
	8:00–6:41	5.0
	6:40–5:44	6.0
	Under 5:43	7.0
1.5 miles	Over 45:01	0
	45:00–30:01	0.5
	30:00–22:31	2.0
	22:30–18:01	3.5

*If you do not find an activity that is applicable to your workout, aerobics points can be estimated by taking total caloric expenditure and dividing by 20.

Distance	Time	Point Value
	18:00–15:01	5.0
	15:00–12:01	6.5
	12:00–10:01	8.0
	10:00–8:35	9.5
	Under 8:34	11.0
2.0 miles	Over 40:01	1.0
	40:00–30:01	3.0
	30:00–24:01	5.0
	24:00–20:01	7.0
	20:00–16:01	9.0
	16:00–13:21	11.0
	13:20–11:27	13.0
	Under 11:26	15.0
2.5 miles	Over 50:01	1.5
	50:00–37:31	4.0
	37:30–30:01	6.5
	30:00–25:01	9.0
	25:00–20:01	11.5
	20:00–16:41	14.0
	16:40–14:19	16.5

Distance	Time	Point Value
3.0 miles	Over 1:00:00	2.0
	1:00:00–45:01	5.0
	45:00–36:01	8.0
	36:00–30:01	11.0
	30:00–24:01	14.0
	24:00–20:01	17.0
	20:00–17:01	20.0
	Under 17:00	23.0
3.5 miles	Over 1:10:01	2.5
	1:10:00–52:31	6.0
	52:30–42:01	9.5
	42:00–35:01	13.0
	35:00–28:01	16.5
	28:00–23:21	20.0
	23:20–20:01	23.5
4.0 miles	Over 1:20:00	3.0
	1:20:00–1:00:01	7.0
	1:00:00–48:01	11.0
	48:00–40:01	15.0

Distance	Time	Point Value
	40:00–32:01	19.0
	32:00–26:41	23.0
	26:40–22:53	27.0
	Under 22:52	31.0
4.5 miles	Over 1:30:01	3.5
	1:30:00–1:07:31	8.0
	1:07:30–54:01	12.5
	54:00–45:01	17.0
	45:00–36:01	21.5
	36:00–30:01	26.0
	30:00–25:44	30.5
5.0 miles	Over 1:40:01	4.0
	1:40:00–1:15:01	9.0
	1:15:00–1:00:01	14.0
	1:00:00–50:01	19.0
	50:00–40:01	24.0
	40:00–33:21	29.0
	33:20–28:35	34.0
	Under 28:34	39.0

Distance	Time	Point Value
6.0 miles	Over 2:00:01	5.0
	2:00:00–1:30:01	11.0
	1:30:00–1:12:01	17.0
	1:12:00–1:00:01	23.0
	1:00:00–48:01	29.0
	48:00–40:01	35.0
	40:00–34:19	41.0
7.0 miles	Over 2:20:01	6.0
	2:20–1:45:01	13.0
	1:45:00–1:24:01	20.0
	1:24:00–1:10:01	27.0
	1:10:00–56:01	34.0
	56:00–46:41	41.0
	46:40–40:01	48.0
	Under 40:00	55.0
8.0 miles	Over 2:40:01	7.0
	2:40:00–2:00:01	15.0
	2:00:00–1:36:01	23.0
	1:36:00–1:20:01	31.0

Distance	Time	Point Value
	1:20:00–1:04:01	39.0
	1:04:00–53:21	47.0
	53:20–45:44	55.0
9.0 miles	Over 3:00:01	8.0
	3:00:00–2:15:01	17.0
	2:15:00–1:48:01	26.0
	1:48:00–1:30:01	35.0
	1:30:00–1:12:01	44.0
	1:12:00–1:00:01	53.0
	1:00:00–51:27	62.0
	Under 51:26	71.0
10.0 miles	Over 3:20:01	9.0
	3:20:00–2:30:01	19.0
	2:30:00–2:00:01	29.0
	2:00:00–1:40:01	39.0
	1:40:00–1:20:01	49.0
	1:20:00–1:06:41	59.0
	1:06:40–57:10	69.0

Outdoor Cycling		
Distance	**Time**	**Point Value**
2.0 miles	Over 12:01	0
	12:00–8:01	0.5
	8:00–6:01	1.5
	Under 6:00	2.5
3.0 miles	Over 18:01	0
	18:00–12:01	1.5
	12:00–9:01	3.0
	Under 9:00	4.5
4.0 miles	Over 24:01	0
	24:00–16:01	2.5
	16:00–12:01	4.5
	Under 12:00	6.5
5.0 miles	Over 30:01	2.0
	30:00–20:01	3.5
	20:00–15:01	6.0
	Under 15:00	8.5
6.0 miles	Over 36:01	2.7
	36:00–24:01	4.5
	24:00–18:01	7.5
	Under 18:00	10.5

Distance	Time	Point Value
7.0 miles	Over 42:01	3.4
	42:00–28:01	5.5
	28:00–21:01	9.0
	Under 21:00	12.5
8.0 miles	Over 48:01	4.1
	48:00–32:01	6.5
	32:00–24:01	10.5
	Under 24:00	14.5
9.0 miles	Over 54:01	4.8
	54:00–36:01	7.5
	36:00–27:01	12.0
	Under 27:00	16.5
10.0 miles	Over 1:00:01	5.5
	1:00:00–40:01	8.5
	40:00–30:01	13.5
	Under 30:00	18.5
11.0 miles	Over 1:06:01	6.2
	1:06:00–44:01	9.5
	44:00–33:01	15.0
	Under 33:00	20.5

Distance	Time	Point Value
12.0 miles	Over 1:12:01	6.9
	1:12:00–48:01	10.5
	48:00–36:01	16.5
	Under 36:00	22.5
13.0 miles	Over 1:18:01	7.6
	1:18:00–52:01	11.5
	52:00–39:01	18.0
	Under 39:00	24.5
14.0 miles	Over 1:24:01	8.3
	1:24:00–56:01	12.5
	56:00–42:01	19.5
	Under 42:00	26.5
15.0 miles	Over 1:30:01	9.0
	1:30:00–1:00:01	13.5
	1:00:00–45:01	21.0
	Under 45:00	28.5
20.0 miles	Over 2:00:01	12.5
	2:00:00–1:20:01	18.5
	1:20:00–1:00:01	28.5
	Under 1:00:00	38.5

Swimming		
Distance	Time	Point Value
200 yards	Over 6:41	0
	6:40–5:01	1.25
	5:00–3:21	1.67
	Under 3:20	2.5
400 yards	Over 13:21	0
	13:20–10:01	2.5
	10:00–6:41	3.33
600 yards	Over 20:01	0
	20:00–15:01	3.75
	15:00–10:01	5.0
	Under 10:00	7.5
800 yards	Over 26:41	0
	26:40–20:01	6.0
	20:00–13:21	7.67
	Under 13:20	11.0
1,000 yards	Over 33:21	0
	33:20–25:01	8.25
	25:00–16:41	10.33
	Under 16:40	14.5

Distance	Time	Point Value
1,200 yards	Over 40:01	0
	40:00–30:01	10.5
	30:00–20:01	13.0
	Under 20:00	18.0
1,400 yards	Over 46:41	0
	46:40–35:01	12.75
	35:00–23:21	15.67
	Under 23:20	21.5
1,600 yards	Over 53:21	0
	53:20–40:01	15.0
	40:00–26:41	18.33
	Under 26:40	25.0

Rope Skipping			
Time	70–90 rpm	90–110 rpm	110–130 rpm
5:00	1.5	2.0	2.5
10:00	3.0	4.0	5.0
15:00	5.5	7.0	8.5
20:00	8.0	10.0	12.0
25:00	10.5	13.0	15.5
30:00	13.0	16.0	19.0

Handball/Racquetball/Squash/Basketball/ Soccer/Hockey/Lacrosse

0.75 point per 5 minutes; do not count breaks and timeouts.

Golf (no motorized cart)

1.5 points per 9 holes

Tennis/Badminton (Doubles)

0.5 point per 15 minutes

Tennis/Badminton (Singles)

0.5 point per 5 minutes

Waterskiing and Downhill Snow Skiing

0.5 point for every 5 minutes of actual skiing

Cross-country Skiing

1.5 points for every 5 minutes of skiing

Ice or Roller Skating

1.25 points for every 15 minutes; for speed skating triple the point value.

Volleyball

0.5 point for every 5 minutes

Fencing

1 point for every 10 minutes

Football

0.5 point for every 5 minutes of actual play

Wrestling/Boxing

2 points for every 5 minutes

Circuit Weight Training

1 point for every 5 minutes

Super Circuit Weight Training
1.25 points for every 5 minutes

Mini-trampoline
1.25 points for every 5 minutes

Aerobic Dance and Other Exercise Programs Conducted to Music
1 point for every 5 minutes

Schwinn Air-Dyne Ergometer (using arms and legs)								
Workload	Time							
	5	10	15	20	25	30	35	40
1.5	0.7	1.4	2.1	2.8	3.5	4.2	4.9	5.6
2.0	1.0	2.1	3.3	4.2	5.2	6.3	7.4	8.4
2.5	1.4	2.9	4.4	5.8	7.2	8.7	10.2	11.6
3.0	1.9	3.9	5.8	7.8	9.8	11.7	13.6	15.6
3.5	2.5	5.0	7.5	10.0	12.5	15.0	17.5	20.0
4.0	3.2	6.3	9.4	12.6	15.8	18.9	22.0	25.2
4.5	3.8	7.7	11.6	15.4	19.2	23.1	27.0	30.8
5.0	4.6	9.3	14.0	18.6	23.2	27.9	32.6	37.2

By now you should have a good grasp of the range of advanced aerobic activity available to you. Furthermore, you should be moving toward a firm decision about the aerobic exercises that best fit your needs and interests as you improve your fitness in the future. But aerobic fitness

An Aerobic Variation: The Cooper Glide™ Model

The Cooper Glide is, in effect, a half-walk/half-jog movement—closer to a walk than a jog. The aerobic effect is similar to that associated with a race-walking style, but there is no requirement to learn a special race-walking technique. Also, to translate this exercise into Aerobic Points, refer to the walking section of the Aerobic Points Chart.

Here's how it works:

Using the aerobic walking guidelines in the chart on page 172 of this chapter, bend your knees slightly and "slide" or "glide" along, but without breaking into a jog. One foot should be on the ground at all times. But with the bend in your knees, you can allow your body to "rise and settle" as you take each step, much as you would do with a jog.

This movement technique allows you to quicken your pace and increase your heart rate with greater control than you can do with an ordinary walk. Of course, the more you can increase your heart rate, the more aerobic conditioning benefit you'll get from the exercise session.

Another benefit of the Cooper Glide is muscular. Because your legs are slightly bent throughout the exercise, the leg motions will exercise your quadriceps muscles ("quads") on the front of your thighs more than a regular jog.

The degree to which a Glide style will increase your heart rate is a highly individual affair because it depends on your level of aerobic conditioning and also on the pace you set for yourself. But here's an example of how the technique has worked for one of our patients, a middle-aged male in good aerobic condition:

When he moved at a Glide rate of twenty-four to twenty-six total footfalls per ten seconds (or when his left foot struck the ground twelve to thirteen times), he could generate a heart rate of 115 to 120 beats per minutes. When he increased his pace to twenty-eight to thirty-two footfalls per ten seconds (fourteen to sixteen ground-strikes with his left foot), his heart rate increased to 125 to 135 beats per minutes.

Finally, this Glide technique is highly flexible: it can be employed throughout an entire aerobic exercise session, or it can be included as a kind of interval-training method during a regular walking or jogging session. In other words, you might walk for ten minutes; then "glide" at a more intense pace for two to five minutes; and, finally, return to your walking pace.

moves you only halfway to your ultimate goal of *total* fitness. Just as important, an advanced program must also help you to become *strong*, both in your muscles and your bones. And this strength challenge becomes ever more pressing as you pass fifty years of age.

The Secret of Strength—at Any Age

You've already been introduced to a simple strength-building program with the calisthenics exercises described in the previous chapter. And quite frankly, if you follow this program, continuing to add gradually to the number of repetitions and sets you do, you'll progress quite nicely toward a stronger set of muscles and bones. Certainly, both of us periodically return to calisthenics at home or in hotel rooms when we've lacked the time or opportunity to go to the gym.

But many people these days want to extend their bodies further with resistance and weight training using various types of equipment, and for the most part, that's the approach the two of us take during a typical week. But because an improper use of equipment can lead to serious injuries, it's important for you to keep some basic guidelines in mind.

GUIDELINES FOR RESISTANCE TRAINING

Although several of the following guidelines will be incorporated into the circuit training program described later in this chapter, you should be aware of—and observe—all of them to ensure the effectiveness and safety of your workout:

- Consult your physician prior to beginning any resistance or strength exercise, including circuit training.
- Warm up for five minutes prior to beginning a resistance training routine, using aerobic exercise such as treadmill walking, elliptical cross training, or cycling.
- Train your larger muscle groups (legs, chest, and back) before you work on your smaller muscle groups (shoulders, arms, and calves).
- As needed to improve your strength level, include additional repetitions: 1 to 3 sets of 12 to 15 repetitions.
- Engage in strength work two to three times per week on nonconsecutive days.
- Set your resistance for each exercise at 65 percent of the maximal load you can lift or pull (if possible, use a personalized exercise prescription by a certified trainer or other fitness specialist).
- Increase your weight or resistance load when you can complete 12 to 15 repetitions and 3 sets with minimal effort.
- Perform stretching exercises at the end of each exercise session for five minutes. Hold each stretch for fifteen to twenty seconds. (See "The Standard Cooper Stretching Routine," on page 148 of Chapter 7.)

One of the most effective and popular strategies we've found for advanced strength work is a circuit training program that we've designed. One of the major advantages of this approach is that you can actually get an aerobic benefit as you increase your muscle strength.

The Cooper Circuit Training Program

Our circuit training program involves this combination of strength (resistance) training and cardiovascular endurance (aerobic) training:

- A *resistance/strength component,* which will comprise about half your workout time.
- An *aerobic component,* which will make up approximately the other half.

GUIDELINES FOR SPECIFIC CIRCUIT TRAINING EXERCISES*

You have two choices as to your exercise intensity in following a circuit training program:

Choice #1: Strength-Only Circuit. In this less demanding approach, rest for thirty seconds after you complete each resistance/strength exercise.

Choice #2: Super Circuit. In this more demanding approach, add an extra aerobic component in your training, such as by jumping rope, or by stepping up and down on a step or low bench, at a rate of twelve to fifteen times in thirty seconds. Or you might do aerobic calisthenics such as running in place or jumping jacks for the thirty-second period.

Note: Beginners or those unaccustomed to an advanced strength workout should start with *Choice #1: Strength-Only Circuit.* Later, they

---

*The order of these exercises is the usual order for a circuit training program, beginning with large muscle groups and moving to small muscle groups. Also, movements for each of these exercises (which we assume will be done on the weight/resistance training equipment you have available at your gym or club) should be executed in accordance with guidelines established by a competent trainer or gym supervisor.

can advance to *Choice #2: Super Circuit* as their conditioning improves. Also, keep in mind that regardless of which of these two choices you make, your circuit training session should include *both* a major resistance component *and* an aerobic component, as indicated in the "Cooper Circuit Training Program" chart at the end of this section. In other words, the *Choice #2: Super Circuit* approach will simply add to, or intensify, the existing aerobic component of the workout.

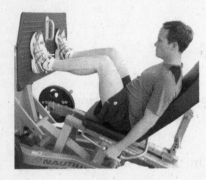

1. Leg Press

Time: 30 seconds.

Goal: 8–15 repetitions. Select your resistance or weight load so that you can do the minimum number of repetitions without undue strain.

- Sit in the exercise chair provided, with seat adjusted so that the knees are bent at an angle no smaller than 90 degrees.
- Extend your legs so that the legs are straight.
- Return to the starting position. This constitutes one repetition.
- Movements should be slow and controlled.

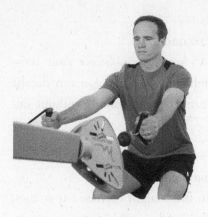

2. Cable Squat Row

Time: 30 seconds.

Goal: 10–15 repetitions. Select your resistance or weight load so that you can do the minimum number of repetitions without undue strain.

- Draw in your abdominal muscles and hold them in tight during the exercise.
- Squat holding the handles attached to the weight machine, with your arms extended.
- As you stand, pull the weight handles toward your abdomen, so your elbows are bent and pulled back against your sides.
- One squat-and-stand movement constitutes one repetition.
- Movements should be slow and controlled.

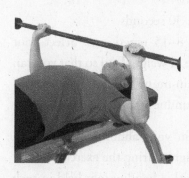

3. Chest Press

Time: 30 seconds.

Goal: 8–15 repetitions. Select your resistance or weight load so that you can do the minimum number of repetitions without undue strain.

- Lie on your back on an exercise bench so that you can push the weighted bar up from your chest to an arms-extended position above your chest, and then back again. One repetition involves one cycle of pressing the weight up above your chest and then returning it to the near-chest position.
- Keep your abdominals drawn in and held tight.

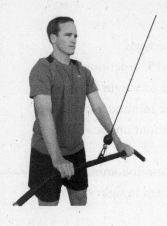

4. Lat Extension

Time: 30 seconds.

Goal: 8–15 repetitions. Select your resistance or weight load so that you can do the minimum number of repetitions without undue strain.

- Draw in your abdominals and hold them tight during the exercise.
- Hold on to the straight exercise bar at chest or chin level, with overhand grip, arms extended, and elbows straight.
- Pull the bar downward to the front of your hips with your hands.
- Return the bar to the starting position. One down-and-up motion constitutes one repetition.

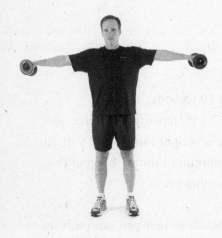

5. Standing Lateral Raise

Time: 30 seconds.

Goal: 8–15 repetitions. Select your resistance or weight load so that you can do the minimum number of repetitions without undue strain.

- Draw in your abdominals and hold them tight during the exercise.
- Start with a hand weight held in each hand at the side of each hip. Your legs should be in a partial squat stance.
- Raise weights straight out to the sides to shoulder height. Keep elbows straight.
- Return weights to starting position next to hips. This movement constitutes one repetition.

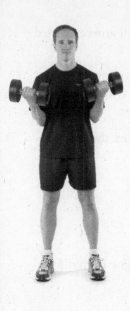

6. Standing Biceps Curl

Time: 30 seconds.

Goal: 8–15 repetitions. Select your resistance or weight load so that you can do the minimum number of repetitions without undue strain.

- Draw in your abdominals and hold them tight during the exercise.
- Grasp free weights with an underhand grip, palms up, arms extended. Keep a normal, erect posture during the entire sequence of movements.
- Your elbows should remain still as you raise your hands, either alternately or at the same time, toward your chest.
- Return to starting position. This up-and-down movement constitutes one repetition.

7. Triceps Extension

Time: 30 seconds.

Goal: 8–15 repetitions. Select your resistance or weight load so that you can do the minimum number of repetitions without undue strain.

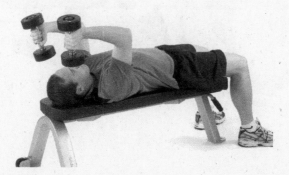

- Lie flat on your back on an exercise bench. Your abdominal muscles should be drawn in and held tight throughout the exercise.

- Begin by holding a hand weight in each hand, with arms extended above the chest and elbows straight.
- Move the weights back behind your head by lowering only your hands and forearms. Your elbows should remain still as you raise and lower your hands.
- Return your arms and the weights to the extended starting position. This sequence constitutes one repetition.

8. Abdominal Crunch

Time: 30 seconds.

Goal: as many repetitions as you can do before fatigue prevents you from performing.

- Your head, chest, shoulders, and hands should rise together with each upward crunch movement.
- The heel of one foot may be placed on top of the toes of the other foot for the first 15 seconds. Then reverse this position for the last 15 seconds.

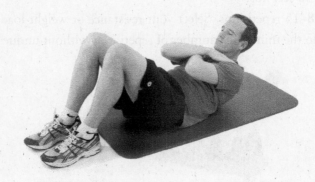

Here is a suggested practical daily circuit training schedule that combines both the above resistance training principles *and* an aerobic component. You can use this chart (see page 196) either for regular circuit training or for super circuit training. Note that the aerobic component of this particular program should be done *in addition to* the aerobic component in the super circuit approach. Also, the exercises should be done in the order indicated, with resistance training before aerobic work.

ADVANCED FITNESS TRAINING— WITH A WEIGHT-LOSS ANGLE

If you're overweight or legitimately concerned about your weight or body-fat percentage, you may want to place a special emphasis on a program that will enhance your weight-loss efforts. To achieve this goal, it's necessary to return to some of the points made in the 30-60-90 discussion on page 161 of the previous chapter.

As you'll recall, U.S. health experts reported that it would take about ninety minutes of activity each day to achieve both fitness conditioning *and* maintenance of weight loss achieved through a calorie-cutting diet. In fact, if you do manage to do ninety minutes of this type of activity every day, you'll almost certainly lose pounds as a result of the exercise alone. And the more intensely you exercise—as with the interval training techniques mentioned in the box on page 202—the more likely it will be that the exercise will take off excess weight.

As with any advanced aerobic regimen, you'll want to try this plan only if you're in reasonably good shape as a result of pursuing another fitness program *and* if you've passed a rigorous gold-standard preventive-medicine exam within the last year.

You'll notice that we've included something physical to do every single day to promote good habit formation. Also, we've injected plenty of variety to keep your interest level up. And we've sprinkled a number of short add-ons into each day's schedule to give you the option of doing extra moderate-intensity activity to achieve greater weight loss.

THE COOPER FITNESS CIRCUIT TRAINING PROGRAM*

	Week 1	Week 2	Week 3	Week 4
Warm-up (slow version of any aerobic exercise)	5:00 minutes	5:00 minutes	5:00 minutes	5:00 minutes
Resistance training†	8:00 minutes (1 set)	16:00 minutes (2 sets)	24:00 minutes (3 sets)	24:00 minutes (3 sets)
Aerobic training‡	10:00 minutes	15:00 minutes	15:00 minutes	20:00 minutes
Cooldown (same as warm-up)	5:00 minutes	5:00 minutes	5:00 minutes	5:00 minutes
Stretching	5:00 minutes	5:00 minutes	5:00 minutes	5:00 minutes
Total Program Time	33:00 minutes	46:00 minutes	54:00 minutes	59:00 minutes

*If time is a factor, Week 1 or Week 2 will give you a good workout. For greater conditioning effect or training for competition, Weeks 3 and 4 should be your goals.
†Remember that resistance training can involve either 1) the regular Choice #1: Strength-Only Circuit, with rest periods between each exercise; or 2) the more demanding Choice #2: Super Circuit, with short aerobic sessions (thirty seconds) between each exercise.
‡These aerobic exercises—which are to be done *in addition to* the short aerobic activity in the Super Circuit—may include any endurance activity, such as treadmill walking, treadmill jogging, outdoor walking, outdoor jogging, outdoor running, elliptical cross training, stationary cycling, outdoor bicycling, cross-country skiing, cross-country skiing simulator training, or swimming.

If you do decide to engage in all the basic exercise and the optional activities, you'll find that you're doing a daily average of ninety minutes of moderate-intensity activity during the entire seven-day period. This amount of exercise should be enough to help you maintain any weight loss you've already achieved through dieting, and perhaps lose a few pounds as a result of the extra exercise alone.

Tyler on Training Intensity

In general, I've seen greater long-term fitness success among those who emphasize *regularity* in exercise, rather than intensity. Or to put this another way, it's best to lower any expectations you may have about being transformed quickly from a couch potato into a superbly conditioned athlete, especially if you are middle-aged and just starting out with a program.

Certainly, as a former intercollegiate athlete, I understand the excitement of fine-tuning your body for athletic competition. But if you're a relative beginner or haven't been used to engaging in competition, you're much better off concentrating on working out most days of the week with a moderate or light program. It's a Herculean feat for some people just to walk a few times a week, ten to fifteen minutes at a time.

On the other hand, if you're feeling ambitious after you've spent at least six weeks getting into shape, you may want to try something more challenging, such as increasing the intensity of your workout through a form of "interval training" (also, see Ken's comments on interval training). In brief, interval training involves mixing pace variations in a workout, both to prevent boredom and to raise your level of performance.[3] For example, if you're a jogger, you might increase your pace for a minute or so, usually until you feel yourself really "pushing it." Then, you return to your normal jogging pace, or even walk for a few seconds or minutes until your breathing returns to normal.

I've done "tons" of interval training during my years of track training, and, when performed safely, the technique can be useful and enjoyable. But before you try this approach, you must be absolutely sure that you're in reasonably good shape and that you have no underlying heart or cardiovascular problems.

DAY ONE

- Walk *30 minutes* in the morning at a moderate-intensity pace of about 3.5–4.5 mph (13.5–17.5 minutes per mile).
- *Optional:* Park far enough away from your office so that you have to walk *10 minutes* to get there.
- *Optional:* Walk *10 minutes* around your office as you're talking on the phone.
- *Optional:* Walk *15 minutes* to a restaurant for lunch, and then walk *15 minutes* back.
- *Optional:* Walk *10 minutes* from your office to your car at the end of the day.

Total basic activity time: *30 minutes*

Total basic plus optional activity time: *90 minutes*

DAY TWO

- Do *30 minutes* of strength training—such as the circuit training program or the calisthenics program suggested in Chapter 7. (You'll note that the times on those programs vary. But remember, you're free to break the rules!)
- *Optional:* Park far enough away from your office so that you have to walk *10 minutes* to get there.
- *Optional:* Walk *10 minutes* around your office as you're talking on the phone.
- *Optional:* Walk *15 minutes* to a restaurant for lunch, and then walk *15 minutes* back.
- *Optional:* Walk *10 minutes* from your office to your car at the end of the day.

Total basic activity time: *30 minutes (i.e., the strength training session)*

Total basic plus optional activity time: *90 minutes*

DAY THREE

- Swim *30 minutes* in the morning. At first, you might use a side-stroke or a combination of sidestroke and overarm crawl. As you get into better shape, you can switch to a continuous overarm stroke. As an alternative, you might try bicycling or some other aerobic activity.
- *Optional:* Park far enough away from your office so that you have to walk *10 minutes* to get there.
- *Optional:* Walk *10 minutes* around your office as you're talking on the phone.
- *Optional:* Walk *10 minutes* from your office to your car at the end of the day.
- *Optional:* Devote *30 minutes* at home to doing housework or yard work. Divide the 30 minutes up any way you like.

Total basic activity time: *30 minutes*
Total basic plus optional activity time: *90 minutes*

DAY FOUR

- Devote *30 minutes* of the time you usually spend watching TV, working on the computer, reading, or just sitting around to a series of strength and stretching exercises.

    For example, you might take three 5-minute breaks to do some stretching (see pages 148–154 for suggestions); some repetitions with hand weights (see pages 193–194); and then some abdominal crunches and push-ups (or modified push-ups; see pages 141–143).

    Finish this sequence off with one 15-minute session walking around while you talk on the phone. *Note:* As you can see, this sequence provides some alternate-day strength training, as well as some very light aerobic activity.

- *Optional:* Park far enough away from your office so that you have to walk *10 minutes* to get there.
- *Optional:* Walk *10 minutes* around your office as you're talking on the phone.

- *Optional:* Walk *10 minutes* from your office to your car at the end of the day.
- *Optional:* Play *30 minutes* of modified "bounce volleyball." (See "Creative Exercise Requires Breaking Some Rules" in Chapter 7.) As an alternative you might play badminton, touch football, doubles tennis, or some other aerobic sport.

Total basic activity time: *30 minutes*
Total basic plus optional activity time: *90 minutes*

DAY FIVE

- Walk *30 minutes* in the morning at a pace of about 3.5 to 4.5 mph.
- *Optional:* Park far enough away from your office so that you have to walk *10 minutes* to get there.
- *Optional:* Walk *10 minutes* around your office as you're talking on the phone.
- *Optional:* Walk *15 minutes* to a restaurant for lunch, and then walk *15 minutes* back.
- *Optional:* Walk *10 minutes* from your office to your car at the end of the day.

Total basic activity time: *30 minutes*
Total basic plus optional activity time: *90 minutes*

DAY SIX

- Walk *15 minutes* with the family to a restaurant for lunch, and then walk *15 minutes* back.
- *Optional:* Play *30 minutes* of slow-break basketball (see our discussion of "Breaking the Rules" in Chapter 7). As an alternative, you could engage in some other activity that provides an aerobic or endurance benefit.
- *Optional:* Park far enough away from your supermarket so that you have to walk 10 minutes each way to get to the door—for a total of *20 minutes.*

- *Optional:* Walk *10 minutes* around your office as you're talking on the phone.

Total basic activity time: *30 minutes*

Total basic plus optional activity time: *90 minutes*

DAY SEVEN

- Do *30 minutes* of strength training—such as the circuit training program or the calisthenics program suggested earlier in this chapter (see Chapter 7). (Note that the times on those programs vary, but you're free to break the rules.)
- *Optional:* Park far enough away from your house of worship or favorite restaurant or coffee shop so that you have to walk *20 minutes* round-trip to get there.
- *Optional:* Walk *10 minutes* around your home as you're talking on the phone.
- *Optional:* Do *30 minutes* of vigorous yard work or housework.

Total basic activity time: *30 minutes*

Total basic plus optional activity time: *90 minutes*

One final note: these advanced fitness models are rooted in the assumption that it's important for you to pay *daily* attention to developing your physical-activity habit. But if you find that some days you can't put in even the minimum thirty minutes of daily activity, don't despair. Just do what you can.

For example, there's nothing wrong with walking only ten minutes on a particular day if that's all the time you can spare. *But be absolutely sure to do something.* No matter how insignificant or small a particular physical activity may seem, the smallest effort will contribute to a big, powerful habit.

Such actions, if pursued with regularity over time, will contribute to those biological changes in your brain and body associated with the "feel-good" secretions of the relaxation response. They will also protect you from the risk of health- and life-threatening disease and, as a bonus, they will contribute to weight loss.

But for most of us, losing weight will require that combination strategy we've referred to several times—exercise plus dietary control. Now, let's take a closer look at how this approach can work in practice.

Ken on Interval Training

Interval training is a conditioning technique appropriate *only* for experienced conditioned athletes who have been cleared by a thorough preventive-medicine exam. The approach involves mixing different speeds or intensities of activity in order to improve performance. This approach will not only increase aerobic capacity, but will also help your body burn up more calories—and lose excess weight.

For example, when the great distance runner Frank Shorter was training for the Olympic Marathon, he would run at least a hundred miles per week, with most of the workout involving regular distance conditioning. But he would also mix in runs with quarter-mile intervals (440 yards or 400 meters) in sixty-two to sixty-five seconds. After one of these fast interval runs, he would walk for one minute, and then repeat the fast interval run. During a typical workout, he might do as many as ten of these consecutive "wind sprints," which were designed to build up his *anaerobic* capacity, or his ability to run at high speeds while tolerating a high oxygen "debt load." This means that he would condition his body to perform at very fast, high-performance levels when he was, in effect, out of breath.

In contrast, your *aerobic* capacity, which provides most of the health and longevity benefits, involves the ability of your cardiovascular and respiratory system to maintain an *extended,* higher rate of breathing and oxygen processing. Developing such an aerobic capacity requires endurance training—or "a method of physical exercise for producing beneficial changes in the respiratory and circulatory systems by activities that require only a modest increase in oxygen intake" (the definition I contributed to the *Oxford English Dictionary,* 1986 edition).

An anaerobic interval training strategy is typically employed only to improve stamina and performance in preparation for an athletic event and is limited primarily to competitive athletes. Even though this approach can add variety and interest to a fitness program, I strongly discourage this kind of high-intensity interval training for anyone who is not in top aerobic shape or who has an underlying health problem, such as coronary disease. For these reasons, I have always insisted on a complete preventive medicine exam and a preconditioning program of at least six weeks before anyone tries a more demanding program, such as interval training.

Nine

■ Start-up #3—Go on a
■ One-Thing Weight-Loss
Eating Plan

We've said that it's better to be fat and fit than to be skinny and unfit. But there's an even better way—*be both lean and fit.*

Being physically fit certainly overcomes a multitude of medical sins. But getting rid of excess weight also adds significantly to your health and longevity. Even if you're modestly overweight, your risk of dying sooner increases—and the risk multiplies if you're obese.[1]

But if you choose to shed extra weight with the One-Thing Weight-Loss Eating Plan, you'll find you not only get rid of the pounds but also promote better health and longevity. So what exactly is this One-Thing Weight-Loss Eating Plan?

> ### Tyler on the Origins of the One-Thing Weight-Loss Eating Plan
>
> As I was sitting in one of my morning classes in medical school, trying to shake off a serious case of first-lecture drowsiness (a price for the late night before), I heard two words that shook me awake:
>
> *"One thing!"* the lecturer declared.
>
> He was talking about the easiest, simplest way to start losing weight—and to render complicated diets obsolete. All that's required, he suggested, is to pick one thing: one food or drink that's adding a lot of extra calories from fats, sugars, or alcohol to your menu. Then, kick that item out of your life!
>
> The chances are that if *you* take this one step, you'll immediately eliminate hundreds of unhealthy calories from your diet. And soon, the calories you're no longer consuming will translate into your loss of excess weight (one pound of fat = 3,500 calories). Furthermore, assuming the food or drink you cut is loaded with bad fats or sugars, you'll lower your risk of life-threatening conditions, such as cardiovascular disease and diabetes.
>
> And just imagine what will happen if you cut one *more* unhealthy thing out of your diet—and another and another, each week for five straight weeks. This line of thinking has led us quite naturally to what we call the One-Thing Weight-Loss Eating Plan.

The One-Thing Weight-Loss Eating Plan in a Nutshell

The One-Thing Weight-Loss Eating Plan is based on a comment that intrigued Tyler during a lecture in medical school (see his account in the accompanying box). In brief, this weight-loss strategy involves a simple but powerful ten-week eating plan:

- **Weeks #1–5:** *Cut out the five most unhealthy foods and drinks in your diet.* As you eliminate one unhealthy food or drink each week, focus on products high in trans fats,* saturated fats, sugar, or alcohol.
- **Weeks #6–10:** *Add healthy foods*—such as extra fruits and plenty of vegetables; a daily intake of whole grains like oatmeal; and healthy fats, including the omega-3 fatty acids found in certain cold-water fish, monounsaturated fats in many nuts, and the plant stanol esters in "functional foods" like Benecol spread, or sterols in Take Control spreads. These functional foods have been specially designed—according to recent scientific findings showing the cholesterol-lowering impact of high amounts of plant stanols and sterols—to help protect you from life-threatening diseases, such as cardiovascular conditions and cancer.

The psychological advantages of this diet are rooted in the reality that most people can't just change their *entire* eating plan "cold turkey." On the other hand, most people can manage to cut just one thing out at a time. The approach we're suggesting gives you the chance to say, "I may not be able to make a wholesale change in my diet, but I can stop eating at least one thing right now." Then, a week later, you'll be in a position to say, "Okay, now I think I can eliminate one *more* thing."

The health advantages of this strategy are also far-reaching (see the accompanying list of benefits). But before you can actually proceed with cutting foods, it's important to understand a little more about the "unhealthy foods" that will be eliminated.

---

*Trans fats are fats that are chemically altered through the process known as hydrogenation (or partial hydrogenation). Food manufacturers use this process to give packaged foods a longer shelf life and make fat reusable more times in deep fat frying.

The Multiple Benefits of the One-Thing Weight-Loss Eating Plan

- Reduce your heart attack and stroke risk significantly if you lose weight—because excess weight has been associated with cardiovascular disease.[2]
- Lower your risk of coronary heart disease by 1) decreasing trans fats and saturated fats; 2) increasing fruits, vegetables, and whole grains like oatmeal; 3) including omega-3 fatty acids (in such fish as salmon, halibut, sardines, and canned light tuna);[3] and 4) adding monounsaturated fats found in nuts, olive oil, and canola oil, as well as in the functional food spread Benecol.
- Lower your risk of cancer of the pancreas, one of the deadliest of all cancers—if you eat a diet rich in fruits and vegetables.[4]
- Lower your risk of ovarian and pancreatic cancer by eating more broccoli and red chili peppers.[5]
- Lower your risk of cancer of the colon if you restrict your consumption of processed meats and those high in saturated fats.[6]
- Lower the risk for kidney stones if you avoid obesity and weight gain.[7]
- Lower C-reactive protein (a marker of vessel inflammation and coronary heart disease) and improve insulin resistance (a risk for diabetes)—if you're an obese person who loses weight.[8]
- Lower your risk of dying from cardiovascular disease if you keep a low waist-to-hip ratio (about 0.8), rather than a high ratio (greater than 1.0).[9] In other words, that extra roll around the middle will kill.
- Decrease your risk of breast cancer if you maintain an ideal weight before, during, and after menopause.[10]

What Are the "Unhealthy Foods"?

You can identify unhealthy foods and drinks by applying these two simple standards:

- First, foods that are high in saturated fats or trans fats are "unhealthy."
- Second, foods and drinks that are high in simple sugars (not complex carbohydrates found in vegetables and fruits) or alcohol are "unhealthy."

These guidelines will get you off to a good start toward significant weight loss and risk reduction. But before you actually begin, let's take a closer look at the worst of the worst—*trans fats*. What exactly are they, and why are they so harmful?

THE WORST OF THE WORST: TRANS FATS

Food manufacturers often use a process known as hydrogenation to create a partially hydrogenated vegetable oil or fat to extend the shelf life in packaged, commercially baked goods. This technique alters the chemical structure of the foods by saturating the double molecular bonds of unsaturated fats with hydrogen so as to make the fat solid at room temperature. In this state, the fat is able to withstand higher frying temperatures, and able to be reused more often.

The result is a biochemical oddity called trans fats or trans fatty acids, which researchers such as Dr. Walter Willett of the Harvard School of Public Health have indicted as a major risk factor for many serious diseases—especially cardiovascular conditions such as heart attacks, strokes, and hypertension. Scientific studies have also implicated trans fats in diabetes, certain cancers, and asthma.

Landmark studies, such as the Harvard Nurses' Health Study, have caused leading researchers to levy charges like these against trans fats:[11]

- The risk for heart disease *doubles* when you add only 30 calories of trans fats (3 to 4 grams) to your diet each day. (This is the equivalent of consuming one serving of fast-food French fries or a doughnut.[12])
- Trans fat consumption is responsible for *one heart disease death every fifteen minutes.*
- More than fifty thousand untimely heart disease deaths each year can be traced to the consumption of trans fats.
- Even a tiny intake of trans fats and saturated fats—which may be contained in a small cookie or a couple of crackers daily—will result in a *relentless increase in girth over months or years as a result of the intake of extra calories.*

A study by the Harvard School of Public Health involving seventeen thousand men found that by adding only 2 percent in trans fats (barely a cookie, cracker, or a few French fries) to the daily diet over nine years resulted in the expansion of the average waistline by one-third of an inch.[13] Also, trans fats tend to attach other types of fat to the waist in a form known as visceral fat.

- According to other recent research, trans fats pose a *more dangerous risk of disease and early death than do ordinary saturated fats—* which are quite dangerous in their own right.
- Leading researchers call trans fats the *"secret killer."*

With such dramatic charges, it's no wonder that trans fats have increasingly come under fire in recent years. In fact, the FDA moved decisively to require manufacturers, after January 1, 2006, to include on their nutritional labels the exact amounts of trans fats in their products.

The 2006 American Heart Association dietary revisions recommend limiting trans fats to less than 1 percent of total calories per day.

Fortunately, food manufacturers have made wide-ranging changes designed to conform to the new trans fat labeling rules. But even so, several trans fat–related problems remain. Here are five you should be aware of:

First, some foods still contain plenty of trans fats. According to a number of experts, stick margarine continues to be a "major culprit," with trans fat amounts that may range from 1.5 to 2.5 grams per serving.[14] Also, various frozen foods and quick mixes may still contain trans fats.

Second, some of our foods—especially commercially made desserts, cookies, crackers, and other packaged foods—may say "0 trans fats" on the label. But they may still be loaded with saturated fats, which pose a high risk for elevated cholesterol and cardiovascular disease. In some cases, in a kind of unhealthy-fat shell game, palm kernel oil, palm oil, and coconut oil, which contain large amounts of saturated fats, have been substituted for trans fats in order to meet the new government standards. This situation has led to the substitution in many foods of *fully* hydrogenated oils known as "interestified fats," which are being tabbed as the deadliest fats of all: they raise total and "bad" LDL cholesterol; lower "good" HDL cholesterol; increase the total/HDL ratio; and increase blood sugars, a feature that can lead to diabetes. So whenever you see "saturated fat" on a label, think "unhealthy fat."

Third, the government requirements allow food manufacturers to put "0 trans fats" on their package labels as long as the amount of trans fats is less than 0.5 gram per serving. But if a serving is listed as four crackers and you eat eight crackers, you may have consumed a total of 3.2 grams of trans fats (e.g., if the amount of trans fat per cracker is 0.4 gram). So consuming larger-than-listed serving sizes can sneak in to upset your fat-control efforts.

Fourth, many fast foods, including shakes, fried foods like French fries, and butter- or margarine-drenched movie popcorn, are loaded with trans fats and saturated fats, not to mention hundreds or even thousands of extra calories that put on extra pounds.

Fifth, for those concerned with weight loss or weight maintenance, *all* fat (even the "healthy" monounsaturated and polyunsaturated omega-3 fats) contains more calories per gram than does protein or carbohydrate. Specifically, 1 gram of fat of any kind contains 9 calories, while 1 gram of protein or carbohydrate contains only 4 calories. So unless you make a concerted effort to control your *total* fat intake, you're going to continue to have a big problem with any serious weight-loss efforts.

Note: Total elimination of *all* saturated fats is not recommended because saturated fats are used in the manufacture of "good" HDL cholesterol. It's for this reason that the American Heart Association says that 7 percent of caloric intake can be in the form of saturated fat.

Now, with this information in hand, let's take a closer look at how you can do your own unhealthy food and drink analysis as a final preparatory step before launching your One-Thing Weight-Loss Eating Plan.

DOING YOUR OWN UNHEALTHY FOOD AND DRINK ANALYSIS

The only way to be reasonably sure about the quantity of unhealthy fats you personally are consuming is to perform a quick "unhealthy food and drink analysis" of your diet. And the easiest, most effective way to do this—without becoming obsessed with performing nutritional research on every food you eat—is to rely on this three-step strategy:

Step #1: First, spend some time reflecting on your eating habits during the last week. Keep a food record in a notebook of the foods and drinks you've consumed at various meals and between meals over that seven-day period. (It's a good idea to put the notebook in a place where you can refer to it later.)

Be honest with yourself here! It's important to identify those really unhealthy foods you've been eating so that you can be sure to cut them later. (Our patients go through a similar procedure by completing a three-day food record for a registered dietician when they come in for a complete evaluation at the Cooper Clinic.)

Step #2: Using the master list you've compiled in Step #1, check the saturated fat, trans fat, sugar, and alcohol on the labels of the ten foods and five beverages you consume most often.

Step #3: From your often-consumed list in Step #2, identify the five foods or drinks that you eat *at home or at restaurants* that have the highest saturated fat, trans fat, sugar, or alcohol content. You can quickly select candidates for foods you prepare at home by checking the food labels. Choose the five foods containing saturated fat, trans fat, sugar, or alcohol that have the highest calorie count per serving. Your elimination of these foods will promote the most weight loss.

Targets of weight-loss opportunity at restaurants and fast-food facilities include any fried foods like French fries, high-fat meats, cheese, and foods with added batter or high-fat sauces. Instead, choose foods that are dry-grilled or otherwise prepared to minimize the addition of fats. If you want to engage in a little research, and the restaurant is part of a food chain or otherwise has a high profile, you should be able to gather nutritional information rather easily either from the restaurant itself or from a Web site. If you're still in doubt about which restaurant food to eliminate, check to see if the food seems greasy, fried, breaded, or covered with sauce. If it has any of these characteristics, put it toward the top of your "cut" list.

Finally, you should be aware that a major bonus of cutting these bad foods and drinks, both at home and in restaurants, will involve a "piggy-back effect": by eliminating just one food or drink high in fats, sugars, or alcohol from your diet, you'll cut many additional calories contained in that food.

For example, suppose you're visiting relatives for a few days, and you're offered a slice of New York–style cheesecake. Or maybe they brought the cake with them when they came to see you. That single serving will contain 2.5 grams of trans fat *plus* 16 grams of saturated fat—for a total of 18.5 grams of really unhealthy fats (about 167 calories: 18.5 grams × 9 calories/gram = 167 calories).

Along with those 167 calories of unhealthy fat, you'll also take in an additional 313 calories of assorted sugars, fats, and other nutrients, for a total of 480 calories for that single piece of cheesecake. Multiply 480 calories by seven servings over the course of a multiday holiday, and you'll find you've taken in 3,360 extra calories—just shy of an extra pound of *body* fat around your middle (3,500 calories adds 1 pound).

Some Guidelines on Unhealthy Drinks: Making decisions about which drinks are bad or worse than others can be a little tricky, but here are a few guidelines to consider:

- *Eliminate colas.* A 12-ounce cola may contain 150 calories of simple sugars. If you order a large cola, that could involve many more calories. So it's best to cut out regular cola consumption entirely and substitute water or a diet cola instead.
- *Avoid alcohol.* One glass of dry wine contains more than 200 calories. So if you typically have two glasses of wine with your evening meal, you'll consume more than 400 calories per evening. To resolve this problem, cut out the wine entirely and replace it with calorie-free sparkling water or club soda with lime for a savings of 400 calories. If you must have wine, limit yourself to one glass. That will save 200 calories if you're usually a two-glass person.
- *Limit sugar.* The equivalent of one tablespoon of granulated sugar added to coffee or tea will add about 50 calories to your daily intake.

  Of course, some people really pour the sugar into their coffee or tea, and in those cases, getting rid of a cup is an easy weight-control decision. But even if a tablespoon of sugar doesn't seem like a lot to you, keep in mind that if you drink more than one cup per day, your sugar consumption may soar. A possible solution is to use a sugar substitute.

Now, with this information in hand, let's move on to the core of the One-Thing Weight-Loss Eating Plan, which involves spending five weeks cutting out your five most unhealthy foods and drinks, and then five more weeks adding healthy foods back into your diet.

Caution: This eating plan is intended to provide general weight loss and health-enhancing benefits, but *not* to replace another type of diet that your physician or registered dietician may have recommended for a particular health condition, such as heart disease, hypertension, or diabetes. If you currently have such a health condition, be sure to consult with your physician before you embark on this One-Thing Weight-Loss Eating Plan strategy.

The First Five Weeks: Cut Five Unhealthy Foods or Drinks

This initial five-week phase of the One-Thing Weight-Loss Eating Plan principle is quite simple: on the first day of each new week, eliminate an unhealthy food or drink. Then spend the rest of the week getting used to the change. You don't have to worry about anything in your diet except that one item you've just eliminated. Then you follow the same procedure for the second week, the third, and so on. Here's how it works:

WEEK #1

On the first day of your first week, weigh yourself undressed in the morning, and record your weight and the date in the journal that you've been using to record typical eating habits, including unhealthy foods and drinks.

Plan to weigh yourself at least once a month after this, and record the weights and dates. Of course, there's nothing wrong with weighing yourself more often if you like. But it's important not to become discouraged as your weight fluctuates up and down from day to day. Those short-term movements are to be expected. But your important weight markers will be your monthly weigh-ins.

Now you're ready for your most important action on your first day:

Eliminate the *one unhealthy food or drink* that you've already identified, which has the highest saturated fat, trans fat, sugar, or alcohol content—or all of the above. One serving of this product should also contain a fairly high calorie content, but don't worry if you find on the food label that you're eliminating only 200 to 300 calories with this elimination. Your overall goal is to assemble a *collection* of your most unhealthy foods and drinks. As you get rid of these foods, the total calories you cut will add up significantly.

Be ruthless! Even if your refrigerator or food pantry is full of that unhealthy food, toss it out. Don't rationalize by saying, "That food cost a lot of money! I'll just finish up what's on hand and then stop buying any more after that." The chances are you'll just continue with your old, ingrained eating habits. So act now!

Finally, at this point, don't substitute any new foods or drinks for the one you've thrown out. The time for wise additions will come during the second five weeks of the program.

WEEK #2

Now eliminate *a second unhealthy food or drink* from your at-home diet—again, without substituting any new food for the one removed.

WEEK #3

Study your unhealthy-food list again and choose a *third unhealthy food or drink* that's high in calories from saturated or trans fats, sugar, or alcohol. Finally, go ahead and kick that one out.

WEEK #4

Eliminate *one unhealthy food or drink* from your meal plan—without substituting any new foods.

WEEK #5

First, weigh yourself—remember you're approaching the end of your first month on this One-Thing plan. Then, cut *one more unhealthy food or drink* from your diet.

At the end of this five-week period, you should find that you have lost four to six pounds. With those unwanted pounds gone, along with the five unhealthy foods or drinks you've eliminated, you're ready to move to the next phase of the One-Thing Weight-Loss Eating Plan program: the addition of healthy foods.

The Second Five Weeks: Add Five Healthy Foods or Drinks

Now that you've lost a few pounds and gotten into the habit of eating fewer foods that are putting your health at risk, you're in a position to adjust your diet to include foods that have the power to enhance your health and promote longevity. During this second five-week phase, you'll begin to add, one by one, various foods that scientific research has proven to have the power to reduce your risk of various diseases. Also, you should continue to weigh yourself monthly.

During this second five-week add-on phase, feel free to be flexible in a number of ways. For example, we expect you to be influenced by your personal preferences for certain types of food and drink. Some people, for instance, may like to eat a lunch that features yogurt and fruit, but no poultry or meat. Others may want a sandwich or salad with turkey or chicken. Any of these choices is fine as long as you *continue* to avoid intake of calories from the five unhealthy foods you eliminated in the *first* five weeks.

Also in the interests of flexibility, you can exercise discretion in making your specific "cuts" during the first five weeks. For example, there's nothing wrong with adding more than one daily serving of some of the vegetables or fruits mentioned below. Here are three reasons for this leeway for vegetables: 1) they are typically quite low in calories; 2) they are quite filling and thus effective in staving off hunger pangs; and 3) they contain important, disease-fighting nutrients.

Another common illustration we encounter is that immediately after many people cut out an unhealthy food, such as stick margarine, they crave some sort of substitute healthy spread. An excellent product in this situation would be the low-calorie "light" version of the functional food spread Benecol, which actually has the power to lower cholesterol.

Now here are some of the healthy food possibilities for you to consider adding during the second five-week period.

WEEK #1: ADD HEALTHY VEGETABLES AND FRUITS.

Your goal should be to increase your total intake of fruits and vegetables to the range of five to nine per day. As we like to say at the Cooper Clinic: Five is fine, but nine is divine. So long as you choose whole fruits and especially whole vegetables, you'll limit your calories with these foods—and at the same time fill up your stomach.

Produce items such as broccoli, cantaloupe, apples, oranges, cauliflower, bananas, carrots, and various berries will maximize your protection against cardiovascular disease, cancer, and other health threats. In addition, as mentioned above, vegetables can help stave off hunger because even though most tend to be low in calories, they still tend to be very filling, and thus able to hold hunger pangs at bay.

Also, many fruits, vegetables, and whole-grain foods add insoluble fiber to the diet—a much needed nutrient that will enhance digestion, prevent constipation, and lower the risk of various health conditions, including diverticulitis (inflammation of outpouches that may develop in the colon).

The whole-grain connection. All-important *soluble* fiber can also be found in many vegetables and fruits, as well as in whole-grain foods. At least one of these whole-grain foods, oatmeal, has been shown to provide special cardiovascular benefits. For example, 1½ cups of cooked, old-fashioned oatmeal eaten daily has been shown to lower "bad" LDL cholesterol. (The red heart symbol of the package will alert you to this benefit.) So when you're adding "healthy" foods into your diet, keep oatmeal in mind.

A hint about fruit drinks. It's best to pick whole fruits with plenty of fiber, rather than fruit drinks. A pure fruit drink, such as orange juice, may have important nutrients, but it's easy to drink one cup of juice (120 calories) without having the sense of being "full"—and then proceed to drink another cup or two. This practice can quickly translate into 240 to 360 or more calories. In contrast, eating a whole orange, which contains plenty of fiber, will fill you up and also will provide only 60 to 70 calories.

We actually know a man who went on a kind of "orange juice diet." Thinking that he was enhancing his health, he typically would drink several glasses each day—until he checked a nutritional chart. He suddenly understood how he had put on an extra eight pounds in the previous couple of months when he saw that he was consuming an extra 400 to 500 calories each day as a result of this "healthy" drink. So he switched to whole oranges and quickly shed the pounds. A bottom-line message here: calories do count!

WEEK #2: ADD AN OMEGA-3 "COCKTAIL."

We recommend that twice a week (and more often, if you like) you consume grilled fish containing omega-3 fatty adds. The recommendations in this category—which are low in mercury and can actually be eaten daily—include salmon, sardines, herring, light canned tuna, halibut, and lake trout.

To avoid dangerous mercury intake from fish, you should stay away from swordfish, king mackerel, shark, and tilefish. Besides the omega-3 fish listed above, other seafood low in mercury content includes shrimp, catfish, flounder, sole, clams, scallops, oysters, tilapia, anchovies, and king crab. Among the seafood with a low to moderate mercury rating are lobster, blue/Dungeness crab, pollack, mahimahi, Atlantic cod, red snapper, and bass.

What's so good about omega-3 fats? Omega-3 fats are very *good* fats, which can protect you from cardiovascular disease and provide other health benefits, such as relief from arthritis. Research has shown that one serving of such fish each week will not only lower your risk of heart problems, but can also slow age-related mental decline by 10 percent annually. And it gets better the more you eat: on average you can lower mental decline 13 percent annually with two fish meals per week.[15] Fish oil has also been shown to reduce the heart rate and may lower the risk of irregular heartbeats.[16] But omega-3 fish-oil supplements have been approved by the FDA only for lowering triglycerides, a fat in the blood associated with cardiovascular disease.

The American Heart Association's 2006 guidelines revisions recommend that you eat omega-3 fatty fish two times per week for a total of eight ounces weekly to get the recommended amount.

Note: A good way to measure a single serving of fish, meat, or poultry is to pick a portion the size of the palm of your hand (3 to 4 ounces).

WEEK #3: ADD SOME MONOUNSATURATED FATS DAILY.

Monounsaturated fats are found in such foods as nuts, peanut butter, olive oil, avocados, and canola oil. These will not only promote satisfaction after a meal or snack, but may also raise "good" HDL cholesterol and lower "bad" LDL cholesterol.

Caution: Because all fats contain high levels of calories, you will need to *limit your portion sizes* of these foods. For example, you should restrict yourself to only one ounce (or one-quarter cup) of nuts daily in order to keep your calorie intake from these foods under 200 calories.

WEEK #4: ADD FAT FROM A "FUNCTIONAL FOOD."

Benecol and Benecol Light spreads, for instance, are specially manufactured, margarine-like spreads that contain plant stanol esters. If you eat four tablespoons daily (200 calories for the "light" version, containing 1.7 grams of plant stanols per two servings, or a total of 3.4 grams for four servings), Benecol actually has the ability to lower your cholesterol levels. Scientific studies have shown that taking recommended amounts of Benecol can reduce levels of "bad" LDL cholesterol by about 10 to 14 percent.[17] In other words, these products go beyond the low-fat tub spreads that merely act as substitutes for margarine spreads with a higher content of saturated and trans fats.

Other products that work in a similar fashion to Benecol contain plant sterols. For example, one to two servings of the spreads Take Control and Take Control Light (1.7 to 3.4 grams of plant sterols) can lower "bad" LDL cholesterol by 10 to 17 percent according to scientific studies.[18] Because plant sterols have been identified in atherosclerotic plaques, there has been a theoretical concern that increasing plant sterol levels in the blood could increase the risk of developing atherosclerosis. But experts currently believe that the increase in sterol levels in the blood with intake of 2 grams per day of plant sterols is negligible. Also, no consistent relationship between plant sterol levels and cardiovascular risk has been shown. Consequently, national and international groups that endorse the use of plant sterols for cholesterol reduction do not distinguish between the sterols and stanols in terms of the benefits or risks.

In a sense, these functional-food products, consumed in recommended amounts, operate as a kind of medicinal supplement by lowering cholesterol through a separate mechanism from that employed by statins. Statins actually influence the production of the body's cholesterol in the liver, while the plant stanol/sterol esters operate in the intestines to block the recirculation of cholesterol from the bowels back into the bloodstream.

WEEK # 5: ADD A SNACK WITHOUT TRANS FATS.

If you're careful—and avoid consuming more than one serving at a time—it's okay to add non–trans fat snacks a few times during the week. They include such products as a variety of non–trans fat Frito-Lay chips carrying the "Smart Spot" seal of approval; Pepperidge Farm natural whole grain German dark wheat bread; Thomas' multigrain English muffins; and Athenos hummus spreads (e.g., spicy three-pepper, or artichoke and garlic). Because new products like these regularly appear in supermarkets, you should periodically check the labels on packaged foods for new items to add variety to your menu.

A word of caution about overdoing a good thing: Even as you add these "good" snacks or other foods to your eating plan, be very careful not to overdo it. Eating several muffins with no trans fats and relatively low saturated fats may add back as many or more calories as you cut during the elimination phase in the first week of your program.

Here are some guidelines to keep in mind to help you avoid this "back-door-calorie" trap:

- Give priority to vegetables and fruits over all other "healthy" foods.
- Consider eating oatmeal, a whole-grain cereal, daily (225 calories).

- Add no more calories from additional "healthy" foods than the total number of calories that you eliminate from "unhealthy" foods. *Exception:* It's okay to add extra vegetables if you like because they tend to be low in calories, high in nutrients, and very filling. For example, two extra-large fruits will include lots of fiber and add only 240 calories to your daily intake. But beware those high-calorie fruit drinks.
- Eat at least eight ounces of omega-3 fatty fish per week.
- Choose one ounce or one-quarter cup of your favorite nuts daily as a snack (approximately 200 calories).
- If you need to lower your cholesterol level, you'll need four servings of Benecol Light daily (200 calories).

Remember the "Action Supplement" to an Effective Weight-Loss Eating Plan

As mentioned in the previous chapter, *every* effective, long-lasting weight-loss regimen *must* include a strong physical activity component—for several important reasons.

First, physical activity burns calories, and that, by itself, will translate into weight loss. Let's assume that you've already started a fitness program that includes only the minimum of daily activity indicated earlier. But you want to ratchet up that activity level, in part to help you with your weight-loss efforts. Here is a suggestion that we call our "20 percent solution."

The 20 percent solution. Those who are currently exercising at about the minimal amount required to maintain a healthy state of fitness (the equivalent of about an hour and a half of walking weekly) but who want to exercise more to lose weight are prime candidates for this strategy.

The main idea is to select a favorite activity and add it to your current exercise program so that you increase your weekly activity levels by 20 percent. Typically, that will enable you to burn an extra 100 to 150 calories over and above your current expenditure.*

For example, a 150-pound person could do an extra twenty minutes of vigorous dancing—say a fast-moving Latin salsa or merengue without a break—which will use up about 140 calories. A 200-pound person doing the same type of dancing will expend even more energy—about 190 calories. Or for those inclined toward less exotic activity, a 150-pound person chopping wood for twenty minutes will burn more than 140 calories, while a 200-pounder will use up more than 190 calories.

If you walk just one extra mile at a leisurely pace for twenty to twenty-five minutes, that will expend about 60 calories. By walking a little faster (4.0 to 4.5 miles per hour), you will expend about 100 calories per mile. Even one hour of gardening that you introduce into your weekly schedule will use up 220 calories.

Playing a moderate game of tennis for about a half hour will burn 250 calories, while putting an hour of square dancing on your social calendar will expend 350 calories. On the other hand, lying down for a half hour in front of the TV will burn a measly 40 calories.

The Metabolism Factor: The additional physical activity will also raise the level of the body's metabolism, or energy-using capacity, by causing the heart and cardiovascular system to shift into a higher-intensity "work mode." Your body actually continues to burn calories at a higher rate after you stop an activity.

Also, because exercise of all types increases and tones the body's muscles, you'll be more inclined—*if* you're in good shape—to use those muscles and burn additional calories. In other words, those who are stronger and more aerobically fit are *predisposed* to engage in active, physical tasks and challenges. Consequently, you'll be more likely to respond to an invitation to take a walk, work around the house, or mow the lawn (250

---

*For a more extensive list of how different exercises and activities burn calories, see Chapter 7, page 160.

calories per hour, using a hand-pushed power mower). Body fat, which is a passive tissue that operates as a drag on the body, doesn't serve the same active, motivational, calorie-burning function.

The Health-and-Longevity Bonus: Finally, remember those studies—including our landmark 1989 Cooper Clinic report in the *Journal of the American Medical Association*—that have shown that doing just a little exercise can have dramatic effects on health and longevity. That *JAMA* study of more than ten thousand men and three thousand women showed that those with low levels of physical fitness had more than twice the death rate of people with just a moderate level of fitness. Also, being physically fit was associated with a lower death rate from all diseases, including diabetes, cancer, and heart disease.

After completing this ten-week start-up phase, you'll be well on your way to losing the amount of weight necessary to reach your ultimate objective. But as you move forward, it's important to keep your eye on the weight-loss ball to ensure that you'll indeed achieve the goal you've set for yourself.

ACHIEVING YOUR ULTIMATE WEIGHT-LOSS GOAL

With the ten-week start-up phase of your One-Thing Weight-Loss Eating Plan behind you, you may decide that you want to continue following that same plan until you've achieved your weight-loss goal. This phase of the plan may span another five weeks, or ten weeks, or longer, depending on how much weight you want to lose. The signal that you're on the right track will be your continuing, regular loss of weight.

But if you reach a weight-loss plateau, where your weight stays the same, you may have to up the ante by extending your original five-week elimination program. Generally speaking, if your weight-loss efforts stall, try one of these strategies:

- If you want to lose a total of eighteen to twenty-five pounds (including the six to twelve you've already lost), repeat the elimination part of the plan for another five weeks. That is, cut one *additional* unhealthy food from your diet each week for five more consecutive weeks.

  But if you start losing weight again before the second five weeks are up, don't bother to eliminate any more foods. Instead, just continue at the level of food consumption you've reached until you reach your desired weight. The usual time period to eliminate this much weight will be about sixty days.

- If you want to take off twenty-seven to thirty-six pounds, continue with your food elimination strategy for as long as necessary. The usual period to achieve this level of weight loss will be about ninety to one hundred twenty days. *Note:* It usually takes longer for women to lose weight than for men.

- If you need to shed additional pounds, extend the time period as required. (For a dramatic example of just how much you may be able to lose, see the amazing account of Rick Salewske in Chapter 15.)

After you've finished making these additional food cuts, it's perfectly acceptable for you to add one extra "healthy" food for each food you've eliminated. But if you do, be sure you follow the principles for adding foods described above in the second five-week phase of the basic One-Thing Weight-Loss Eating Plan program. When you're adding foods at this stage, it's always wise to give first priority to extra vegetables and fruits, which can bring your total to the "divine nine" mentioned earlier.

Regardless of the total weight-loss time period you choose, you should find that you'll be able to lose approximately one to two pounds per week—depending on the calorie content of the foods you've eliminated. Also, you'll probably find that you can lose more weight than this at first if you're trying to lose a great deal of weight, say forty to fifty pounds or more. Furthermore, you'll achieve this result without counting calories, without complicated new recipes, and without convoluted meal plans. At the same time, you'll begin to make significant inroads in reducing your risks for many life-threatening diseases.

The One-Thing Weight-Loss Eating Plan works because it promotes the sound nutritional principles that we observe at the Cooper Clinic—principles that everyone on it should understand.

THE NUTRITIONAL FOUNDATIONS OF THE ONE-THING WEIGHT-LOSS EATING PLAN

Nutritionally, the One-Thing Weight-Loss Eating Plan is designed to move your basic eating plan closer to the three general guidelines for *fat, complex carbohydrates,* and *protein* mentioned below. A plan that conforms to these criteria, which our registered dieticians at the Cooper Clinic follow, will revolutionize your eating habits and improve your health.

But you don't have to worry about doing complex calculations to get the numbers exactly right. Just apply the One-Thing principles, and you'll move toward the guidelines. The short summary at the end of each category below, entitled "Link to the One-Thing Weight-Loss Eating Plan," will remind you how this diet is helping you reach the recommended nutritional percentages, as advised by the Institute of Medicine's Food and Nutrition Board (September 2002).

Fat—20–35 percent of daily calories

- *Link to the One-Thing Weight-Loss Eating Plan:* As you eliminate unhealthy foods, you'll focus on getting rid of those with saturated fats (e.g., whole milk, butter, visible fat on meats, and high-fat cheese) and trans fats (e.g., stick margarine, commercial baked goods, fried foods at restaurants or fast-food facilities).

    Your ultimate goal is a diet with trans fats reduced to less than 1 percent of your total daily calorie intake. Also, saturated fats should comprise less than 7 percent of your total daily calories (2006 AHA guidelines). When you do consume fats, you should eat mostly monounsaturated fats (e.g., nuts and olive or canola oil), polyunsaturated fats (corn oil), and omega-3 fats (salmon and light canned tuna).

Complex carbohydrates—45–65 percent of daily calories

• *Link to the One-Thing Weight-Loss Eating Plan:* As you eliminate unhealthy foods and drinks, you'll focus on getting rid of items with a very high sugar or alcohol content, such as desserts, cola drinks, sugary beverages, various sweet snacks, beer, wine, and mixed drinks.

Also, as you begin to *add* good foods in the second five-week period, you'll select more fruits, which contain natural fruit sugars, and vegetables and whole grains packed with complex carbohydrates. Your goal will be to eat five to nine servings of fruits and vegetables every day. In addition, you should include a serving of whole grains, such as a cereal like oatmeal, whole-grain bread, brown rice, or whole-wheat pasta. These choices will take you up into the 45–65 percent range.

Protein—10–30 percent of daily calories

• *Link to the One-Thing Weight-Loss Eating Plan:* Each day, you'll eat one or two servings (three to six ounces) of poultry, omega-3 fish, or lean meat. A good balance during a seven-day period for lunch and evening meals would be two servings (eight ounces per week) of fish such as salmon, halibut, or lake trout; four to five servings of poultry (not fried, with visible skin removed); and less than twelve ounces weekly of lean meat, like filet mignon or pork tenderloin.

Note: Once again, a three- to four-ounce single serving of lean meat, poultry, or fish is about the size of the palm of your hand.

Finally, remember that regular exercise is an essential "diet supplement," able both to enhance your health and longevity and to promote faster, more efficient weight loss. Now, to see how easily the One-Thing Weight-Loss Eating Plan strategy can be implemented, consider the experience of Ted, who had reached a tough resistance point in his efforts to lose weight.

A ONE-THING WEIGHT-LOSS EATING PLAN SAGA

Ted's weight had been creeping up a couple of pounds a year for about four years, until he found that, at 162 pounds, he was fourteen pounds above his best level. The signs were showing up not just on his bathroom scale, but also in his inability to button well-tailored trousers and collar buttons.

He had tried several popular weight-loss plans, but none seemed to work for him. So he embarked on the five-week One-Thing Weight-Loss Eating Plan strategy. His program proceeded this way:

During the first week, Ted cut from his diet a serving of commercially packaged, saturated and trans fat–laden cookies each day (6 unhealthy fat grams per day, or 42 grams per week).

For the second week, he eliminated his typical snack serving: ten Ritz crackers a day, which contained 2 unhealthy fat grams per day, or 14 grams per week.

The third week, he cut out three small bags of regular potato chips he usually consumed each week (9 unhealthy fat grams per week).

During the fourth week, he eliminated three tablespoons of butter a day that he used as a spread (21 unhealthy fat grams per day, or 147 grams per week).

The fifth week, he stopped drinking a twelve-ounce cola a day (150 high-sugar calories a day, or 1,050 calories per week).

To enhance his weight-loss efforts, Ted decided to extend his elimination program for another week. (Remember, this One-Thing Weight-Loss Eating Plan is flexible.) So during the sixth week he dropped his customary two orders of fast-food French fries each week—for a total additional reduction of an extra 16 grams of unhealthy fat per week.

In the end, through this simple elimination strategy, Ted reduced his weekly consumption of unhealthy fats by 228 grams, which amounted to a total of 2,052 calories weekly in bad fats alone. Also, by cutting out that one cola per day, he eliminated another 1,050 calories per week (mostly simple sugars). Furthermore, the total calories (unhealthy fats and sugars plus other calories) contained in the foods he had cut brought his *grand total* of eliminated weekly calories to more than 5,000 calories per week—a level that enabled him to drop about 1.5 pounds each week (one pound of fat = 3,500 calories).

As a result of his reduced bad-food intake, Ted lost more than eight unwanted pounds in a little more than one month. Before he finished his sixty-day target period—the time he had established to achieve his ultimate weight-loss goal—he was down to 147 pounds, or one pound less than his targeted weight loss of fourteen pounds. But just as important, he lost those pounds by removing from his menus only high-risk, unhealthy fat and high-sugar foods, which are responsible for some of our most lethal health conditions.

The health benefits showed up immediately when Ted went in for his annual checkup a couple of months after losing the weight. His total cholesterol had dropped by thirty points—with his "bad" LDL cholesterol accounting for most of that reduction. Also, his "good" HDL cholesterol had increased by four points. Finally, his blood pressure reading had declined from 140/85 to 124/72, undoubtedly as a direct result of his weight loss and the elimination of the bad fats in his diet.

Ted continued with the second phase of the One-Thing Weight-Loss Eating Plan by adding five extra fruits and vegetables over the next five weeks. (He had been mainly a meat-and-potatoes man before starting the diet. As such, he usually consumed only two or three fruits or vegetables during a typical day.) But he was able to maintain his weight loss because adding these foods into his diet provided him with complex carbohydrates, which accounted for only about half the calories of the fats he had tossed out.

FROM TEN WEEKS TO LIFE:
MAINTAINING YOUR LOSSES

After you've taken off your unwanted pounds, what happens next?

When all the weight you wanted to lose is gone, you'll be ready for the maintenance phase—which will continue for the rest of your life. Here are some options:

- You can continue on the exact same program you've established with the One-Thing Weight-Loss Eating Plan; or
- You can continue to eliminate other trans fats from your diet—a great choice for those who want to minimize their risk of various diseases, and at the same time accelerate their weight loss (see above how Ted added a sixth week of food elimination); or
- You can judiciously substitute other "healthy" foods *without* trans fats, saturated fats, or simple sugars back into your daily menus.

  But when you substitute, keep these principles in mind: always prefer vegetables, fruits, and whole grains when you are considering additions. Also, be sure that you really do *substitute* by cutting high-fat or high-sugar foods you're now eating before you add in the good foods. In other words, don't just add extra foods without making eliminations. If you do, you'll put on extra pounds—no matter how nutritious those new foods are. (The safest approach is to follow the basic elimination-substitution guidelines described in the ten-week start-up phase of the eating plan.)

The great thing about this maintenance stage is that you really don't have to do anything new unless you want to. As long as you stay at your ideal weight, your health will benefit from the One-Thing Weight-Loss Eating Plan you've already set in place.

Of course, if you find your weight starting to edge up in the months or years ahead, you'll have to return to the drawing board to see what's going wrong. It may be that you've started adding a little extra food to your serving sizes. If that's the case, all you have to do is cut back on that extra intake. Or you may have added some additional food or drink—such as cheese and crackers as an appetizer, or an additional half-glass of wine each evening, or a biscotti after lunch. A little thought and analysis should help you identify the nutritional culprit—and get rid of it without delay.

Or as you get a little older, you may find that you're exercising a little less often or less intensely. Maybe you're now walking half the time during your daily half-hour workout instead of jogging the entire thirty minutes. Reducing exercise time or intensity will also reduce the calorie burning—and put you at risk of gaining weight.

But these are just fine-tuning issues. So watch your weight closely; if you see at some point that it has begun to creep up, that will be a sure sign that you need to tweak your program a little to put your eating plan back on track.

Finally, to show you how deeply personal this program is for us, let's take a journey back through time with Ken—who will explain in his own words how his life was saved by something akin to a One-Thing Weight-Loss Eating Plan strategy.

Up to this point, we've discussed the three foundational components of the Start Strong, Finish Strong approach to good health and long life—a gold-standard physical exam, a personal fitness regimen, and a simple diet, with powerful weight-loss and health-enhancing benefits. But there's more: a wise supplement strategy should also be part of your complete health-and-longevity program.

How Ken Saved His Life with a
One-Thing Weight-Loss Eating Plan

As a young man, I was quite athletic, a hard, wiry 170 pounds at my "fighting weight." In fact, the University of Oklahoma awarded me a track scholarship, and I regularly worked out and competed in intercollegiate meets as a miler.

But after I graduated from college and entered medical school, the pressure of studies and my own lack of motivation about personal fitness started me on a downhill physical slide. My basic assumption at that point in my life was, "Nothing's really important except my medical studies!"

For one thing, I felt I had no time for exercise, and so I became quite sedentary. Also, being the typical Oklahoma boy coming of age in the 1940s and 1950s, I developed a taste for fried chicken, other deep-fried specialties, and especially those huge quantities of grease-dripping, French-fried potatoes we could order at drive-ins. I can still recall how my mouth would water when the waitress walked over to my car and placed those aromatic hamburgers and fries on the little tray they always attached to the window outside the driver's side of the car.

At the time, I had no idea what I was doing to my body. For example, with the fries, nobody ever told me that fast-food places may use the same grease forty or more times in a row without cleaning the frying pans and cooking surfaces—and manage to keep the stuff from going rancid by using partially hydrogenated plant oils. (I've been amazed to hear reports that this practice is typical in many fast-food establishments today.)

More important, in those days no one knew that all this food processing produced the most destructive form of fats on earth—the so-called trans fats that emerge from the hydrogenation process. Maybe I would have thought twice if I had known that by ingesting this poison, I was significantly increasing my risk of high cholesterol, hypertension, heart disease, diabetes, certain cancers, and a host of obesity-related diseases. Although scientists have confirmed in recent years that "trans fats prolong shelf life, but shorten human life," nobody told me because nobody knew.

As a result of this couch-potato lifestyle, by the time I had graduated from medical school and finished my internship, my weight had shot up from 170 to 200. Then, I entered the army as a physician and married my wife, Millie, who turned about to be too good a cook. The result was that by age twenty-nine, I had hit my all-time top weight of 204 pounds.

Now, that may not sound like a lot for a man who is six foot one inch. But as I say, at my fighting weight I was wiry—and I remember all too well those rolls that had appeared on my stomach, backside, and thighs. At the time, we didn't have sophisticated techniques like underwater weighing to determine the precise percent of body fat. But I know now, after years of observing and treating overweight patients, that my body fat had reached about 30 percent of my total weight.

To realize the significance of this deterioration, you have to understand something about body fat percentages. Our studies at the Cooper Clinic have shown that a minimally healthy man should have less than 19 percent body fat. Yet I was in a category that put me in about the top fifth percentile for my age group. (Lest you think that sounds okay, look again. The number means that 95 percent of the male population below age thirty had less body fat than I did.)

As my weight increased and my fitness level plummeted, my blood pressure crept up—to a level that approached full-blown hypertension. It didn't help matters that I almost never exercised. Also, stress was building on me as I became frustrated with my work with the army: I had actually begun to inquire about transferring to more interesting duty with the air force.

In other words, at age twenty-nine I found myself an obese blob, thirty-four pounds overweight, with borderline hypertension and a highly stressful, sedentary lifestyle. If the Ken Cooper today had done a physical exam on the Ken Cooper of those days, the diagnosis might have gone something like this: "Young man, you're a ticking time

(continued)

bomb—with multiple risk factors that scream, 'Early heart attack or stroke!'"

In fact, before any doctor could get hold of me, I *did* suffer a cardiac event after a particularly rigorous waterskiing session. After an intense, high-speed slalom run, for which I was totally unprepared physically, I nearly collapsed, nauseated and dizzy. Most likely, I had a cardiac arrhythmia, or irregular heartbeat—which isn't the same thing as a heart attack, but in a severe form the condition can lead to death.

Needless to say, that experience got my attention—and led to what I can only describe as a "fitness conversion." Over the next year, under the guidance of a physician-mentor in the military, I embarked on an exercise and diet program that gradually returned me to a fit condition—and a much lower body fat percentage at a weight of 170 pounds.

An important part of this program—much more important than I realized at the time—was that I was encouraged to reduce the fats in my daily diet. In those days, we of course knew that all fats carry 9 calories per gram, while carbohydrates and protein contain only about 4 grams. So it was logical for most weight-loss plans to concentrate on cutting out fats. But what we *didn't* know was that by cutting down on fats, *we were also reducing those fats that are the most dangerous to our health— trans fats*—as well as minimizing the second-most dangerous kind of fats, saturated fats.

In particular, I started eliminating or limiting—one by one—my intake of fast-food French fries, other fried foods, and visible fat on steaks and chicken. Also, I began to avoid second and third helpings and extra-large servings of entrées and rich desserts. At the same time, I added more fruits and vegetables to my daily menu.

In effect, I began my weight loss and my recovery of health and fitness with a variation of what we have called the One-Thing Weight-Loss Eating Plan, and I've continued with this strategy most of my life. Over the years, some variation on this program has worked for me and for many others—and I predict it will work for you as well.

Ten

■   **Start-up #4—Follow**
■   **a Wise Supplement**
    Strategy

What's the point in consuming food supplements over and above a healthful, balanced diet? Certainly, if you follow the eating guidelines in the previous chapter, you'll get solid nutrition that can help maximize your health and longevity. But sometimes we need a helping hand with our food plan, and that's why we regard supplements as one of the key components of twenty-first-century medicine.

Here are just a few of the practical benefits we've seen among participants at the Cooper Aerobics Center, friends and family members in our personal experience, and patients in our practice:

- *Folic acid (folate)*, a member of the B-vitamin complex, when taken in daily doses of 400 mcg, can lower blood levels of homocysteine, which is an emerging marker for possible heart disease.[1]

  "Karin" came to us with a homocysteine reading of 19 micromoles per liter—a level that placed her at very high risk of cardiovascular disease. But after only three months of folate therapy—involving daily intake of 400 mcg of an inexpensive, over-the-counter folic acid tablet—her homocysteine reading dropped to 9, where she was now at low risk. (She also took daily doses of vitamin B_{12} to ensure that the folic acid wouldn't mask pernicious anemia, which is related to a deficiency of vitamin B_{12}.)

- *Fish oil* containing omega-3 fatty acids can provide many cardiovascular benefits, including reduction of potentially dangerous irregular heartbeats (arrhythmias). [2]

"Eric" complained periodically of a strange sensation in his chest involving a feeling that he was "out of breath" or even that his heart had momentarily stopped beating. In fact, he was diagnosed as experiencing irregular heartbeats—a condition that apparently ran in his family.

Resting and stress electrocardiograms and a sonogram revealed no physical problem, such as a coronary blockage or abnormality in heart valves. So he was told to start taking a daily dose of 2,000 mg of a fish oil supplement that contained significant amounts of important omega-3 acids: 760 mg of EPA and 440 mg of DHA. Within a couple of weeks, the tendency to have irregular heartbeats was corrected almost completely.

- *Zinc* can shorten the duration of the common cold—from seven days to one or two, according to some studies.[3]

Many of our patients have found that taking over-the-counter zinc lozenges containing 15 mg of zinc every two hours, or using zinc nasal gels, has resulted in shorter colds.

- *Antioxidants, including vitamins C and E,* may improve immune function—and help decrease the frequency of the common cold.[4]

After she started taking multivitamin tablets with values similar to those listed in the chart in this chapter on page 239, "Ariel," an eighty-year-old resident of an assisted-living facility, found that the number of colds she caught declined from about four to only one or two per year. Her experience is consistent with that reported in studies of respiratory infections among nursing home residents and other elderly patients.

Supplements are certainly not replacements for a good diet, proper exercise, and stress management. But proper supplementation is a kind of "health insurance" that enables us to fill gaps in the diet. More specifically, some of us may require an extra nudge to ensure that we get important nutrients, which may be overlooked in a daily diet. Others may need an additional dose of nutrition that can provide added protection against certain life-threatening conditions, such as heart disease or prostate cancer. Still others may want to increase the odds that they *may* be protected by certain supplements, even though the current evidence may point in different directions.

As we embark on a discussion of this topic, keep in mind this last point: research is sometimes sparse or contradictory on some supplements. A basic principle on which we operate is that if there is a reasonable chance that a supplement will improve health or guard against disease—*and* there is significant evidence that the supplement *won't* do harm—then it's perfectly acceptable to incorporate that supplement into your food plan. Now, what supplements should be candidates for your Start Strong, Finish Strong program?

We have divided the supplements we'll be considering into three broad groupings, which you'll immediately see reach beyond the usual understanding of supplements as "vitamin pills." They include the following categories:

- General vitamins and minerals
- Over-the-counter medical supplements
- Functional food supplements

As a result of scientific investigations done by the Cooper Institute and other research centers, we have become convinced about the potential benefits of these additions to your diet.[5] In fact, we continue to fine-tune these categories and dosages, and encourage their practical use by patients as part of our Cooper Complete supplement program. Now here's what you need to know about the first of these three supplement categories—the general vitamins and minerals.

General Vitamins and Minerals— an Overview

To provide you with a reference point for the more detailed discussion of vitamins and minerals that follows, we have included some charts that should provide helpful overviews. These are based on our extensive research relating to the Cooper Complete nutritional supplements that are studied at the Cooper Institute.

Specifically, the first chart includes our complete set of basic vitamins and minerals *without* iron, and the second contains the complete set *with* iron. The reason for the difference is that women in their childbearing years need supplemental iron, as deficiencies are common. Also, men and women of any age who are anemic or are advised by their physician to take iron in a supplement form should consider the chart with iron.

The third and fourth charts contain our recommendations for calcium and omega-3. We have listed these separately because the recommended dosages of both are sufficiently large that they can't be included in one typical vitamin pill. With our Cooper Complete supplements, for example, the complete basic set of vitamins and minerals is contained in one tablet, with a daily dosage recommendation of eight tablets. But both calcium and omega-3 supplements are packaged and taken separately.

CHART #1: COMPLETE BASIC VITAMIN AND MINERAL SUPPLEMENTS—IRON-FREE

(for men and women, including postmenopausal women, who have *not* been prescribed iron supplements by their physician)

Supplement Facts

The daily dosage provides:

Ingredients	Daily Amount	% Daily Value
Vitamin A (mixed carotenes)	3,000 IU	60
Vitamin C (ascorbic acid)	500 mg	833
Vitamin D (cholecalciferol)	1,000 IU	250
Vitamin E (d-alpha tocopherol succinate)	400 IU	1,333
Vitamin K (phytonadione)	25 mcg	31
Thiamine (vitamin B_1 as HCl)	3 mg	200
Riboflavin (vitamin B_2)	10 mg	588
Niacinamide (vitamin B_3)	20 mg	100
Pyridoxine (vitamin B_6)	10 mg	500
Folic Acid	400 mcg	100
Cyanocobalamin (vitamin B_{12})	400 mcg	6,666
Biotin (d-biotin)	300 mcg	100
Pantothenic Acid (vitamin B_5 as d-calcium pantothenate)	10 mg	100
Iodine (potassium iodide)	150 mcg	100
Magnesium (oxide)	400 mg	100
Zinc (oxide)	15 mg	100

Ingredients	Daily Amount	% Daily Value
Copper (copper gluconate)	2 mg	100
Selenium (rice bran chelate)	100 mcg	142
Chromium (amino acid chelate)	100 mcg	83
Potassium (potassium phosphate)	400 mg	11
Choline (choline bitartrite)	500 mg	*
Coenzyme Q_{10} (ubiquinone)	50 mg	*
Lycopene	10 mg	*
Lutein (FloraGLO)	6 mg	*

*Percent Daily Value not established

CHART #2: COMPLETE BASIC VITAMIN AND MINERAL SUPPLEMENTS—WITH IRON
(for men and women, including premenopausal women, who *have* been prescribed iron supplements by their physician)

Supplement Facts
The daily dosage provides:

Ingredients	Daily Amount	% Daily Value
Vitamin A (natural mixed beta-carotene and other carotenoids from d-salina)	3,000 IU	60
Vitamin C (ascorbic acid)	1,000 mg	1,666
Vitamin D (cholecalciferol)	1,000 IU	200
Vitamin E (d-alpha tocopherol succinate)	400 IU	1,333
Vitamin K (phytoadione)	25 mcg	31

Ingredients	Daily Amount	% Daily Value
Thiamine (thiamine hydrochloride)	3 mg	200
Riboflavin (vitamin B_2)	10 mg	588
Niacinamide (vitamin B_3)	20 mg	100
Vitamin B_6 (pyridoxine hydrochloride)	25 mg	1,250
Folic Acid	400 mcg	100
Vitamin B_{12} (cyanocobalamin)	400 mcg	6,666
Biotin (d-biotin)	300 mcg	100
Pantothenic Acid (vitamin B_5 as d-calcium pantothenate)	10 mg	100
Iron (iron carbonyl)	18 mg	100
Iodine (potassium iodide)	150 mcg	100
Magnesium (magnesium oxide)	400 mg	100
Zinc (zinc oxide)	15 mg	100
Selenium (rice bran chelate)	100 mcg	142
Copper (copper gluconate)	2 mg	100
Chromium (amino acid chelate)	100 mcg	83
Potassium (potassium phosphate)	400 mg	11
Choline (choline bitartrite)	400 mg	*
Lycopene	10 mg	*
Lutein (FloraGLO)	6 mg	*
Coenzyme Q_{10} (ubiquinone)	50 mg	*

*Percent Daily Value not established

CHART #3: CALCIUM RECOMMENDATIONS
(adults, age 18 and older)

Supplement Facts

The daily dosage provides:

Ingredients		Daily Amount	% Daily Value
Calcium (from calcium citrate)	*Men:*	500 mg	50
	Women:	1,000 mg	67–83%

Note: This dosage contains 50 percent of the daily value for men; the other 500 mg for men should be obtained from the diet. Also, for women 250 to 500 mg should come from dietary sources. Also, because calcium should be taken with a complete multivitamin containing vitamin D, that vitamin is not included in this recommendation. Finally, as studies show, calcium citrate is the type of calcium supplement best absorbed by the body.

CHART #4: OMEGA-3 FISH OIL RECOMMENDATIONS
(adults, age 18 and older)

Supplement Facts

A daily dosage of 2 softgels provides:

Ingredients	Daily Amount	% Daily Value
Omega-3 (EPA/DHA) Fish Oil (providing 1,000 mg of EPA and 200 mg of DHA)	1,000–2,000 mg	*

Other ingredients

Gelatin, glycerin, and water

*Percent Daily Value not established

Note: The addition of vitamin E in these supplements isn't necessary if you're taking a daily multivitamin with the larger amounts of vitamin E recommended in this chapter (see the "Complete Basic Vitamin and Mineral Supplements" charts #1 and #2).

With these overviews in mind, let's now take a closer look at the reasoning and science behind these recommendations.

General Vitamins and Minerals— in Depth

VITAMIN A (INCLUDING BETA-CAROTENE AND OTHER CAROTENES)

The best form of this vitamin is a "provitamin," beta-carotene, along with natural mixed carotenoids. As a provitamin, beta-carotene can be regulated by your body and converted into vitamin A in the amounts your body needs. Vitamin A as beta-carotene can bolster your immune system and help maintain the health of your eyes, skin, teeth, bones, and mucous membranes.

Beta-carotene has been linked to a lower risk of cataracts, heart disease, and various cancers (rectal cancer, melanoma, and bladder cancer). Also, beta-carotene (in the amount of 5,000 IU per day) and other carotenoids have been connected to decreased risk or even reversal of age-related macular degeneration, which is the leading cause of blindness in Americans over sixty-five.[6]

It's best to avoid full-blown vitamin A (as retinol) because, in this form, too much of the substance can become toxic. Also, high intake of retinol has been associated with an increased risk of hip fractures in both men and women.

Another concern to keep in mind relates to beta-carotene and smoking. Two studies published in 1994 suggested that very large doses of beta-carotene were associated with increased risk for lung cancer and heart disease in smokers. Although these results need further clarification, it would be wise for smokers either to avoid this supplement—or to quit smoking.

Recommended daily dosage: 3,000 IU

% Daily Value*: 60

VITAMIN C (ASCORBIC ACID)

Important in your body's formation of collagen, vitamin C is a vital substance for the growth and repair of body tissue cells, gums, blood vessels, bones, and teeth.

Vitamin C is also an antioxidant that has been proven to reduce early cataracts by 77 percent and to lower the rate of moderate cataract development by 83 percent in women between the ages of fifty-six and seventy-one. These women took 1,000 mg of vitamin C daily for ten years.[7]

Another study showed that vitamin C (1,000 mg) combined with vitamin E could block the detrimental effects of a fatty meal (900 calories with 50 grams of fat) on blood circulation.[8]

According to still another study, 500 mg daily of vitamin C, taken for one month, can reduce blood pressure. Also, individuals with high blood levels of vitamin C have a significantly reduced risk of stroke, as compared with those who have low blood levels of vitamin C.[9]

Recommended daily dosage: 500 mg

% Daily Value: 833

---

*The "% Daily Value" figure for each of these entries refers to the amount recommended by government and medical authorities for proper nutrition in a 2,000-calorie daily diet. The reason that our recommended dosages are often much higher than the % Daily Value is that various scientific studies have suggested that larger amounts of certain vitamins and minerals may be protective against disease.

VITAMIN D (CHOLECALCIFEROL)

Vitamin D helps get calcium and phosphorus to those parts of the body where they can promote bone growth in children and regenerate (or "remineralize") bone in adults. Although just ten minutes of direct sunlight can provide the required amount of this vitamin, almost 38 percent of American adults are deficient in it, according to the *New England Journal of Medicine.*

Another report, in *Cancer, Epidemiology, Biomarkers, and Prevention,* found that of the 5,000 women studied, those with higher sunlight exposure, plus at least 200 IU of vitamin D, had a lower risk of developing breast cancer.

Finally, a recent meta-analysis of sixty-three studies conducted between 1966 and 2004 indicated that vitamin D lowers the risk of colon, breast, and ovarian cancer. The lead author of the study, Dr. Cedric Garland from the University of California at San Diego Moores Cancer Center, said, "The benefit of vitamin D is as clear as the harmful link between smoking and lung cancer."[10]

Recommended daily dosage: 1,000 IU
% Daily Value: 250

VITAMIN E (D-ALPHA TOCOPHEROL SUCCINATE)

A powerful antioxidant as well as a blood thinner (anticoagulant), vitamin E as an antioxidant fights the destructive effects of free radicals, or unstable oxygen molecules, in the body. (Excess free radicals have been linked to a higher risk of heart disease and cancer.) Unfortunately, 30 percent of U.S. adults are deficient in vitamin E, according to the Centers for Disease Control and Prevention.

In various studies, vitamin E has been associated with a reduced risk of cardiovascular disease because of its ability to neutralize the oxidation of "bad" LDL cholesterol. (The oxidation of LDL is a major factor in the buildup of blood-vessel plaque, which in turn leads to atherosclerosis and heart attacks.)

Other studies have linked vitamin E to a lower risk of cancer, cataracts, decreased immunity, and exercise-induced damage to the body's DNA.[11]

We recommend the d-alpha tocopherol form of vitamin E, which has been shown to be three to five times more potent than the synthetic, dl-alpha tocopherol.[12]

Recommended daily dosage: 200–400 IU

% Daily Value: up to 1,333

VITAMIN K (PHYTONADIONE)

This nutrient, which is found in the small intestine, combines with protein to facilitate blood clotting. Vitamin K is also essential for the synthesis of proteins found in plasma, bone, and the kidneys. Low intakes of vitamin K may increase the risk of hip fracture in women, according to a 1999 report in the *American Journal of Clinical Nutrition.*

Recommended daily dosage: 25 mcg

% Daily Value: 31

THIAMINE (VITAMIN B₁ AS HCI)

Thiamine helps in the metabolism of carbohydrates, bolstering of the nervous system, skin health, and physical growth. A thiamine deficiency may result in beriberi, which causes fatigue, calf muscle pain, constipation, upset stomach, neuritis (inflammation and deterioration of nerves), or mental problems such as depression. Those at particular risk are alcoholics and people who eat large amounts of white-flour products.

Recommended daily dosage: 3 mg

% Daily Value: 200

RIBOFLAVIN (VITAMIN B$_2$)

Important for healthy skin and vision, riboflavin may also help in the metabolism of the body's sugar (glucose) and fatty acids. A deficiency of riboflavin may emerge as eye irritation, including sensitivity of eyes to light; dry or scaly skin; cracking lips; and swelling of the legs.

Recommended daily dosage: 10 mg
% Daily Value: 588

NIACINAMIDE (VITAMIN B$_3$)

A form of niacin, niacinamide can promote a healthy nervous system, healthy skin, and proper gastrointestinal functioning. Plus, niacinamide lacks the side effects associated with niacin or nicotinic acid, such as flushing.

On the other hand, unlike niacin or nicotinic acid, niacinamide doesn't have the ability to lower cholesterol. (Because of possible side effects, niacin or nicotinic acid, which can be bought over the counter, should be taken only under the supervision of a physician.)

Recommended daily dosage: 20 mg
% Daily Value: 100

PYRIDOXINE (VITAMIN B$_6$)

An important function of vitamin B$_6$ is to ensure that certain biological processes, including fat and protein metabolism, occur as they should.

In conjunction with vitamin B$_{12}$ and folic acid, vitamin B$_6$ has been shown to lower homocysteine,[13] an amino acid in the blood that has been associated with damage to cells lining the vessel walls. This process can play a significant role in the development of atherosclerosis ("hardening of the arteries") and coronary artery disease. Furthermore, lower levels of vitamin B_6 and folate have been associated with an increased risk of atherosclerosis.[14]

Recommended daily dosage: 10 mg
% Daily Value: 500

FOLIC ACID (FOLATE)

Folic acid, also called folate, part of the vitamin-B complex, is essential to the formation of red blood cells and also aids in protein metabolism.

Women of childbearing age should be sure to take at least 400 mcg of folic acid daily to help prevent neural-tube defects in their unborn children.

Many studies have shown the ability of folic acid to lower homocysteine, a marker for cardiovascular disease. Higher levels of folic acid intake (at least 400 mcg daily) may help prevent the buildup of vessel plaque by reducing total homocysteine levels.[15] In addition, long-term use of multivitamins, including folic acid, may substantially reduce the risk of colon cancer.[16]

Recommended daily dosage: 400 mcg
% Daily Value: 100

CYANOCOBALAMIN (VITAMIN B_{12})

A member of the vitamin-B complex, B_{12} plays a major role in the metabolism of proteins, fats, and sugars. This nutrient facilitates the absorption and conversion of folic acid into its active form.

An extremely important function of B_{12} is to help maintain the fatty sheath (myelin) that protects the nerves. A deficiency in the vitamin can result in memory loss, confusion, and decreased reflexes, along with other nervous disorders. In addition, a deficiency may result in pernicious anemia, which can be masked if you are taking high doses of folic acid. As a result, it's important always to take vitamin B_{12} and folic acid together.

Studies have also found that taking a combination of *three* nutrients— vitamin B_{12}, folic acid, and vitamin B_6—is associated with the most significant decrease in homocysteine, an important marker for cardiovascular disease.[17]

Recommended daily dosage: 400 mcg
% Daily Value: 6,666

BIOTIN

Biotin, another component of the vitamin-B complex, is involved in the breakdown of proteins, the metabolism of carbohydrates, and the formation of fats. This substance works with vitamin B_2 (riboflavin), B_6, niacin, and vitamin A to promote healthy skin. A deficiency of biotin is rare because the intestines can manufacture it from other food.

Recommended daily dosage: 300 mcg
% Daily Value: 100

PANTOTHENIC ACID
(VITAMIN B_5 AS D-CALCIUM PANTOTHENATE)

Once called vitamin B_5, pantothenic acid helps build cells, maintain normal growth, develop the nervous system, and synthesize antibodies. The substance is also vital to the proper functioning of the adrenal glands and is essential for converting fat and sugar to energy.

Recommended daily dosage: 10 mg
% Daily Value: 100

IODINE (POTASSIUM IODIDE)

The thyroid gland uses iodine to produce the hormone thyroxine. Thyroxine, in turn, helps regulate energy production, body temperature, breathing, and muscle tone. It also assists in tissue development and breakdown. Usually, adequate intake occurs through the use of commonly consumed iodized salt.

Recommended daily dosage: 150 mcg
% Daily Value: 100

MAGNESIUM (MAGNESIUM CHELATE)

Magnesium, a mineral, assists in helping nerve and muscular impulses and muscular contraction. It is also necessary for the metabolism of calcium, vitamin C, phosphorus, sodium, and potassium.

Recommended daily dosage: 400 mg

% Daily Value: 100

ZINC (ZINC CHELATE)

A trace mineral,* zinc is essential for normal growth, pregnancies, and transmission of our genetic material. As an enzyme component, the substance is also required in the eyes, liver, kidneys, muscles, skin, testes, and other organs. The highest concentrations of zinc are in the bones, the prostate gland, and the eyes.

In addition to zinc's role in these bodybuilding and maintenance functions, there is some evidence that when taken at the onset of an upper respiratory illness, zinc may reduce the severity of such infections.

Caution: Megadoses of zinc may inhibit the immune response, according to research from the USDA's Nutrition Center at Tufts University.

Recommended daily dosage: 15 mg

% Daily Value: 100

COPPER (COPPER GLUCONATE)

Copper plays a major role in the metabolism and conversion of iron into hemoglobin—an important component of red blood cells. Copper also protects the bones against deterioration and osteoporosis (loss of bone mass).

---

*A "trace mineral" refers to a mineral found in extremely small amounts in the body. But even though amounts may be minuscule, the mineral's importance to bodily functioning may be large.

In addition, it functions as an antioxidant, or an antidote to free radicals in the body. Free radicals have been associated with a number of health conditions, including cardiovascular disease and cancer.

Adequate supplies of copper in the body have been linked to lower levels of total cholesterol and higher levels of "good" HDL cholesterol.

Recommended daily dosage: 2 mg
% Daily Value: 100

SELENIUM (SELENIUM CHELATE)

Selenium is a trace mineral that works with vitamins C, E, and beta-carotene to provide your body with a strong antioxidant defense.

One study, conducted with older men who were followed for 6.4 years, showed that selenium supplementation can reduce the frequency of lung, colon, rectal, and prostate cancer.[18]

Recommended daily dosage: 100 mcg
% Daily Value: 142

CHROMIUM (AMINO ACID CHELATE)

Chromium, a trace mineral, is necessary for proper functioning of insulin, a major player in the metabolism of sugar and is involved in the body's use of protein and fat.

Studies have suggested that high doses of chromium picolinate that accumulate in the tissues may damage chromosomes, including DNA, a process that is associated with the development of cancer.

Recommended daily dosage: 100 mcg
% Daily Value: 83

POTASSIUM (POTASSIUM PHOSPHATE)

Potassium works with sodium to regulate the body's overall fluid balance and also to normalize heart rhythms. It is also necessary for good muscle contraction and rapid transmission of nerve impulses throughout the body.

Low potassium intake may help cause high blood pressure. As a result, those who are unable to reduce their sodium intake may take steps to prevent and treat hypertension by increasing levels of potassium in their diet.[19]

Recommended daily dosage: 400 mg

% Daily Value: 11

CHOLINE (CHOLINE BITARTRITE)

Choline, part of the vitamin-B complex, helps the body utilize fats and cholesterol. It's also involved in producing a chemical that aids memory.

Recommended daily dosage: 500 mg

% Daily Value: not established

COENZYME Q_{10} (UBIQUINONE)

Coenzyme Q_{10}, also known as ubiquinone, acts as a catalyst to convert food into energy. Found in every cell in the body, this nutrient has stimulated interest because of its potential as an antioxidant. Various studies have indicated that coenzyme Q_{10} could help protect the body against tissue damage from heart attacks, heart disease, retina deterioration, breast cancer, and other diseases.

In a 1985–1993 study conducted at the University of Texas Medical Branch, Galveston, researchers used coenzyme Q_{10} to treat more than four hundred patients with various forms of cardiovascular disease, including enlarged heart, hypertension, mitral valve prolapse, and heart valve disease. Those with heart disease showed a significant improvement in their heart function, and their overall medication requirements dropped considerably. The researchers concluded that coenzyme Q_{10} is a safe and effective treatment for a broad range of cardiovascular diseases.[20]

Recommended daily dosage: 50 mg

% Daily Value: not established

LYCOPENE

Lycopene—a carotenoid found in tomatoes, red grapefruit, and watermelon—is the substance that gives these foods their red color.

This nutrient has been linked to lower rates of prostate cancer. A six-year study published in 1995 revealed that men in such countries as Greece and Italy were the most likely to eat tomato-based produce and the least likely to develop the cancer.[21] Other studies have shown that those who intake from 6.4 to 10 mg of lycopene per day—a level that can also be obtained from two to four servings of tomato sauce a week—have the lowest risk of prostate cancer. In addition, certain findings have suggested that lycopene can help maintain a healthy heart and cardiovascular system.

Recommended daily dosage: 5–10 mg

% Daily Value: not established

LUTEIN (FLORAGLO)

Natural carotenoids, such as beta-carotene, lutein, and zeaxanthin, are effective in decreasing the risk or even reversing the development of age-related macular degeneration (AMD), according to the *Journal of the American Medical Association*.[22] Macular degeneration is the leading cause of blindness in Americans over age sixty-five.

Recommended daily dosage: 6 mg, or 10 mg for those with a family history or diagnosis of AMD. Also, we recommend the FloraGLO type of lutein, which is the purest form of lutein available and is also highly absorbable.

% Daily Value: not established

CALCIUM (CALCIUM CITRATE)

An adequate daily intake of calcium—from 1,000 to 1,500 mg per day for women and 1,000 mg for men—is absolutely essential to promote good bone development and ward off the onset of osteoporosis (bone-thinning) with age. The lower amount for men takes into account some preliminary studies that suggest a potential for an increased risk of prostate cancer with higher intakes of calcium.

Various studies have suggested that calcium citrate is the type of calcium supplement that is somewhat more likely to be absorbed well by the body.

The daily dosages recommended below assume that if you fail to take in the full recommended amount of calcium through your diet, you will take in the balance of the required amount through an appropriate supplement.

Recommended daily dosage: For women, a total of 1,200 to 1,500 mg in diet or supplement form. For men, a total of 1,000 mg in diet or supplement form. Also, remember that vitamin D helps regulate your body's utilization of calcium; so make sure you are getting 1,000 IU of vitamin D daily.

% Daily Value: 100

OMEGA-3 FATTY ACIDS

Omega-3 fatty acids, which are found naturally in oily fish like salmon, light canned tuna, and sardines, may also be obtained through fish-oil capsules. Our specialists at Cooper Concepts believe that omega-3 fish-oil capsules may be the single most important supplement you should take. Omega-3s are not just "good" fats: based on a tremendous volume of solid research (more than 8,500 published articles), they may qualify as "great" fats.

The omega-3 fatty acids are categorized as "essential"; because our bodies can't make them, we must consume them to remain healthy. They are present in the membranes of every cell in our body and have been shown to benefit the heart, brain, eyes, and immune system. Those who suffer from rheumatoid arthritis, lupus, or any other autoimmune disease should consider taking omega-3 acids because of their anti-inflammatory properties. These acids may also decrease asthma attacks and help those with macular degeneration of the eye.

The most beneficial omega-3s are the "long chain" acids known as EPA (eicosapentaenoic acid) and DHA (docosahexaenoic acid). You can get these from certain types of fish (salmon, halibut, light canned tuna, sardines) or from fish-oil supplements. Both EPA and DHA are so important that you should strive for a combination of at least 1,000 to 2,000 mg of the two acids every day.

For pregnant and breast-feeding women, and also children under ten years of age, experts suggest a product with more DHA than EPA. For everyone else, a product with more EPA than DHA is appropriate.

How do you choose the right fish-oil supplement?

The first rule: always be sure to read the label of any omega-3/fish-oil supplement very closely. Most products that you find at the grocery store or pharmacy offer only a 30 percent concentration of EPA/DHA. But higher-quality products contain a 50 to 60 percent concentration. Most fish-oil products go through a strict purification process, and as a result you should find very little, if any, risk of contamination from mercury or PCBs from these products.

Plant sources of omega-3 fatty acids include walnuts, flax oil, and canola oil. But they provide the "short chain" omega-3s (i.e., ALA, or alpha linolenic acid). Unfortunately, however, humans don't convert ALA to EPA and DHA very efficiently. ALA is certainly better than no omega-3 product at all, but it's not nearly as beneficial as EPA/DHA from fish-oil supplements.

Recommended daily dosage: For most people, capsules containing a total of approximately 1,000 mg of EPA and 200 mg of DHA. For breast-feeding or pregnant women or children under ten, the amounts of EPA and DHA should be reversed.

A word of caution: Because of suggestive results in a number of medical investigations, fish-oil supplement labels will typically carry a warning that fish oil should be avoided by those who are allergic to fish. Also, those who are advised to consult a physician before using fish-oil supplements include pregnant or lactating women; those with heart disease, diabetes, or a bleeding disorder; and those who are taking blood-thinning medications or aspirin.[23]

% Daily Value: not established

Also, increased intake of omega-3 fatty acids may cut the risk of co-lorectal cancer in men who are *not* taking aspirin by 66 percent, according to a 2007 report in *Cancer Epidemiology, Biomarkers and Prevention.*[24]

Some Cooper Thoughts on Fish-Oil Supplements

Omega-3 supplements containing the proper amounts of EPA and DHA can have a multitude of health benefits, including the reduction of triglyc-erides in the blood, prevention of cardiac arrhythmias, and the supply-ing of "brain food" that promotes more efficient mental functioning.

Another benefit of fish oil is moderate anticoagulation in the blood, but this benefit may be double-edged. On the one hand, fish oil could help prevent the formation of dangerous blood clots. On the other hand, those patients taking aspirin or blood thinners such as Coumadin have found that fish oil provides just one anticoagulant too many. The complexity of this issue leads us to different approaches in our patient-care strategies:

Ken: When my patients take fish oil, I'm less inclined to place them on aspirin, especially if they have a tendency toward gastrointestinal bleeding. The potential of GI problems is much less with fish oil than with aspirin. Also, fish oil that has been "de-burped" no longer has the aftertaste of many such supplements.

Tyler: Because of the proven benefits of aspirin, I usually suggest both aspirin and fish oil. But each patient must be evaluated individually.

Over-the-Counter Medical Supplements

As indicated above, some supplements may have some use in counter-ing symptoms of certain diseases. Zinc, for example, relieves the symp-toms and the duration of upper respiratory complaints, and niacin (under a physician's supervision) lowers cholesterol. Others, such as those mentioned below, have gained growing support in the medical community as measures to prevent or relieve other medical problems.

ASPIRIN

Various studies have indicated that low doses of aspirin can lower the risk of heart disease, stroke, and various cancers, including those of the colon, stomach, prostate, rectum, breast, and esophagus.

But at this point there appear to be gender and age differences in the benefits. Men taking low doses of aspirin are less likely to suffer heart at-tacks, but this same benefit doesn't apply to women aged forty-five to sixty-four. On the other hand, women who took low-dose aspirin (100 mg every other day) as part of the women's health study were 24 percent less likely to suffer an ischemic stroke (from blockage of an artery) than those who didn't take aspirin. Furthermore, older women—those over sixty-four—who took the low-dose aspirin were 30 percent less apt to have an ischemic stroke, and also were 34 percent less apt to suffer a heart attack.[25] In other words, older women enjoy even greater benefits from aspirin therapy.

Warning: Taking aspirin increases the risk of experiencing stomach bleeding and hemorrhagic (bleeding) stroke. In addition, aspirin is *not* recommended for those patients on blood thinners, such as Coumadin, or those who have a propensity to bleed easily. So be sure that you con-sult with your physician before you go on any aspirin therapy.

Recommended daily dosage: 81–162 mg (1–2 small-dose or "baby" aspirin)

% Daily Value: not established

GLUCOSAMINE AND CHONDROITIN

Two amino sugars that occur naturally in the body, glucosamine and chondroitin work to lubricate the joints and promote flexibility. Another substance sometimes included is bromelain, an extract from the pineapple stem that is useful for reducing muscle and tissue inflammation.

Researchers publishing in the *Journal of the American Medical Association* reviewed fifteen trials that studied the impact of glucosamine and chondroitin on osteoarthritis ("wear-and-tear" arthritis). They found that the compounds are safe and have some effectiveness in treating osteoarthritis symptoms.[26]

Further support for the ability of these supplements to relieve arthritis pain emerged in a 2006 report in the *New England Journal of Medicine,* which involved the study of more than 1,600 patients with arthritis of the knee.[27] The researchers concluded that the supplements appear to relieve knee pain associated with moderate-to-severe arthritis, but don't help with pain associated with milder forms of arthritis.

Caution: If you take chondroitin and glucosamine—or any other supplement, for that matter—be sure to inform your physician so that he or she can be alerted to possible interactions with other drugs or to possible allergic reactions. At least one study has indicated that exacerbation of an asthma condition may have resulted from these supplements.[28] Also, some of the glucosamine-chondroitin supplement labeling uses boldface to indicate that the bottle contains shellfish shells, including those of shrimp—a warning that those with shellfish allergies should be aware of.

Recommended daily dosage: 1,500 mg of glucosamine (HCI) and 1,200 mg of chondroitin sulfate. Bromelain may be included in the amount of 100 mg.

% Daily Value: not established

IRON (IRON CARBONYL)

Iron plays an integral role in the formation of hemoglobin, the substance that helps red blood cells transport oxygen from the lungs to the rest of the body, and is especially important for women in their childbearing years, children, young adults, and athletes who exercise at a high intensity for longer periods of time. Those in these high-risk categories are often deficient in iron and should make a special effort to include in their diets foods like red meats that are high in iron and to consider the inclusion of iron supplements.

Recommended daily dosage (for those in high-risk categories): 18 mg

% Daily Value: 100

Functional Food Supplements

"Functional foods" are those that have been designed and manufactured from certain nutrients that have been shown to have significant health benefits—but that aren't available through normal agricultural channels. Those with the most solid scientific authority behind them tend to be the ones that lower cholesterol or otherwise balance blood lipids.

BENECOL

This margarine-like spread contains plant stanols derived from the tall oil wood pulp of pine trees. Studies have shown that plant stanols, or phytostanols, can dramatically lower total cholesterol and "bad" LDL cholesterol through a mechanism that involves blocking the return of cholesterol to the bloodstream through the intestinal walls.[29]

In a landmark Finnish study, those who took the stanols daily experienced an average reduction in the total cholesterol of 10.2 percent, and a

14.1 percent decrease in their LDL cholesterol. Also, taking more of the stanols (2.6 grams versus 1.8 grams daily) resulted in a greater reduction.

The stanols can also be obtained in softgel form at www.benecol.com.

TAKE CONTROL

This cholesterol-lowering spread contains plant sterols, or phytosterols, which are derived from soybeans. Studies have shown that Take Control is as effective as Benecol in lowering cholesterol through the blocking mechanism mentioned above.[30]

OTHER CHOLESTEROL-LOWERING FUNCTIONAL FOODS

It's also possible to make use of the sterol/stanol mechanism by purchasing such products as Heart Wise Orange Juice (8 ounces contains 120 calories and 1 gram of phytosterols). Another possibility is Cocoa Via, a crunch bar containing 80 to 90 calories and 100 mg of flavanols, plus 1.5 grams of phytosterols. Flavanols have been linked to improved cardiovascular health through the promotion of better platelet activity and a decrease in oxidation of "bad" LDL cholesterol.

Supplement Red Flags

For the most part, supplements won't harm you, and they may help you—significantly. But it's important to keep in mind certain danger areas involving some supplements.

First, it's always possible to get too much of a good thing. For example, you may feel that because you're a woman of childbearing age, you really need a lot of iron. So you proceed to overdose on the iron, far above the amounts indicated in this book or any other responsible source of recommendations. Such excessive intake can result in iron poisoning or other side effects.

The same thing can happen with zinc, for example, if you take too much in an effort to ward off the onset of a cold. Among other things, too much zinc has been linked to a suppression of the immune response. The main lesson in all this is that if you and your physician decide that a particular supplement may be right for you, go ahead and take it—but *stick to the recommended dosages.*

Another concern is that because each human body responds differently to medications, it's important to know what your particular physical vulnerabilities are—and to avoid supplements that may put you in danger. For example, if you frequently get nosebleeds, bleeding ulcers, or other bleeding conditions, you should avoid aspirin. In any event, you should take it only with the approval of your physician.

Still another red flag is grapefruit. If you are currently on prescription medications, including drugs to control high blood pressure, you should avoid this fruit because it enhances the effect of certain drugs. That is, you may be taking a 20 mg dose of a particular drug, but the grapefruit can cause that drug to enter your system more quickly and have a more powerful effect on your body than would be the case if you weren't consuming grapefruit.

Excessive amounts of vitamin A can also be toxic (that's why we recommend beta-carotene, which, as a precursor of vitamin A, is more subject to your internal bodily regulations). But as indicated above, even beta-carotene has been identified as possibly dangerous for smokers—so keep this risk in mind if you smoke.

Other supplements in doses beyond what we recommend may actually have a kind of "backfire effect," by putting you at higher risk for the very health conditions you hope they will prevent. For example, excessive doses of vitamin E (far beyond the daily 400 IU amounts we recommend) have been linked to an increased risk for cardiovascular disease. Yet ironically, cardiovascular disease is one of the main health challenges that lower doses of vitamin E may help prevent.

In addition, the purity of supplements is always an issue because their manufacture isn't regulated in the same way that regular medications are. To help protect yourself against impure products—or products that claim to be giving you a stated amount of a particular vitamin, mineral, or other nutrient when they're really delivering something else—you might look for a *direct guarantee of purity and potency on the label*. Such a claim, if intentionally untrue, could get a manufacturer into big trouble.

Finally, you should be aware of the potentially harmful effects of combining or overdosing on over-the-counter painkillers. Aspirin, ibuprofen (Motrin, Advil), and acetaminophen (Tylenol) usually remain safe and effective when used as directed, but many patients may take more than the recommended doses or mistake a package offering an "extra" dosage for a regular dosage.[31]

For example, overdoses of acetaminophen can cause serious liver damage and even death. Aspirin, ibuprofen, and other nonsteroidal anti-inflammatory drugs (NSAIDs) can increase the risk of gastrointestinal bleeding, kidney injury, and various other gastrointestinal problems, such as diarrhea and nausea, even when the correct dose is taken. These risks have also been linked to thousands of deaths each year. The FDA is now placing warnings on these drugs, advising against combining them. So always read the labels and follow the recommended dosages.

Ken on the Supplement Industry and Research

To understand supplements and make wise choices among the many products, it's important to know a few things about both the industry and the research.

I know, for instance, that many people believe the supplementation industry is not regulated. But actually, that's not true. The multibillion-dollar-per-year industry is very well regulated through a law known as D.S.H.E.A., the Dietary Supplement Health and Education Act of 1994.

Still, there's a problem: the Food and Drug Administration (FDA) has limited resources to enforce the regulations. Manufacturers are expected to "do the right thing," such as meet label claims or properly represent potential benefits. For the most part, they do abide by the rules, though occasionally a manufacturer will attempt to cut corners.

My biggest complaint about the supplement industry is that manufacturers are not required to do any research on their own products. Because good, solid scientific investigation takes time and significant resources, there seems to be a heavy reliance on what I refer to as "borrowed" or "stolen" science—i.e., research conducted by other organizations on a particular nutrient or nutrient combination, which is then applied by nonresearching companies to their own products.

This disconnect between research and specific products is the primary reason we started the Cooper Complete line of nutritional supplements in 1998 (www.coopercomplete.com). We wanted to provide products that were guaranteed pure and potent, and also to subject them to rigid scientific investigation. Believe it or not, linking research to a specific product is a rare phenomenon in the supplement industry.

Over the years, we have developed our own internal models and protocols, which we hope will eventually become the industry standard. Working with a team of consultants from four leading universities, we rely on the latest scientific research to help formulate products. We also subject the products we study to ongoing double-blind, placebo-controlled clinical trials. All of our formulations are "dynamic"—a term that means if we learn something that indicates we can improve upon an existing formulation, then we make this change immediately.

Published research involving our original Cooper Complete multivitamin and mineral product (four tablets taken twice daily) is an example of the strong position we and others have taken in support of proper supplementation. Specifically, the researchers found that the supplements are well absorbed and substantially lower homocysteine (–17 percent), LDL-cholesterol oxidation (–14 percent), and C-reactive protein (–32 percent). These results, which are available through links

(continued)

on our Web site, have been reported in the *American Journal of Medicine* (December 2003) and in the *Journal of the American College of Nutrition* (November 2003). New research on our Cooper Complete Basic One product, taken with the Advanced Omega-3 essential fatty acid supplement, has been shown to lower homocysteine, triglycerides, and C-reactive protein. Those results have been submitted for publication as this book goes to press.

Designing Your Personal Supplement Program

It would be nice if we could give you a list of essential supplements, then a second-tier list of recommended but nonessential supplements, and so on. But unfortunately, that isn't possible, since each person has different nutritional health needs and weaknesses. That's the main reason that we recommend—and produce—multiple vitamin and mineral products that include the variety of nutrients listed earlier in the overview charts on pages 239 to 241 of this chapter.

For more specific use of supplements, you and your physician will have to do an evaluation of your current risk profile and then choose the supplements that may help lower your risk. Here's an illustration relating to cardiovascular disease:

A Heart Protection Strategy: If you know you are at relatively high risk for cardiovascular disease, such as heart attacks or strokes, you will want to put the following three groups of supplements at the top of your list. It's actually possible to obtain all of these supplementation groups in as few as four tablets daily.

HEART PROTECTION, GROUP I (1 TABLET DAILY)

Supplement Facts

The daily dosage (can be included in 1 tablet) provides:

Ingredients	Daily Amount	% Daily Value
Vitamin A (mixed carotenes)	2,000 IU	40
Vitamin C (ascorbic acid)	150 mg	250
Vitamin D (cholecalciferol)	1,000 IU	250
Vitamin E (d-alpha tocopherol succinate)	200 IU	666
Thiamine (vitamin B_1 as HCl)	1.5 mg	100
Riboflavin (vitamin B_2)	2 mg	118
Niacinamide (vitamin B_3)	20 mg	100
Pyridoxine (vitamin B_6)	10 mg	500
Folic Acid	400 mcg	100
Cyanocobalamin (vitamin B_{12})	400 mcg	6,666
Pantothenic Acid (vitamin B_5 as d-calcium pantothenate)	10 mg	100
Magnesium (oxide)	200 mg	50
Zinc (oxide)	15 mg	100
Selenium (rice bran chelate)	100 mcg	143
Chromium (chromium amino acid chelate)	100 mcg	83
Lycopene	5 mg	*

*Percent Daily Value not established.

HEART PROTECTION, GROUP II (2 TABLETS DAILY)

A daily dosage of 2 softgels provides:

Ingredients	Daily Amount	% Daily Value
Omega-3 (EPA/DHA) Fish Oil (providing 760 mg of EPA and 440 mg of DHA)	2,000 mg	*
Vitamin E (d-alpha tocopherol succinate)	6 IU	20

Other ingredients:
Gelatin, glycerin, and water

*Percent Daily Value not established

HEART PROTECTION, GROUP III: (1 TABLET DAILY)

Supplement Facts
A daily dosage of 1 fast-melt tablet provides:

Ingredients	Daily Amount	% Daily Value
Coenzyme Q_{10} (ubiquinone)	60 mg	*

This product contains *no* yeast, wheat gluten, soy protein, milk/dairy, corn, sodium, sugar, starch, artificial coloring, preservatives, or flavoring.

*Percent Daily Value not established.

In addition, for heart protection you should consider taking:

- Low doses of aspirin daily (81–161 mg)
- Benecol or Take Control as an alternative to regular margarine or other spreads

Of course, heart protection is only one possibility for a supplement strategy. If you're mostly concerned about bone thinning, for instance, or you feel you're at risk for osteoporosis (everyone over fifty should put himself or herself in this category), you'll want to look closely at your calcium intake, along with vitamin D and magnesium. Or if you feel you are at particular risk for prostate cancer, you should focus on such supplements as lycopene and selenium. Still other combinations of supplements would be appropriate for those at risk for macular degeneration, various cancers, diabetes, or other health conditions.

Finally, keep in mind that *there is no certain outcome* with supplements, no matter how pure or accurate the labeling is. Much of the research in this area is still in progress, and sometimes a new study will seem to contradict older studies. With supplements, we're basically introducing you to a game of odds—a life-or-death game that *may* improve your chances of avoiding a particular health condition.

The basic rule is to be sure that you play the game wisely. In other words, *don't* overdose; *don't* follow a particular regimen without consulting with your physician; and *do* examine closely with your physician possible interactions between your supplements and other medications. So long as you use your head, why not play the game? After all, in the end a supplement or group of supplements may actually help save your life.

Eleven

■ Start-up #5—Do
■ Serious Smoke Control

"Don" was a regular cigarette smoker, a pack-a-day man for years. His philosophy of life went like this: "Okay, so I'll die five years earlier. But that's okay with me because I'll enjoy smoking until I go."

Unfortunately, Don's experience didn't proceed as he expected. He suffered a heart attack in his midfifties and had to undergo a bypass operation. He survived, but that wasn't the end of his problems. A few years later, he developed emphysema as a direct result of his life of smoking. Soon, he was carrying around an oxygen tank just so he could breathe.

Don died twelve years after his heart attack and seven years after he was diagnosed with emphysema. He was clearly a person who had made some very bad health choices that prevented him from finishing strong. Or to use an image we employed in an earlier chapter, he failed to "square off the curve" of his life.

Another potential tragedy of Don's decision about smoking is that he exposed his family members to a sidestream of smoke for decades. The health results of that exposure have yet to be determined. But given the flood of recent research showing the dangers of secondhand smoke, the chances are that Don's habit could negatively impact the health of one or more of his loved ones well into the future.

The lesson we can take away from Don's experience is twofold:

First, you can never plan your life's "end game": you can't assume that you can control your health risks so as to arrange a quick, clean, somewhat earlier end to your life. There is absolutely no way to know for certain whether you'll die quickly or be relegated to years of suffering and debilitation before your end finally arrives. This fallacious way of thinking, which is common among smokers, has also infected the thinking about various health issues and may affect many others in addition to the person who has chosen to act foolishly—as the account in the accompanying box suggests.

Ken on the Folly of Taking Silly Health Risks

You can never assume that you can take an unnecessary health risk and somehow predict how that risk will play out.

For example, as I was delivering a lecture on preventive medicine at U.C.L.A. a few years ago, I mentioned at one point the importance of always wearing a helmet when riding a bicycle or motorcycle. Yet during the question-and-answer session, an irate student accused me of infringing on his rights.

"If I don't want to wear a helmet—and I'm thrown off my motorbike, land on the curb, and get killed—that's my right, not yours! You don't have any right to infringe upon my rights!" he declared.

"Son, I've been practicing medicine for thirty years," I replied, "and far too many times I've seen young people fail to wear a helmet and get into an accident—but then they *aren't* killed. They are knocked unconscious and end up in a coma for months or years. They go through their health insurance and savings and end up as wards of the state.

(continued)

> "If they do finally regain consciousness, brain damage may impair their ability to function. In other words, their indifference to danger and their poorly chosen risk not only rob them of their health but end up costing taxpayers a fortune. So, in such a case, your rights infringe upon my rights—and I have a duty, a responsibility as a citizen, to speak out against your bad choices."
>
> Of course, this argument could be made against those who fail to take any other preventive measure to protect their health—including those who smoke.

Second, whether or not you smoke, you should become acutely aware of certain "marching orders" about the habit—and the impact it may have on you and on others.

Your Marching Orders

There are two simple imperatives you should keep in mind about smoking:

- Don't do it.
- Stay away from those who do.

You shouldn't smoke yourself because of the many health problems associated with the practice: according to one recent study, smokers can expect to live ten fewer years than nonsmokers.[1] Also, even if you don't smoke, you should avoid smokers—because other studies have shown that secondhand smoke, or the smoky atmosphere created by smokers, can be as deadly as smoking itself.

Unfortunately, these two marching orders are easier said than done. Those who smoke know how addictive the habit is, and how hard it is to stop. And the tobacco industry isn't making things any easier. A recent report by the Massachusetts Department of Public Health revealed that from 1998 through 2004, even as public health campaigns to counter smoking were accelerating, the manufacturers increased the amount of addictive nicotine in products sold to the average smoker by 10 percent.[2] Furthermore, the nicotine increase occurred without regard to tobacco brand.

Exacerbating this nicotine-addition problem are the aggressive strategies of the tobacco companies. Despite lawsuits brought against them, they continue to lure smokers into their web through special promotions, such as dollar-off coupons and multipack discounts.[3] Young adults tend to be the most likely to use the coupons, according to research published in the *American Journal of Preventive Medicine*.

The second main problem we face is secondhand smoke. Those who live, work, or socialize with smokers know how uncomfortable, if not impossible, it can be to avoid their smoke and still maintain a relationship. But don't despair. There are a number of ways you can deal with this issue. A good first step is to confront your in-house smoker directly about the horrendous dangers of smoking—not just on the smoker himself but on the people around him whom he respects and loves.

A Guide to Guilt Therapy

For decades, we've known that smoking will kill. Sometimes, that news has been conveyed in widely disseminated but highly personal accounts. For example, most Americans have heard through one medium or another how lung cancer has taken the lives of high-profile cigarette smokers, such as the news anchor Peter Jennings and, much earlier, the legendary journalist Edward R. Murrow.

One of the most shocking victims in recent years was forty-four-year-old Dana Reeve, widow of *Superman* star Christopher Reeve and mother of a teenage son. Her death in March 2006 shook the public primarily because, even though she was a nonsmoker, she died of lung cancer.

Speculation has centered on the possibility that her death resulted from her exposure to passive smoke in nightclubs where she had once performed. In fact, an estimated 10 to 15 percent of lung cancer victims are nonsmokers, and most of those are women.[4]

There has also been no lack of public warning on the topic. During the past thirty years at the Cooper Clinic, for instance, we have included smoking in our various publications and lectures as a major risk factor for cardiovascular disease. Also, we've highlighted the habit as one of the four major causes of aging, along with obesity, sedentary living, and stress.

And of course, the federal government has hammered away at the danger for decades. Most Americans are aware that the U.S. Surgeon General years ago began to require cigarette manufacturers to include a prominent warning on packages about the hazards of smoking to your health. Even more dramatic, the 1982 Surgeon General's report stated: "Cigarette smoking is the major single cause of cancer mortality in the United States." The American Cancer Society has affirmed this statement as being just as true today as it was more than twenty years ago.[5]

Such warnings seem to have had some positive impact. Smoking among teenagers, for example, has decreased significantly after peaking in 1997. In that year, 38 percent of high school seniors smoked. The percentage has steadily declined back to the range of about 29 to 30 percent, the percentage that prevailed up to the early 1990s.[6]

But such numbers among teenagers are still far too high, especially among young women, and they bode ill for the future because of the difficulty of breaking the powerful nicotine habit. Smoking also continues among about 50 million American adults, with slightly more men than women trapped in the habit. The high incidence of smoking has been consistently linked to a high percentage of the 150,000 deaths a year from lung cancer.

And of course, in addition to lung cancer, hundreds of thousands die from smoking-related heart disease, stroke, and a variety of other lethal conditions. The American Heart Association warned in a response to a World Health Organization Report that by the year 2020, assuming preventive efforts fail, there will be nine million deaths caused by tobacco, compared to nearly five million in 2002.[7]

Because the general warnings have gone unheeded by many people—and because ordinary news reports, no matter how horrendous or touching, often fail to register—we would offer this modest suggestion: *As a powerful medicine to counter the smoking epidemic, smokers should be force-fed a major dose of guilt about what they are doing not just to themselves, but also to their families and loved ones.*

As an initial step in administering this "guilt-therapy" antidote, we would urge you to think hard about the following heartbreaking findings. Feel free to use this scientific research as a kind of "guilt list" to motivate yourself—especially if you are a smoker yourself, or if you are in a family or work environment where smoking is still prevalent and you can have some influence in changing the situation. You might also try laying the list out on the side table where the smoker in your family can see it.

The Smoking Guilt List

- *Cancer of the pancreas:* Smoking has been linked to highly lethal pancreatic cancer, especially in younger people.[8]
- *Male impotence:* Smoking can increase the risk of impotence, especially in younger men.[9]

   In a study of more than 1,300 men, researchers from the Mayo Clinic found that those who smoked were at greater risk of erectile dysfunction (ED) than were either former smokers or nonsmokers. Smokers in their forties, who were the youngest group in the study, had the highest smoking-related risk. They were nearly three times as likely to have ED as the other study participants.
- *Age-related macular degeneration (AMD):* Smoking doubles the risk of developing this degenerative eye disorder—the leading cause of blindness among the elderly—reported a British study of more than 4,000 patients.[10]

- *Anxiety disorders in children:* Cigarette smoking can increase the risk of anxiety disorders in children during late adolescence and early adulthood.[11]
- *Bad nutrition for teen girls:* A female teenager who smokes, or who is at risk to start smoking (e.g., by the example of a parent or influential peer), will likely lack the basic elements of a sound diet—including fruits, vegetables, and dairy products.[12]
- *Hearing loss:* Smokers—and nonsmokers who live with a smoker—have a higher risk of hearing loss than nonsmokers who are not exposed to environmental smoke.[13]
- *Pregnant women and ADD children:* If you smoke when pregnant, your child will have nearly triple the risk of being born with attention deficit disorder, according to a 2005 Danish study.[14] This condition is characterized by inattention, excessive muscular activity, and impulsive behavior.
- *Cardiovascular disease risk in children:* If one parent smokes in the presence of a child, that youngster will have up to a 50 percent higher risk for early signs of atherosclerosis, published in a 2002 Austrian study.[15] (Atherosclerosis is plaque buildup in arteries, associated with heart disease.)

The senior researcher noted that a compound in the blood caused by sidestream smoke "is a very potent blood vessel constrictor and may help create blood vessel spasm and set the stage for blood clot formation."

Furthermore, the Austrian investigators found that smoke from fewer than twenty cigarettes a day by one smoking parent would elevate the harmful compound by up to 50 percent in the children. Also, smoking additional cigarettes will increase the level of the deadly compound even more.

Finally, the study reported that smoking by the mother had a significantly more pronounced influence than that of the father. "We speculate that mothers may have closer contact with their children at home," the head researcher said.

How can this horrendous health impact on children be prevented? The researchers recommend the obvious: *Don't smoke when your children are present.*

• *Even short-term passive smoke damages arteries in young nonsmokers:* Short-term secondhand exposure to environmental tobacco smoke causes changes in the arteries that impede blood flow. The process encourages the development of artery disease even in young, healthy nonsmokers.[16]

In a 2002 Japanese study, the researchers examined the impact of a half hour of exposure to environmental tobacco smoke on twelve nonsmoking men, averaging thirty years of age. None of the men had a history of cardiovascular disease, high blood pressure, or diabetes. The researchers found that after the smoke exposure the men's arteries underwent changes that impeded blood flow and also that the blood levels of a compound associated with atherosclerosis increased significantly.

"These findings may add relevance to the idea that everyone should be protected from even short-term exposure to secondhand smoke," the lead researcher said.

• *Passive smoke promotes heart disease for the family:* Secondhand smoke can increase the heart attack risk for you, your children, and other family members by 45 percent.[17]

In this international Canadian study (the Interheart Study) published in the August 2006 issue of *Lancet,* the researchers determined that any form of tobacco exposure—smoking, passive smoking, or chewing—can increase the risk of cardiovascular disease by up to three times the normal rate. Those with the highest levels of passive exposure to smoke (twenty-two hours or more per week) showed an increased heart disease risk of 45 percent.

The researchers in the Interheart Study summed up their findings this way: "The overwhelming conclusion from this mass of data is [that] tobacco exposure—be it cigarettes, pipes, cigars, or smokeless; secondhand or primary; filtered or nonfiltered, even at low levels—causes a large proportion of heart attacks in men and women around the world."

Studying this "guilt list" yourself—or putting it under the nose of the smokers in your home—may at least spark the beginning of a change in smoking habits. And that may help move smokers beyond guilt to the knowledge that they are finally starting to protect their own health and the health of their loved ones.

What You Can Expect If You Stop

The first component of any effective stop-smoking program is to recognize that quitting has far-reaching health benefits.

For example, light smokers who quit can escape heart disease. In one study, those who smoke ten cigarettes a day or fewer showed no excess cardiovascular risk three to five years after they quit.[18] The message is clear: if you're not a heavy smoker, you have a great chance to allow your blood vessels to heal completely. But you have to quit *now*.

But what if you're a heavy smoker or a person who has smoked for many years, if not decades?

There is no question that the longer you smoke, the more you put yourself at risk. But you can still benefit from quitting, according to the *British Medical Journal*.[19] Specifically, smokers who stop between the ages of fifty and sixty and don't smoke again can eliminate much of their subsequent risk of developing lung cancer. Furthermore, even those who refrain from smoking for less than ten years can lower their risk of getting lung cancer by one-third—and the benefits multiply each year the individual continues to avoid smoking.

The U.S. Surgeon General has summed up the physiologic advantages of quitting this way:[20]

Twenty minutes after quitting, your blood pressure drops, and your hand and foot temperature increases to normal.

Eight hours after quitting, the carbon monoxide level in your blood returns to normal.

Twenty-four hours after quitting, your chance of a heart attack decreases. (Think of it—after only one day.)

Two weeks to three months after quitting, your circulation improves and lung functions increase by 30 percent.

One to nine months after quitting, coughing, sinus congestion, fatigue, and shortness of breath decrease. Physiologically, the cilia, or tiny hairlike structures that rid the lungs of mucus, resume normal functioning. This change enhances the ability of the lungs to clean themselves and reduces the possibility of infection.

One year after quitting, your risk of coronary heart disease is half that of a smoker's.

Even patients with existing heart disease benefit quickly from quitting. German researchers reported in 2004 that heart patients who quit during the first year after a coronary event experienced a 40 percent reduction in the risk of a secondary coronary event.[21] Also, in a 2001 Canadian study, people who had not smoked for two years or less experienced significantly lower rates of congestive heart failure than those who continued to smoke.[22]

Five to fifteen years after quitting, stroke risk is reduced to that of a nonsmoker.

Ten years after quitting, lung cancer death rate is about half that of a continuing smoker's. Also, there's a decrease in risk of cancer of the mouth, throat, esophagus, bladder, kidney, and pancreas.

Fifteen years after quitting, risk of coronary heart disease is the same as that of a nonsmoker.

What about nonsmokers who are removed from an environment full of passive smoke and their prospects for physical healing?

A telling study published by the *Journal of the American Medical As-*

sociation on October 11, 2006, revealed significant benefits for nonsmoking Scottish bar workers after Scotland prohibited smoking in confined public places on March 26, 2006. The researchers studied 105 nonasthmatic and asthmatic nonsmoking bar workers, of whom 77 completed the study. They were evaluated for respiratory symptoms, oxygen capacity, and other factors before and after the introduction of the smoking ban.

The researchers found, among other things, that the percentage of workers with respiratory and sensory symptoms decreased from 79.2 percent to 53.2 percent within one to two months after the ban; lung capacity and functioning improved after two months; asthmatics had less airway inflammation after one month; and quality-of-life scores on a standard medical questionnaire increased significantly.

The researchers concluded: "Smoke-free legislation was associated with significant early improvements in symptoms, spirometry measurements, and systemic inflammation of bar workers. Asthmatic bar workers also had reduced airway inflammation and improved quality of life."[23]

Clearly, then, there are horrendous dangers to you, your children, and other members of your family if you smoke or anyone in the household smokes. Furthermore, there are tremendous health benefits—all solidly established by scientific research—if you quit smoking. But how can you make the leap from these incontrovertible facts to a practical smoke control strategy?

Toward an Effective Smoke Control Strategy

Because nicotine is a powerful, physically addictive drug, it won't be easy to quit smoking—or to convince your spouse or other loved one to stop. But people break the habit every day, and you and your family members can do the same. Here are a few tactics that have worked for others—and that you may find helpful.

TACTIC #1: USE MEDICAL AIDS.

Modern medicine is increasingly devising powerful responses to the smoking problem—beginning with the basic annual physical exam.

As part of a complete physical, every smoker should undergo regular CT scans, such as the ones described in Chapter 5. This scan, which can identify lung cancer lesions as small as a grain of rice, is far superior to the X-ray, which may not detect such cancer until it's the size of an orange. A reported 80 percent of lung cancers are caught in the earliest stages when the CT scan is used.[24] Just undergoing one of the scans, along with a complete gold-standard preventive-medicine physical, will often be enough to motivate the smoker to quit.

Many effective medical treatments are also available to overcome the smoking habit. These include nicotine replacement therapy and related treatments. Specifically, physicians may prescribe sustained-release bupropion (Zyban or Wellbutrin), the nicotine patch, nicotine gum, the nicotine inhaler, and the nicotine nasal spray.[25] The FDA has approved all these methods as appropriate for smoking cessation.

It's also possible that some of the physiologic effects of smoking can be reversed by new treatments that are emerging on the medical scene. For example, studies published by the American Heart Association in 2003 indicated that allipurinol, a drug used to treat gout—when combined with vitamin C and taurine, an amino acid in fish—can reverse abnormal blood vessel response caused by cigarette smoking.[26]

Another study, conducted at the M.D. Anderson Cancer Center in Houston, indicated that a form of vitamin A—9-dcis-retinoic acid—may help reverse some of the lung damage caused by cigarette smoking. The study involved more than two hundred former smokers who had smoked at least two packs of cigarettes a day for at least twenty years. The form of vitamin A used produced improvement in the condition of cellular proteins associated with lung cancer.[27]

Even though some of these studies are quite preliminary and clinical applications may not be available in your area, still be sure to consult with your physician about your taking advantage of them.

TACTIC #2: CREATE A SMOKE-FREE ENVIRONMENT FOR YOUR FAMILY.

In light of the clear evidence we've cited so far about the dangers of passive smoking, you should have plenty of ammunition to protect the nonsmokers in your home—and especially your children.

First, you should make it clear to friends and others who visit that you have created a nonsmoking environment in your home—and any smoking is completely off-limits. If a visitor simply must take a puff, he or she should be asked to do so outside your home. This may mean directing them to the hallway if you live in an apartment (assuming management allows smoking there) or to an unoccupied patio or part of the yard if you live in a single-family home.

Most smokers quickly get the message and don't push the subject. But those who are more aggressive may ask after a meal, or while sitting around the living room, if you mind if they light up.

Your answer should be, "I'd rather you didn't." Then, direct the person to the area where the smoke won't affect you, your family, or other guests. This sort of strictly enforced household smoke control is the only way you'll protect your home from the health threat of smoking by outsiders.

Of course, if your spouse or another loved one smokes—and resists being put outside to pursue the habit—that presents more of a problem. One approach might be to have a heart-to-heart with that individual and, if you get an argument on the grounds that "it's not really hurting anybody," show the person your "guilt list," with those clearly cited and footnoted scientific studies.

To check the actual effect of secondhand smoke, you might consider taking advantage of certain medical detection devices that are becoming available. One of these involves a test kit called TobacAlert, which can detect in human urine as little as an hour's worth of tobacco smoke to which an individual has been exposed in the previous three days.[28]

This device was used by a woman with asthma to detect passive smoke exposure, which she believed came from nicotine residue in her husband's car. Her husband was a regular smoker but smoked outside her presence. The results of the test gave the couple a starting point to discuss other measures to protect her from nicotine.

TACTIC #3: FIND A WAY TO EXERT YOUR WILLPOWER.

If you're a smoker, you should face the facts about your prospects of quitting on your own. According to medical studies, only 5 percent of smokers who try to go "cold turkey" without any assistance actually succeed.[29]

On the other hand, if you seek help from a medical professional who intervenes properly to help you—and to reinforce your willpower—your chances for success will rise to 15 to 25 percent. Interventions that such professionals should use include asking about your tobacco use; advising you to quit; assessing your willingness to make an attempt to stop; assisting you in stopping, such as by referring you to counseling or drug therapy; and following up to see how you're doing.

Another possibility to bolster your willpower is to begin your anti-smoking effort with a piecemeal, rather than an all-or-nothing, approach. If you just feel you can't go cold turkey and you want to ease out of the habit, it may be possible to begin your program by cutting down on the number of cigarettes you're smoking each day. In fact, a 2005 Danish study published in the *Journal of the American Medical Association* showed that among individuals who smoke fifteen or more cigarettes per day, cutting those cigarettes by 50 percent per day can greatly reduce the risk of lung cancer.[30]

On the other hand, it's important to remember that even this type of limited smoking carries a much higher risk of heart disease and other health problems than not smoking at all. Some studies have actually shown that smoking only one cigarette per day can have harmful effects. British researchers, for instance, determined that each cigarette you smoke will cost you on average eleven minutes of your life.[31] And by the way, if you work or socialize in a smoke-filled office, home, or club—and are a nonsmoker yourself—you are in effect smoking one to two cigarettes per day.

So the "50 percent tactic"—cutting your cigarette usage in half each day—should be recognized for what it is: perhaps a helpful first step, but not your final goal. The only way to get rid of the danger of smoking for you and your loved ones is to quit entirely.

You'll probably do an even better job of shoring up your willpower if you utilize the next tactic—enlisting the aid of a support group—as part of your program.

TACTIC #4: CONNECT WITH A SUPPORT GROUP.

Any support group that focuses on encouraging its members to stay off tobacco permanently will greatly enhance your chances for success. Phone counseling can also increase your chances of stopping.

In a 2002 study published in the *New England Journal of Medicine*, researchers focused on the effectiveness of the California Smokers' Helpline, one of thirty-three state-financed telephone counseling programs. Of those participants who used the phone service, 21 percent remained smoke-free, as compared with 10 percent of those who relied on a self-help, stop-smoking kit they were given.[32] Those receiving phone counseling got calls an average of three times over a period of one to two months from trained counselors who helped them set up a plan to quit smoking.

The American Cancer Society manages a number of the state phone lines for smokers and provides information at 1-800-227-2345. Typical assistance from those who man the phones includes personal counseling and information on nicotine replacement therapy, such as the nicotine patch or nicotine chewing gum.

TACTIC #5: EXERCISE.

Exercise operates as a powerful adjunct to other programs designed to improve health. These include weight-loss programs, stress-reduction programs—and smoking cessation.

We have seen tremendous results from those who enter our wellness program as smokers. They often emerge on the other side as militant nonsmokers, committed to abstinence because they have been educated about the dangers of all forms of tobacco use.

The experience of "Mark" is typical. A one-pack-a-day man, he began his health evaluation with our complete preventive-medicine exam. During that checkup, his physician related to him the dire, dangerous realities of smoking. At first, Mark wasn't convinced because he had heard a lot of these warnings in the past. A couple of friends had been nagging him for years.

But when he launched a regular aerobic exercise program, a strange thing happened: he was struck by the utter inconsistency of spending time walking and jogging to increase his lung power yet at the same undercutting his efforts with smoking. The very idea of polluting his positive exercise experience with tobacco smoke seemed repulsive. Also, with the scientific information he had absorbed from his physician and from trainers at the gym, he began to understand for the first time in his life that it would be impossible for him to continue to smoke and at the same time improve his maximum aerobic conditioning—measured by the ability of his lungs and heart to process oxygen during a stress test. All these thoughts and concerns culminated inside him to the point that one day, toward the end of the first month of his exercise program, he just quit—and never looked back.

One scientific study after another reinforces this link between exercise and smoking cessation. For example, one Brown University investigation[33] explored the impact of exercise on a group of sedentary female smokers, who averaged forty years of age. One subgroup of these women remained sedentary but received health education, and another subgroup engaged in intensive exercise three times a week. Their abstinence from smoking was confirmed by saliva nicotine tests.

The researchers found that exercisers succeeded in stopping their smoking more successfully than did the sedentary women. Specifically, 16 percent of the exercisers were still off cigarettes at three months, and 12 percent remained smoke-free after twelve months. In contrast, only 8 percent of the nonexercisers had stopped after three months, and just 5 percent were smoke-free after twelve months.

TACTIC #6: KEEP ADDING TO YOUR "GUILT LIST."

Obviously, the scientific studies we have provided you in this chapter are a kind of snapshot of our current medical understanding. New studies continue to appear—and you should add them to your guilt list to shore up the evidence against smoking.

Some people won't be convinced by such facts, and by themselves, a list of studies, no matter how impressive, usually won't change behavior. But as another strong piece of evidence, these studies contribute to a comprehensive understanding of what stopping can do for you and your family—and to the motivation that's needed to make the needed changes.

TACTIC #7: DECLARE WAR ON THE TOBACCO MANUFACTURERS.

The companies that produce all forms of tobacco—cigarettes, chewing tobacco, cigars, you name it—are enemies of you and your family. There is no other conclusion a reasonable person can reach.

These manufacturers and marketers are doing everything in their power to cause you and your children to become addicted to nicotine. They offer your kids discount coupons and try to titillate them with advertising. They play on the vulnerabilities of your children, on their lack of self-confidence, and on their desire to conform to a group. These companies are out to destroy the health of your family for the sake of earning a buck—so feel free to get angry at them. But direct your anger into productive channels.

For example, don't invest in these companies. Put your broker and your friends on notice that you're now on a soapbox to fight big tobacco financially—and you'd like them to join you.

Also, whenever you have the opportunity, support government action that restricts or eliminates the places or opportunities for tobacco use. Give the tobacco industry no quarter. Vote for measures that would prohibit smoking in public places. Work to make your state a smoke-free one. Support efforts to fund state tobacco-control programs with settlements from lawsuits against tobacco companies.[34]

Also, get behind government-funded multimedia campaigns—paid for with increased excise taxes on cigarettes—to influence young people not to smoke. (The majority of people who smoke begin the habit before they reach age eighteen.) In a 2004 report in the *American Journal of Preventive Medicine*, researchers determined that through such campaigns, funded by a one-dollar increase in the price of a pack of cigarettes, smoking prevalence could be reduced by 26 percent. Also, the campaign would result in an annual savings of 108,466 lives and 1.6 million lost years of lives attributed to smoking.[35] In fact, as of January 1, 2007, a one-dollar tax on a pack of cigarettes became mandatory in Texas.

A corollary of the above point is to *vote for an increase in excise taxes on cigarettes!* Currently, the worst state offenders—the ones with some of the lowest excise tax rates on cigarettes—are Kentucky (state rank number fifty, at 3 cents a pack), and Florida (number forty-one, at 33.9 cents).

The states with the highest excise tax rates include New Jersey (number one, at $2.05 a pack); Massachusetts and Connecticut (tied at number three, at $1.51); New York (number five, at $1.50); and Hawaii (number seven, at $1.30).

Putting an extra tax burden on tobacco will accomplish at least three purposes. First, the added cost will make it harder for the industry to profit from its lethal products. And second, the tax can force the industry to pay for programs designed to bring about its demise.

Third, if you aren't an activist and don't see your way to becoming one, you can still have perhaps the greatest impact of all on the tobacco industry. If you smoke, use the most devastating weapon at your disposal: stop smoking. And then encourage your fellow workers and family members to join you. A grassroots movement, which consists of citizens who know the sordid facts about smoking and are willing to act personally on them, can be the most powerful force of all in stopping the tobacco manufacturers and marketers in their tracks.

Twelve

■ Start-up #6—
■ Counteract Substance
Surprises

Certain common substances that we consume or drink can blindside us—for a number of reasons.

For one thing, we may discover that a substance like alcohol, caffeine, or an over-the-counter drug has a more deleterious impact on us personally than it's supposed to have on the population at large. Or we may not take care to regulate our intake of certain substances and end up taking more than is good for us. When such "substance surprises" occur, they can put us on a sure path to finishing *weak,* rather than finishing *strong.*

The problem often begins with what might be called a "creep effect" produced by powerful stimulants or relaxants. For example, you may seem to be operating quite well on low doses of a substance that may be perfectly legal. In fact, the substance may have received some scientific kudos—as has been the case with alcohol, coffee, and various prescription drugs. But a common human temptation is to try too much of a good thing.

Four substances that raise many questions among our patients—and that may unexpectedly pose serious health issues—are alcohol, prescription and over-the-counter drugs, performance enhancers, and caffeine.*

The Mixed Alcohol Message

Despite some of the positive things about alcohol that have been uncovered by recent research, we typically tell our patients, "If you don't drink, don't start." The reason is, there are just too many dangers associated with drinking to justify starting the practice to garner certain health benefits—benefits that are available through other channels and don't carry the dangers.

On the other hand, if patients do drink in moderation—and shows no signs of abuse or alcoholism—we don't tell them to quit, but we do advise them to be careful. Always monitor your drinking, and *never* exceed the *safe* amounts that the scientific studies have shown can produce benefits without dangers to health.

One of the greatest pitfalls with drinking alcohol is what we have called the "creep effect." In other words, it's quite easy to start off with one drink of wine during an evening meal. But then many people we know are inclined over time to add an extra half glass and then another half glass. That process moves them to consuming two drinks at one sitting, a practice that introduces too many calories, increases the danger of temporary mental and physical impairment, and may threaten good health.

Another common scenario is for a person to have a drink with hors d'oeuvres before the meal—say, a glass of wine, a beer, or a mixed drink. Then, he or she may indulge in *another* predinner drink and *also* have a glass of wine or two with the meal. Obviously, with this approach, the

---

*Problems involving serious addiction to drugs, alcohol, and other substances require medical or other special interventions, which lie beyond the scope of this book. If you feel you or someone close to you has such an addiction problem, you should seek medical treatment and counseling.

drinks can really begin to add up (the four drinks indicated in this case are far above the recommended daily amount—see below).

So what are the healthiest, safest amounts? The current scientific findings suggest guidelines, which differ for men and women.

For Men: Research indicates that the optimum range for a man's protection against all types of death is about one to six drinks *per week*. But under no circumstances should a man who wants maximum health benefits drink two or more drinks *per day*.

Note: One alcoholic drink is often defined as containing 12 to 15 grams (about half an ounce) of ethanol. One drink would then translate into approximately one 4-ounce glass of table wine, one half-pint of beer, or one mixed drink containing no more than one-half to one ounce of 80-proof spirits.

A landmark 1997 study[1] reported that the risk of death from all causes, including heart disease and cancer, was 28 percent lower among men who had two to four drinks per week, in comparison with men who drank less than one drink per week. Also, the risk was 21 percent lower for men who had five to six drinks per week. But you can see from these figures that the benefits go down as you drink more. In fact, for men who had two or more drinks per day, the risk of death went *up by 51 percent*.

A more recent, 2006 study in the *British Medical Journal* found that for heart disease, the risk decreased as the amount of alcohol consumed per week increased.[2] One drink a week resulted in a 7 percent lower risk of heart disease; two to four drinks per week, in a 22 percent lower risk; and five to six drinks per week, in a 29 percent decrease. Also, those who had a drink every day enjoyed a 41 percent lower risk of heart disease than did those who abstained completely.

For unknown reasons, moderate drinking may also provide protection against other diseases, such as diabetes. A March 2005 report in *Diabetes Care* showed that those who indulged in moderate consumption of about one alcoholic drink per day reduced their risk of developing adult-onset (type 2) diabetes by about 30 percent in comparison with nondrinkers. But the risk of diabetes for heavier drinkers increased back to the level for nondrinkers. So again, a clear pattern emerges: if you're a light or moderate drinker, you may experience health benefits. But if you're a three-drinks-per-day consumer, you'll lose all the benefits—and put yourself at greater risk.

Why should drinking result in any health benefits at all?

Scientists have speculated that the benefits of light to moderate drinking may arise from a tendency of alcohol to work against the development of blood clots. Or alcohol may inhibit the tendency of high levels of "bad" LDL cholesterol to contribute to plaque buildup in the arteries.[3] Also, alcohol has been associated with an increase in the levels of "good" HDL cholesterol. But at this point, the explanations that have been offered remain speculative.

For Women: The healthy drinking limit should be no more than one to three drinks *per week.*

In the above *British Medical Journal* study, for instance, women who had one drink per week lowered their risk of heart disease by 36 percent. In other words, women appear to get their maximum protection with up to three drinks per week, but then the protective effect levels off.

There's also some evidence that moderate drinking in women may afford some protection against the risk of cognitive decline that occurs with aging.[4] But an editorial in the *New England Journal of Medicine* offered a word of caution:

> Low-to-moderate alcohol consumption has previously been linked to several positive health outcomes, most convincingly to a decreased risk of coronary heart disease, but alcohol abuse is also linked to a wide range of health and social problems according to both common knowledge and formal study.[5]

This warning can't be overemphasized. Aside from drunk-driving tragedies and other accidents, drinking above the two-drink-per-day limit will threaten the health of both men and women in so many ways that it's hard to list them all.[6] The most common alcohol-related health problem that comes to mind is cirrhosis of the liver. But another, little-known danger was highlighted in a 2004 report by Boston University School of Medicine researchers. They found that people who consumed more than about three drinks per day increased their risk of developing atrial fibrillation (serious heartbeat irregularities) by 34 percent.[7]

In another line of investigations, researchers with the Harvard Nurses' Study have found that consuming more than five drinks per week is associated with a 26 percent increase in breast cancer—unless women consume at least 400 mcg of folic acid per day.*

The Centers for Disease Control and Prevention warned in 2005 that nearly one in three Americans drinks too much, and reminded us that alcohol is the nation's third leading cause of death. In fact, excessive drinking kills 75,000 Americans each year through related injuries and diseases. Clearly, no amount of alcohol is "safe" unless 1) you can easily keep your consumption within medically prescribed limits, 2) you are in no way dependent on alcohol for relaxation or stress relief, and 3) you can quit at will for any length of time.

---

*S. M. Zhang; S. E. Hankinson; D. J. Hunter; E. L. Giovannucci; G. A. Colditz; W. C. Willett. 2005. "Folate Intake and Risk of Breast Cancer Characterized by Hormone Receptor Status." *Cancer Epidemiology, Biomarkers and Prevention*, 8: 2004–8.

Shumin M. Zhang; I-Min Lee; JoAnn E. Manson; Nancy R. Cook; Walter C. Willett; and Julie E. Buring. 2007. "Alcohol Consumption and Breast Cancer Risk in the Women's Health Study." *American Journal of Epidemiology*, 165: 667–676.

Stephanie A. Smith-Warner; Donna Spiegelman; Shiaw-Shyuan Yaun; Piet A. van den Brandt; Aaron R. Folsom; R. Alexandra Goldbohm; Saxon Graham; Lars Holmberg; Geoffrey R. Howe; James R. Marshall; Anthony B. Miller; John D. Potter; Frank E. Speizer; Walter C. Willett; Alicja Wolk; David J. Hunter. 1998. "Alcohol and Breast Cancer in Women: A Pooled Analysis of Cohort Studies." *Journal of the American Medical Association* 279: 535–540.

The "creep effect" associated with alcohol abuse is clearly a major danger that every drinker should understand and avoid. And this effect can become *at least* as dangerous, if not more so, with certain prescription or over-the-counter drugs.

The Creep Effect with Prescription and Over-the-counter Drugs

One of the most common forms of drug abuse starts off perfectly legally, but then gets out of hand. Here's a typical scenario:

As "Beth" moved into her fifties, she began to experience more aches and pains than she had when she was younger. In particular, her lower back would "go out" when she was feeling extra work or family stress. Also, she had developed arthritis in her knee and hands, with attendant pains that bothered her more some days than others.

Because Beth's over-the-counter medications didn't provide sufficient relief, her internist prescribed a strong painkiller, which he directed her to use only when she began to experience pain that interfered with her daily functioning. But like many patients, Beth gradually began to use the prescription drug more often than directed, such as when she was merely *anticipating* a back problem. Typically, this anticipation would occur just before a deadline at work or a big family event. Also, she was able to get extra prescriptions from an orthopedic specialist she was seeing out of state. Unfortunately, she succumbed to the temptation to "stockpile" the drugs, "just in case I need some and my supply has run out," she explained.

With many prescription drugs, it's quite easy for a person like Beth to go overboard, and that's just what happened in Beth's case. She became almost obsessed with trying to get rid of any discomfort she felt anywhere in her body. In other words, she couldn't accept the normal "creakiness" that all older people may feel after sitting for a long time in a chair or upon getting up in the morning. As a result, she sought increasing amounts of the drug to produce her desired *total* painkilling effect.

But as usually happens in such circumstances, Beth began to experience certain side effects, including occasional stomach bleeding that showed up in her stool, and allergic reactions that included swelling in the limbs. Her internist identified the problem and took her off the drug—a remedy that was temporarily more painful than the original pains she had experienced.

The lesson for you to learn from Beth's use of painkillers, or from any use of any other prescription drug, is quite simple: take them only in the amounts and at the times recommended by your physician. Also, if you can put up with some level of discomfort, it may be best to delay taking the drug until you absolutely have to have it. Becoming too free in the use of any prescription or over-the-counter drug is a sure way to jeopardize your health.

Low-Performing Performance Enhancers

Because we see many athletes of all ages at the Cooper Clinic and Aerobics Center—from those in college or professional sports, to elite performers in masters and senior games competitions—we frequently have to field questions like these:

What supplement can I take that will improve my performance or endurance?

Is there a pill or other substance with a short-term effect that will help me in the race this Saturday?

Do you think steroids are all that bad if they're used for a very short time?

How about my using performance enhancers, or growth hormones, or some other such drug to stave off the effects of aging?

There's a fairly easy answer to all such questions: in one way or another, using performance-enhancing drugs for any purpose has a tremendous potential to ruin your life. Our blanket condemnation includes anabolic steroids, testosterone, blood doping substances like DMT, THG, and EPO, and similar drugs—even including excessively high doses of certain ordinary supplements.

Steroids used for any purpose carry side effects that can destroy your health. The problems include shrunken testicles for men, masculine appearance for women, sterility, oily skin, acne, and even the growth of male breasts. Testosterone shots, creams, skin patches, or pills can also *decrease* levels of "good" HDL cholesterol, thereby increasing the risk of heart disease.

Furthermore, these supposedly performance-enhancing drugs won't increase your skill in a particular sport. You'll still be a poor tennis player or golfer if your forehand is technically defective or your putt or drive is inaccurate.

Unfortunately, as masters' and seniors' competitions gain in popularity, the pressure increases to use the drugs to enhance performance in those areas such as track and field competitions, weight lifting, or body-building contests, which can be affected by such drugs as steroids. As a result, testing for drugs has been instituted at many of the high-level events, such as those sponsored by the World Masters Athletics (WMA). The enforcement procedures have become so stringent that sometimes, apparently innocent violations can result in onerous penalties.[8]

One disconcerting story involved a fifty-six-year-old grandmother, an elite American sprinter who hadn't begun to run competitively until she had turned fifty.[9] But then in the late 1990s, during a track meet in England, she broke the world record in the 100 meters for her age group. Almost immediately, her victory was contested, requiring her to undergo drug testing. As a result, she was disqualified and banned from competitions for two years—because she tested positive for anabolic steroids.

But this incident turned out to involve more complicated issues than observers first thought. Along with other medications, the woman had been taking hormone-replacement therapy for her hot flashes, and the particular prescription she was using contained steroids—enough to have caused her to test positive at the meet.

The implications of this decision for the future are confusing because an estimated 64 percent of senior athletes, age fifty and over, use prescription medications—and many of them contain substances that have been banned by international athletic groups. These include various cough medicines, high blood pressure medications, and drugs used to treat osteoporosis, the bone-thinning condition that threatens many older people. In fact, hormone-replacement therapy, such as the prescription taken by the banned grandmother, may be used to combat osteoporosis.

While the temptation to use performance-enhancing drugs may plague athletes of all ages, nonathletes may be drawn into the orbit as they try drugs that have developed a reputation of improving mental abilities. Interestingly, Ritalin, which is prescribed widely for children with attention deficit disorder or other hyperactive problems, has become increasingly popular among aging patients. The reason is that the drug can produce an effect in older people that counters depression and increases energy levels, attention capacities, and the sense of well-being. Part of the positive action of Ritalin with older people is that it triggers the release of the neurotransmitter dopamine, which has been associated with feelings of well-being. Also, Ritalin (methylphenidate) tends to act more quickly than other antidepressants: the drug typically enables patients to overcome their depression within two to five days.[10]

At the same time, however, Ritalin and related drugs carry certain risks. They may produce dangerous irregular heart rates in adults as well as in children. According to a 2005 report from the Food and Drug Administration, about 29 million prescriptions were written for Ritalin in 2004 in the United States. Of those prescriptions, 23 million were for children and the remainder for older people, including the elderly.[11]

So what can we conclude about performance-enhancing drugs or medications for older people?

In general, it's best to avoid them unless your physician prescribes them for a legitimate medical purpose.* This recommendation assumes particular importance if you hope to compete in elite senior competitions. Because of the increasingly sophisticated testing techniques, if you do try to employ blood doping or other performance-enhancing substances, you're likely to be found out—and lose the opportunity to enjoy competing against your peers as you grow older.

Now, let's turn to a "drug" that, contrary to much popular thinking, may actually be good for you—provided it's taken in the proper doses. We're referring to your morning brew.

The Surprising Case of Coffee

A few years ago, dire warnings were being issued about drinking too much coffee. And it's quite true that in certain people excessive caffeine may result in irregular heartbeats or other undesirable symptoms. But for most of us, a cup or two in the morning seems to help get the brain in gear, a phenomenon that recent research has confirmed.

A 2005 report by Austrian researchers at the Radiological Society of North America, for instance, revealed that the caffeine in coffee, tea, certain soft drinks, and chocolate stimulates areas of the brain that control short-term memory and attention. The functional MRI (magnetic resonance imaging) scans done on patients in this study showed that two cups of coffee increased activity in the memory and attention-controlling areas of the brain. The participants in the study also im-

---

*One exception is our recommended use of relatively high doses of antioxidants and other legitimate supplements by elite athletes to counter the production of excessive free oxygen radicals. (See the discussions in Chapter 10.)

proved their performance in remembering a sequence of letters after they consumed 100 milligrams of caffeine (the equivalent of about one cup of coffee).[12]

Recent scientific research has also suggested that coffee may be healthy in other ways, which we might not have expected. For example, a 2005 investigation in the *Journal of the American Medical Association* found that habitual coffee consumption is associated with a "substantially lower risk of type 2 diabetes"—i.e., the "adult onset" type of the disease.[13] Other studies have shown that coffee drinking may decrease the risk of cirrhosis of the liver and liver cancer.[14]

There are also investigations indicating that the risk of cardiovascular disease decreases with coffee consumption. Researchers with the Iowa Women's Health Study, involving evaluation of more than 27,000 women, age fifty-five to sixty-nine, reported that women who drank one to three cups of coffee per day enjoyed a 24 percent reduction in their risk of cardiovascular disease, compared with noncoffee drinkers.[15]

What were the reasons for these benefits of caffeine? The researchers speculated that the antioxidants in coffee may have countered inflammation that is linked to cardiovascular disease.

But with coffee, as with many other foods or supplements, there can apparently be too much of a good thing: when the women in this study drank more than six cups of coffee per day, their benefits decreased, with no significant reduction in their cardiovascular risk.

Also, other possible dangers have been linked to this drink. In another study, those breathing air that approximated oxygen levels at high altitudes experienced a significant decrease in blood flow to the heart during exercise—with just two cups of coffee.[16] In this particular report, the caffeine triggered a 22 percent reduction of blood flow when the subjects exercised at the equivalent of fifteen hundred feet, and a 39 percent reduction at the equivalent of fifteen thousand feet. But the lead researcher said that drinking coffee before doing ordinary exercise should cause no health problems for healthy subjects. Also, he observed that drinking the stimulant at high altitudes was mainly a concern for those with existing coronary artery disease.[17]

Another possible danger of too much coffee is a decline in mental function. At a March 2006 meeting of the American Psychosomatic Society, researchers from Penn State reported that when volunteers were asked to do tough math computations in a stressful environment, they did better when they were given two cups of coffee. But when they received twice as much caffeine as the amount in two cups, their performance on the problems decreased.[18]

 ## Tyler's Soda Overdose

Prior to starting medical school, I was not much of a caffeine drinker. I never liked the taste of coffee, and I avoided soft drinks because of my athletic training. However, when I started to experience the long days and nights associated with medical training, I started drinking diet soft drinks to stay awake.

Initially, I would have just one drink when I felt I needed an energy boost. Over time I found myself wanting a soda when I knew I didn't really need it. In effect, I became mildly addicted to diet sodas, and so I decided to take control.

I made the decision to allow myself only one caffeine drink per day. This plan worked well for me because I found myself "storing up" that one drink until I really needed it—and often the need never arrived. As a result, I would go through a day without any drink at all, until I reached the point where I had control over the situation once again.

As a result of both my personal experience and responses I've observed in my patients, I would caution anyone who doesn't drink coffee, sodas, or other drinks with caffeine to avoid them, in part because it's hard for many people to control their drinking. Excessive consumption of caffeine can result not only in the discomfort of caffeine withdrawal but also, in some people, more serious consequences, such as heart irregularities and potential hypertension.

So my best advice is that if you don't drink caffeinated drinks, don't start. If you do currently drink caffeinated drinks and can limit yourself to the equivalent of two cups of coffee per day, that's fine. But be on guard to avoid overdoses!

So what are we to conclude about coffee drinking from these studies, some of which may seem to be sending some mixed messages? The safest approach seems to be to *limit your coffee drinking to no more than two cups per day*, preferably in the morning hours when there is no chance that the caffeine will interfere with your sleep.

Another rule of thumb that may help you identify your appropriate total caffeine intake is this: the maximum amount of caffeine in milligrams from all sources you consume daily should be no more than your body weight in pounds multiplied by two. So if you weigh 150 pounds, you should consume no more than 300 milligrams of caffeine.

To help you monitor those foods and drinks that contain significant amounts of caffeine, here's a representative list:[19]

- One 5-ounce cup of brewed (drip method) coffee: 100–150 mg (average = 130 mg)
- One 5-ounce cup of percolated coffee: 94 mg
- One cup of instant coffee: 74 mg
- One cup of decaffeinated brewed or instant coffee: 3 mg
- One 12-ounce glass of tea: 70 mg
- One 5-ounce cup of brewed tea: 50 mg
- One bottle or can of caffeine-containing soda: 40 mg
- Two squares of dark chocolate: 20 mg

Also, over-the-counter medications such as those for pain or for countering drowsiness may contain anywhere from 65 mg to 200 mg of caffeine. It's important to check the labels.

Caution: If you have a heart condition or special sensitivity to caffeine, you should abstain from all caffeine-containing foods, beverages, and over-the-counter medications.

Ken's Morning Sip

I've never been a real coffee drinker. But for years, I've followed a morning routine.

When I arrive at the Cooper Clinic, I have a cup of coffee, half regular and half decaffeinated, brought to my desk. Then I nurse it along for about an hour. Although I never drink more than a few sips in total, I find that the stimulant seems to help get my thinking in gear.

Of course, the effect could be completely psychological. In other words, I may just anticipate—and really *believe*—that the coffee will perk me up, and this anticipation may jump-start my mind and body all by itself. Sometimes I suspect this mental explanation is true because I drink so little of the brew. But I suspect, though I can't prove it, that my increased early morning alertness results *both* from my psychological anticipation *and* from the chemical effects of the caffeine.

Obviously, the way not to be surprised by alcohol, caffeine, or another substance is to avoid getting involved in the first place. That's a major reason that we recommend that those who don't drink alcohol now shouldn't take up the habit. On the other hand, we all have to take prescription or over-the-counter drugs at some time in our lives, and so it's unrealistic to think we can avoid such substances entirely. So our advice would be this: be wary whenever you move outside the realm of normal nutrition—and watch for that substance surprise that could put your health or even your life at risk. And be especially careful in times of stress because those are the times when we tend to look for a substance to help relieve the pressures bearing down upon us.

Our last start-up strategy for maximum fitness and health is directly related to this last point—the pervasive health challenge posed by the stress in our lives. If you can learn to head off or at least handle stress, you'll be in a much stronger position to manage your health and maximize your longevity. To see how this works, let's move on to Start-up #7—learning to combat stress with mind-spirit strength.

Thirteen

▪ Start-up #7—
▪ Combat Stress with
Mind-Spirit Strength

Stress is the great epidemic of our age. But unfortunately, we have failed miserably to counter its health effects—for at least two reasons: first, we have refused to recognize the real ravages that stress can wreak in our lives. And second, we have neglected to develop long-term stress-reduction habits.

"Meredith" came into our offices complaining about chronic headaches and backaches and a general feeling of malaise. Her blood pressure was elevated, her "bad" LDL cholesterol was too high, and her treadmill stress test times placed her only in the "fair" category of fitness.

Her energy levels were so low that she consistently fell asleep when she was reading a bedtime story to her five-year-old. And she was always too tired to help her ten-year-old with his homework. A forty-one-year-old single working mother, she felt under constant pressure from her job in a real estate firm and her responsibilities for her two children. In a typical week, she became chronically stressed out as she fielded calls from her children's schools about their homework, health, or other issues and at the same time was trying to show properties to prospective clients.

During her medical exam, she was told that the stress she was experiencing had turned her body into a ticking time bomb. Unless she took steps to correct things, she could almost certainly expect to encounter serious health problems within ten years. And in the interim, she could expect to experience increasing health challenges.

A major part of her prescription was to embark on a start-up fitness program, of the type described in Chapter 7. But her first response was: "I can't afford the time for exercise!"

Her physician's reply: "You can't afford *not* to take the time to exercise!" Then, he proceeded to catalog the many benefits she could expect if she just took the simple step of injecting some regular physical activity into her life.

Finally, after contemplating the advantages she would likely receive from a fitness program—including the antistress effects of regular aerobic exercise—she decided to give the program a try. Now, after six months on the start-up regimen, Meredith has developed a solid exercise habit. Just as important, she has discovered that even though those major stresses are still present in her life, she handles them much better. Getting calls at work about her children doesn't rattle her anymore. It's been weeks since she has fallen asleep reading to her younger child. And she has found that her mind usually even works well enough at the end of the day to help her older boy with his math.

Meredith's reason for seeking medical help—and the "cure" she found—are typical of many, many people we see at the Cooper Clinic. A number of studies have indicated that approximately 75 to 90 percent of visits to doctors' offices are somehow stress related.[1] Also, we know from solid research that many fatal illnesses, such as cardiovascular disease and cancer, often have a stress component.[2] Yet somehow, we often don't link the stress that permeates our lives and the state of our health. As a first step in making this all-important connection, let's consider some of the specific ways that stress ravages our health.

Know Your Enemy:
The Ravages of Stress

Here are a few things we now know about specific health conditions and illnesses that have been linked to stress:

- *Heart attacks:* Within one hour of experiencing negative, stress-related emotions—such as tension, sadness, or frustration—patients in a 1997 study had two to three times the risk of silent heart attacks (myocardial ischemia) compared with those who did not experience stressful emotions.[3]

  Interestingly, Monday is generally considered a highly stressful day because it involves getting back into the routine of work after a relaxing weekend. In fact, a number of studies have established a link with stress, showing that more heart attacks occur on Monday.[4]

- *Potentially deadly heartbeat irregularities:* Heart irregularities such as atrial fibrillation have been linked to patients with psychological stress, including those who are also depressed, hostile, or anxious.[5]

  In one startling study, researchers from Johns Hopkins University found that sudden emotional stress—whether resulting from fear, anger, shock, or grief—can cause heart failure, especially in women.[6] In this particular study, the highly stressful events "stunned" the heart and sent eighteen women and one man to the coronary-care unit at Johns Hopkins University in Baltimore. Unlike a typical heart attack, which may occur as a result of a clot that blocks blood flow to the heart, this condition apparently involves the shocking of the heart with excessive amounts of the body's stress chemicals and hormones, such as adrenaline.

- *Headache, muscle ache, and backache:* Many studies have linked these complaints and chronic pain to stress.[7]

- *Peptic ulcers:* This condition involves the development of a raw area of the stomach, the beginning of the small intestine (duodenum), or upper digestive tract (esophagus).[8]
- *Impaired immune function:* Stress has been implicated in reduced immune function involving common complaints such as colds or other upper respiratory illness, or in more serious conditions such as rheumatoid arthritis and systemic lupus erythematosus.[9]
- *Skin abnormalities and diseases:* Studies have linked stress and various skin conditions, such as psoriasis and acne. Also, excessive stress, such as that caused by exam-time pressure for students, has been associated with a failure of the skin to heal properly from wounds.[10]
- *Cancer:* There are some strong indications, though the evidence isn't conclusive, that stress may be linked to various cancers, such as women's breast cancer.[11]

But despite our *intellectual* understanding that stress may be implicated in these and other health conditions, we often fail to make the leap to *practical* measures that could help us counter the impact of this health threat in our daily lives. So what's our problem with this stress issue—and how can we deal with it?

Why We Fail to Control Stress

In our practice, we have identified several reasons many of us fail to control stress—even though we may be fully aware of the scientific evidence that points directly to stress as the source of many health problems. Four in particular stand out—and one or more may apply directly to your situation.

First, you may simply choose to ignore the impact stress has on your health because you don't think modern medicine is equipped to deal with it. If you have a broken bone, a bleeding cut, a fever, or nausea, you'll tend to those problems because you've been conditioned to believe the answer can be found in the doctor's office, or maybe on a shelf of medications at the local drugstore. But you may not be at all inclined to ask your doctor for help with your occasionally churning stomach, rapidly beating heart, or increased breathing rate.

Second, stress as a concept may seem a little unreal or "mushy" to you. You may even conclude that those symptoms you're feeling are more imaginary than real—that they're "in your head" and not worthy of your attention.

Third, if you're a man, you may feel that worrying about stress is unmanly. You're been taught to "suck it up" and bull your way through the pressures of life. So you cover up your feelings of stress or try to ignore the symptoms you're feeling—the cold sweats, the obsessive worrying, the periodic headaches and backaches, or the roiling gut.

Yet the dangers with this head-in-the-sand mentality are not just serious, they are also potentially deadly. Take the situation confronted by the former coach of the Chicago Bears, Mike Ditka, who was at the top of his field in the extremely high-pressure job of professional football coach.[12] He had none of the risk factors usually associated with heart disease except for one: he appeared to represent a version of the type A personality who was under enormous stress. This stress-vulnerable type is characterized by a tendency to overwork, an intensive competitive streak, high ambition, aggressiveness, a chronic sense of time urgency, and, often, hostility.[13]

Also, he preferred weight lifting to aerobic exercise such as walking, jogging, or cycling. (Even though both types of exercise are important for your overall health and fitness, rhythmic aerobic exercise is more conducive to stress management than high-resistance weight work, stress-reduction experts believe.)

When Ditka suffered a heart attack on November 2, 1989, the risks of a high-stress life hit home with many men, who thought toughing it out in high-pressure, competitive work environments was the masculine thing to do. But of course, learning to *manage* stress is in no way an unmanly exercise; in fact, *real* men are those who recognize the dangers of stress and deal with it decisively.

Fourth, because the medical community is not too adept at teaching patients how to counter stress, you may lack an understanding of the tools at your disposal to deal with it. The next section has been designed to help you with a series of questions that you should ask yourself when you feel under stress. Use it as a checklist to help you identify your stress vulnerabilities—and deal effectively with them.

The Cooper Stress Questionnaire

To complete your Start Strong health-and-fitness program, ask yourself seven "stress questions" at least once a week. If you can answer yes on a regular basis to at least four of these questions, you can assume that you possess important tools to deal effectively with stress. But it's important to be certain that these strengths are not just short-term phenomena; they must become *deeply ingrained habits* if they are to exert their full power in your life.

If you give a positive answer to only three of the questions, your stress-handling capability is probably marginal. And if you respond yes to two or fewer, you're most likely vulnerable to a negative impact of stress on your health.

STRESS QUESTION #1: AM I GETTING REGULAR AEROBIC EXERCISE?

Although poorly managed stress can kill, regular exercise can act as a protective shield against the impact of stress. As we often say at the Cooper Clinic, "aerobic exercise is nature's greatest tranquillizer." Most likely, the physiologic explanation for the power of aerobic exercise involves the release of neurotransmitters, such as endorphins and dopamine, which are natural "drugs of well-being" produced by the body under certain conditions. Also, the soothing impact on your system is probably linked to the well-documented medical phenomenon known as the "relaxation response" (see the further explanation below, under Stress Question #2).

Evidence has emerged in a British study reviewing medical articles over a period of thirty-five years that the risk of having a heart attack as a result of stress can be altered by the level of health and fitness a person is in before the stress strikes.[14] Or to put this another way, when sedentary people are emotionally or physically stressed, they are more likely to be at high risk for a heart attack than those who exercise regularly.

In a related issue, excess stress often leads to emotional dysfunction, such as depression. Yet medical studies have shown that regular aerobic exercise can operate as a highly effective antidote to depression.

In a 2005 report in the *American Journal of Preventive Medicine*, for example, researchers from the Cooper Institute studied eighty adults, ages twenty to forty-five, who had been diagnosed with mild to moderate "major depressive disorder."[15] They found that participants who engaged in the "public health dose" of exercise—or the equivalent of at least thirty minutes of moderate-intensity activity (such as brisk walking) for most or preferably all days of the week—experienced a significant alleviation of the symptoms of depression. This public health dose could be achieved in three to five days a week of activity, as long as the total amount of exercise equaled at least the equivalent of thirty minutes of exercise on most or all days of the week (three to three and a half hours of activity per week).

The message is fairly clear and straightforward: if you want to control the symptoms of stress, such as depression, engage in a weekly total of at least three hours of moderate-intensity aerobic activity (e.g., brisk walking) three to five days per week.

STRESS QUESTION #2: DO I USE MENTAL RELAXATION TECHNIQUES REGULARLY AND EFFECTIVELY?

Relaxation techniques that elicit the "relaxation response" on a regular basis also have the capacity to counter the effects of the stress response. The basic technique, according to the Harvard Medical School experts at the Mind/Body Medical Institute in Boston, works like this:[16]

- Pick a focus word or phrase that has a comfortable, positive connotation for you and, if possible, arises from your deepest personal beliefs. The word or phrase should be short enough to be repeated silently as you exhale. Examples might include "peace and love," "shalom," "God is love," "calm waters," or some other comfortable word or sound.

- For a couple of minutes, breathe regularly and slowly, and concentrate on relaxing every part of your body, from your toes to your face to your fingers.

- For approximately ten minutes, close your eyes and continue breathing regularly while repeating silently on every outbreath the focus word or phrase that you've chosen. When outside thoughts come to mind, turn away from them gently and return to your focus word or phrase.

- During the final minute of the exercise, continue to breathe regularly with your eyes closed, but now allow normal thoughts to enter your mind.

- Finally, open your eyes and proceed with your daily schedule.

The physiologic changes that occur during this type of mental exercise—changes known as the "relaxation response"—operate in direct opposition to the stress response. (For a more detailed discussion of this biology, see Chapter 4.)

Important reminder: Researchers have also determined that the rhythmic nature of aerobic exercise (e.g., regular footfalls with walking or running, regular strokes with swimming, or regular pedaling with cycling) can produce the relaxation-response effect. In other words, you get a double dose of stress reduction when you engage in aerobic exercise—including both mental relaxation and an aerobic-exercise impact.

Another variation that a number of people have found to be helpful is the combination of a mental relaxation technique with aerobic activity. One of our patients, for instance, always repeats a line of a favorite poem or verse of Scripture as he walks or jogs. As a result, he experiences a "double effect" of relaxation arising from both the mental and physical exercise.

STRESS QUESTION #3: DO I KNOW HOW TO "SHIFT GEARS"?

In a variation on the relaxation technique described in Stress Question #2, researchers have determined that breaking a prior, stress-ridden train of thought or mind-set can by itself produce a response comparable to the relaxation response.[17] This process is often called "backing off" or "letting go," and is a highly effective method for jump-starting the creative process when the pressure to perform has caused temporary mental paralysis.

It's common knowledge, for example, that if you're feeling stressed out and mentally blocked as a result of several straight hours of work, you can often get rid of the stress and also the block simply by standing up and walking into another room, perhaps to leaf through a magazine or get a drink of water.

Similarly, taking a break in the middle of the day or after a hard day's work to engage in some entirely different kind of activity will often relieve the stress, in addition to gaining the obvious physical benefits. (See the accompanying box for Ken's approach.)

Ken on Stress-Busting Breaks

Although a great deal of research indicates that those who schedule their exercise time first thing in the morning have the best record of consistency and good habit formation, I prefer to work out at the end of the day.

The reason? I'm always rejuvenated and energized after a long day of work at the desk—and ready to spend quality time with my family in the evening or even do a couple of extra hours of work. But actually, this end-of-day workout is only one part of my daily "stress-busting" routine.

Typically, I'll get to the office around 6:30 a.m. and then have my daily ten to fifteen minutes of stress-controlling "quiet time," including Bible study, prayer, and the occasional reading of one of my favorite devotional authors, such as Chuck Swindoll or Max Lucado.

After that time of personal focus, I'll work steadily until lunchtime, which for me is usually between 2:00 and 2:30 p.m. During that break, I'll get a quick meal at our Aerobic Center restaurant and also spend fifteen minutes walking around the center, talking to club members or staff. This physical break also serves as a mental break, preparing me for a full afternoon of work.

Admittedly, I am sometimes so rushed that I'll have a bowl of soup brought to my desk for lunch. But on those occasions, I never seem to be as productive during the rest of the day.

By about 6:30 p.m., I'm typically feeling rather wound up or tired—the result of a stressful day of making decisions, preparing for our radio program, doing medical research, or pursuing one of my other "careers." It's at this point that an end-of-day workout contributes most to my mind and body. After spending about an hour of fast walking and doing strength work, I'll take a shower and head for home. Most times, this program completely transforms my mind and body, and prepares me for several more alert hours of family or work time before I finally go to bed.

STRESS QUESTION #4: HAVE I DEVELOPED A "POSITIVE DEFAULT" IN MY OUTLOOK ON LIFE?

This is just another way of asking if you are happy most of the time, or usually rather unhappy. If you answer that you're mostly optimistic, your chances of avoiding death from cardiovascular disease increases significantly, according to medical research.

A 2006 article in the *Archives of Internal Medicine,* for example, concluded that "dispositional optimism"—or generally positive expectations about the future of one's life—is associated with lower risk of cardiovascular death.[18] In this study, Dutch researchers followed more than five hundred men, ages sixty-four to eighty-four, over a fifteen-year period. They determined the level of optimism in the subjects through questionnaires.

Part of having a happy, upbeat outlook appears to depend on your innate disposition. In other words, some people are simply born happier than others, or they have been conditioned to be happier as a result of long-term early influences. But we don't subscribe to the idea that it's impossible to change into a happy or optimistic person. In fact, both medical studies and clinical observations suggest a number of strategies you might follow to become happier.

Devote some time every day to laughing.

A University of Maryland study, presented at a 2005 meeting of the American College of Cardiology, found that fifteen minutes of laughter every day "is probably good for the vascular system." The researchers found that blood flowed more feely in the lining of the vessels when healthy volunteers laughed at funny movie scenes. In contrast, their blood flow was restricted when they watched stressful clips.[19]

Avoid or manage situations that make you angry or hostile.

It really doesn't matter what situations irritate you; just the fact that you become teed off is enough to hurt your health. For example, a research presentation from the University of Utah at a March 2006 meeting of the

American Psychosomatic Society showed that hostile women are more likely to suffer hardening of the coronary arteries (atherosclerosis). Furthermore, their artery situation becomes worse if their husbands are also hostile.[20]

A 2002 study from the Boston University School of Public Health reported that men who measured as hostile on a personality test experienced many more heart attacks, chest pains, or other signs of heart disease than those who weren't hostile.[21] The eight hundred men in the study had been followed for forty years and averaged sixty years of age when their hostility levels were measured.

Other observers explain that people with elevated hostility levels tend to have higher blood pressure and heart rate responses when they become angry. Interestingly, this Boston study revealed that the only measurement that predicted heart disease risk more accurately than hostility was low levels of "good" HDL cholesterol.

According to psychiatrist Redford Williams of Duke Medical School, an independent 1999 study of his LifeSkills hostility-management seminars showed that it's possible to simultaneously lower hostility levels *and* blood pressure readings. The participants were taught to get perspective on situations that make them angry by asking four questions:

Is this important?
Is this anger appropriate?
Is this action modifiable?
Is it worth it to take action?[22]

If you're feeling hostile, you might ask yourself these same questions.

STRESS QUESTION #5: AM I GETTING ADEQUATE SLEEP?

In our overly busy, overworked society, sleep often gets short shrift as a way of sheltering ourselves from the fallout of stress. We have friends and patients who relate with some pride how well they operate on four or five hours of sleep—as though depriving themselves in this way is a sign of their stamina, strength, and high energy.

In fact, getting too little sleep can be a significant risk factor for a host of health problems, including hypertension. Researchers from Columbia University's Mailman School of Public Health reported in the April 2006 issue of *Hypertension* that men and women thirty-two to fifty-nine years of age who got five hours of sleep a night or less were about 60 percent more likely to develop high blood pressure than those who slept six to eight hours. But getting more than eight hours of sleep a night had no effect on blood pressure levels. The researchers followed more than 4,800 men and women over a ten-year period.

STRESS QUESTION #6: AM I GETTING ADEQUATE NUTRITION?

In general, a balanced diet will give you a strong defense against the ravages of stress.[23] But in addition, there are certain types of foods and supplements that have been associated with stress protection.

First of all, increasing your intake of antioxidants—including vitamins E, C, and beta-carotene—will help counter the production of excess free radicals in your body during stress. Free radicals are unstable oxygen molecules that have been associated with an increased risk of cardiovascular disease, cancer, and other serious health conditions. Other antistress nutrients include riboflavin (vitamin B_2) and pantothenic acid (once known as vitamin B_5). (For recommended dosages of these vitamins, see Chapter 10.)

The best way to get these nutrients is through your food. For example, you may be able to take in adequate amounts of vitamin C if you consume daily helpings of oranges, cranberry juice cocktail, cantaloupe, and Brussels sprouts. But unfortunately, most of us don't include adequate amounts of these antistress vitamins in our diets—hence the need for supplementation. Also, we simply can't take in enough of certain important antioxidants, such as vitamin E, through the diet; in the case of E,

400 IU per day would require eating more high-calorie almonds and hazelnuts than our waistlines could bear.

STRESS QUESTION #7: HAVE I DEVELOPED A PHILOSOPHICAL PERSPECTIVE ON LIFE?

Sometimes, when a hugely stressful event hits you, it may take more than a relaxation technique or exercise to help you recover. In such catastrophic situations, a more profound philosophical perspective may be necessary.

What kinds of pressures can trigger overwhelming stress? The greatest stressors of life have been enumerated in a life-events monitoring list known as the Holmes-Rahe Social Readjustment Scale. The stressful events include, in descending order of impact on the individual, the following: death of a spouse; divorce; separation from a living partner; a jail term; death of a close family member; a serious personal injury; being fired from a job; and retirement. Also, marriage and menopause may be included toward the top of this list.[24]

Numerous scientific studies have supported the validity of Holmes-Rahe in the decades since it was first devised. For example, researchers from the U.S. Centers for Disease Control and Prevention reported at an Orlando conference in February 2005 on a study of nearly 35,000 women, a number of whom had been fired from their jobs. Those who were terminated were more likely to suffer heart disease than either employed women or those who chose not to work but to stay at home. In general, the employed women had the best physical and mental health, while the fired women reported the worst.[25]

When such catastrophes strike, those who can place the stress into a broader context are much more likely to cope effectively. But such a perspective usually doesn't come quickly or easily. Thinkers of all ages have recognized that in most cases, it's necessary to develop habits of personal philosophy over time, in ways similar to those we have discussed for developing firm health-and-fitness habits.

Developing a Philosophical Perspective

In developing philosophical habits, we must begin to apply many of the principles we explored in Chapters 3 and 4, beginning with the principle of moving beyond thought to action.

THE ALL-IMPORTANT PRINCIPLE OF ACTION

As we saw in Chapter 4, probably the most fundamental truth about habit-formation emphasized by William James is that you can't just *think* about desired habits or *wish* them to come to pass. Instead, the sages have long said, you have to *act* on your good intentions if you want to develop a strong personal philosophy that can be used to protect you against stress or any other negative outside force.

This idea comes across clearly in a frequently quoted nineteenth-century saying of uncertain authorship—which goes like this:

> *Sow a Thought, and you reap an Act;*
> *Sow an Act, and you reap a Habit;*
> *Sow a Habit, and you reap a Character;*
> *Sow a Character, and you reap a Destiny.*

Such observations may give the impression that developing good habits is primarily a matter of engaging in a lot of unpleasant, tedious, hard work—but that's not really the case. It's just that those who have considered this issue over the centuries have come to understand that New Year's resolutions and other good intentions designed to improve our character and personality are doomed to fail unless they are bolstered by a practical, action-oriented daily program to put them into effect.

For a case study in how a hard-earned philosophical habit can be used as a stress-reducing strategy, consider the following autobiographical account of how Tyler dealt with a particular crisis in his life. As the story unfolds, you'll also see how strategies suggested by several of the other six stress questions discussed above—namely, regular exercise, "shifting gears," and a "positive default" mind-set—came into play.

Tyler on Catastrophic Stress

I sometimes wonder if Holmes and Rahe had younger people in mind when they devised their social readjustment scale—or if they were just dealing with those fifty and older. If I had been collaborating with them, I think I might have included a couple of additional stressful life events typically encountered by those in their late twenties, thirties, or even early forties. I'm thinking in particular of those events related to the struggle over choosing the ultimate direction of one's life.

Like most other younger adults I know, the source of greatest stress in my late twenties and early thirties involved understanding my life's purpose and direction, including the nature of my career. Several categories from the older Holmes-Rahe scale would have applied to my situation—such as stresses related to changing my role in business or work; changing work responsibilities; leaving college; changing my living conditions; and moving to a new residence. But I would also add items like "trying to find my permanent life purpose" and "settling on a career." I can see now that, taken together, all these stressors catapulted me up into a high-pressure category that made me a candidate for stress-related health problems.

Whatever your age, until you resolve the issue of personal purpose—and relieve the attendant stress—you're likely to behave like a rudderless ship. Such uncertainty and aimlessness open the door to making bad choices in relationships, taking unwise risks, and, in the end, increasing your vulnerability to depression and other emotional ills.

I know from experience that a lack of focus about a career can many times translate into a failure to follow wise health habits. I've often witnessed frustrated, directionless young people—sometimes close friends

(continued)

of mine—become involved in ill-advised personal behavior, such as destructive sex, perilous physical risk-taking, drug use, and alcohol abuse. More often than not, after the initial endorphin rush, these thrill-seeking young men and women recognize the fleeting satisfaction of their unwise choices and see that they haven't found real purpose in life. As a result, they often sink into depression or are racked by anxiety.

My own uncertainties about my ultimate life's direction may serve as an object lesson, but I'll readily admit that in some ways I'm an odd case. After all, I appeared to be on an inevitable track to become a physician from the get-go. I had grown up in a family where my father was a world-famous physician; my sister worked in health care and was an accomplished collegiate athlete; and my mother had authored books on fitness and well-being. For as long as I can remember, health, medicine, and fitness have been prime topics of discussion around the dinner table.

To seal the deal on my probable future, my grandfather, uncle, and many other relatives had been physicians or dentists. In fact, there had been no "Mister" Cooper going back three generations in my ancestral line—all had been "Doctor." So understandably, the unspoken assumption around our house was, "Tyler will follow in his father's footsteps. . . . Tyler will become a doctor. . . . Tyler will take his 'rightful' place at the Cooper Clinic."

But as any independent-minded young person knows, nothing in this life is quite that simple or automatic. It might have *seemed* quite logical to any outsider that I would become a doctor. But in my heart of hearts, I wasn't at all sure that was the life I wanted to lead. In fact, as I moved through college, I became quite convinced that medicine would *not* be my career. I did quite well in all my business courses at Baylor, but when it came to premed courses like biology, I bombed out. I didn't like them and didn't do particularly well at them. So I decided: Medicine is out the window!

But to be honest, the decision to dump my dad's life's work didn't create a lot of angst for me. My main focus in college had not been on making medicine my career but rather on big-time sports. As a scholarship recruit for the varsity track and cross-country teams, I was named captain of our Baylor teams, was selected All-Southwest Conference, and barely missed All-American in cross-country. I even came fairly close to Olympic qualifying time in one event.

After I graduated, everything changed for me, as it did for many of my college classmates. Without my team at my side practically every waking moment, I faced a major void in my life—and a sense of stress began to overwhelm me. Athletic achievement had been all-important to me, but I didn't have the option of becoming a professional runner. So what was I going to do with my degree? I didn't have a clue.

When I finally sat and jotted down a few options, several possibilities floated through my still-maturing twenty-three-year-old brain. These included:

- Running for a certain semiprofessional track team;
- Joining the navy and maybe trying to become a SEAL, as I had been inspired by a good friend who was one;
- Returning to the Cooper Clinic and Aerobics Center in a business management role and getting an MBA later, or
- Becoming a ski bum in Colorado for a year or so and reflect on the meaning of my life.

Now, I liked that last idea. Even though my dad wasn't too thrilled with the ski option, I knew I had to get away from home to think more clearly. For one thing, I found myself becoming increasingly uncomfortable because my view of work and play diverged from his. As I interpreted our differences, his secret to success involved working long hours and never goofing off—and I couldn't go along with that.

Anyhow, feeling that I needed to work out some things on my own, I told my folks I wanted to spend some time on the slopes in Colorado as a way to clear my head—and establish myself as my own man. Amazingly, even though I thought my dad might have some issues with my decision, he was completely supportive, though he made it clear he

(continued)

would provide no financial backing. So I headed for the Rockies and, I hoped, for a clear vision of my future.

When I arrived in the Vail–Beaver Creek area, I linked up with a man I had been told about while at a sports camp that summer. He was running a "discipleship house" in East Vail that catered to young people who were trying to find their way in life—and stay away from the drugs, alcohol, and other habits that plague singles living near a ski resort. To earn money for food, rent, and incidentals, I worked at odd construction and janitorial jobs and ran ski gondolas up and down the mountains when snow season arrived.

After a while, I started volunteering as a guide for blind skiers. They had impressed me ever since I was a kid, and this was a great chance for me to understand a little better what it must feel like to fly down the slopes without any vision. I continued to be amazed that they could accomplish this feat with great skill and without an ounce of fear. I wanted to live life like that, without being afraid of what I couldn't see.

Usually, I worked six days a week—that is, until the snow started falling. Then, I'd cut back on the work and use the money I'd saved to do some skiing of my own. But all the while, I was sensing this weight of trying to figure out what I was supposed to do with my life. Then, one cold December day, when I was closing down a ski gondola that I had been running at the top of one mountain, I moved too quickly in turning the crank that released the hand brake. The machinery spun out of control and crushed my finger. Even though I was wearing heavy gloves, the pain was overwhelming. I cringed, looking around for help, but everyone had already gone.

Fortunately, I had access to a snowmobile, and so I was able to get down the mountain quickly and then head for a medical clinic. The doctor, an orthopedist, quickly confirmed what I already knew: my finger was broken, snapped in half. I finally left his office with my hand tightly wrapped in tape and gauze and hoped for better days. But even with my injured finger—and my reduced ability to do physical labor— I didn't want to leave Vail. So I stayed, did the best I could doing work that didn't require ten good fingers, and kept reflecting.

When I returned to the orthopedist's office a couple of months later to have my hand checked, I was a lot more relaxed. So this time, I found myself looking around his office as I waited for him to finish with another patient. As my eyes fixed on several little crayon drawings he had been given from kids in the area, I noticed that many had short captions:

"Thank you, Dr. Smith, for fixing my arm."

"Thanks for making my leg well."

"Thanks for helping me play basketball again."

Something nudged me inside—not a major revelation or a lightning bolt, but maybe a light mental snowflake. I thought, "I want to do something with my life that will let me give tangibly to people every day—to make their lives better."

Then I asked myself, "How can I do that?"

Then a thought came: "You're in a doctor's office, aren't you?"

I decided that maybe I had never really given medicine a fair chance. Certainly, I hadn't studied hard enough to do well in the one or two premed courses I had taken. But now, I was older and more focused.

"Maybe I should try it again," I thought.

When I finally decided to return to Dallas, after a five-month stint trekking in Australia and New Zealand, my mind was made up. I took a job on the business side of the Cooper Clinic so that I could take night classes at local universities to cover premed requirements. Two years later, I began applying to medical schools—and entered the University of Texas Medical School in San Antonio.

I think I can say without contradiction that I was the least-prepared person in my entering class. I had completed the absolute minimum premed course requirements, while many of the other students were science majors, had master's degrees in biochemistry, or had actually worked in health-service jobs, such as physical therapy and nursing.

The entire four-year medical school experience was a tough, uphill climb for me—and my confidence in my abilities slipped month by month. At one point at the end of my third year, I faced a crucial com-

(continued)

prehensive exam that would enable me to enter my final, fourth year and go on to qualify for my M.D. But the fear of failure paralyzed me—and I had a lot of trouble with that exam.

I found myself thinking: "What if I don't get through medical school—how would I stand the embarrassment?"

As my fears increased, so did a growing cloud of depression.

"Why is God letting this happen to me?" I wondered.

After failing on the crucial final exam, I found myself alternating between crying episodes and overwhelming feelings of anxiety, and I knew I desperately needed advice and help. So I called a young woman whom I was dating at the time and asked her to come over to my apartment. When she arrived, I was lying practically catatonic on the sofa. I could hardly talk to her about my fears, which had virtually immobilized me. As I remember, I said almost nothing to her, just a couple of disconnected words and moans. It was the lowest point in my life.

Finally, my girlfriend convinced me to go to dinner with her, and as we sat in the restaurant, something began to happen inside. I started getting angry—not at medical school or at God, but at myself. When I finally arrived back home and my girlfriend had left, I exploded. In retrospect, I think she had decided that she didn't want to become the target of the anger she could see building in me.

"You're a coward!" I shouted at myself. "Stand up like a man! Who cares what others may think if you fail. Don't let your life be ruined because you're petrified that you won't measure up to the expectations of others!"

Then I thought about my dad.

"There's nothing he's afraid of," I told myself, reflecting back on the challenges he had faced over the years. "He's shown he hasn't been afraid of his career falling flat, or opposition from the medical establishment, or going broke—or anything else."

I had been amazed to learn that my father had walked away from the military when he was close to retirement—with a five-year-old daughter and a pregnant wife. Against all odds, he had set up the first treadmill stress-test facility in Dallas. He had also stood up to the Dallas medical establishment after they threatened to run him out of town when he advised patients about the benefits of preventive medicine and lifestyle changes to reduce coronary risks. Also, I could still remember seeing him on his knees, praying but hanging as tough as could be when the Dallas economy tanked in the early 1990s and he was pushed to the brink of bankruptcy. As I meditated inside the dark emotional tunnel where I now found myself, I trusted that his example might inspire me and help carry me through to the light I could now see glimmering in the distance.

This inner dialogue continued into the next day, as I sat around the apartment and then drove here and there about the city. While riding around, I listened to one of my favorite bands, U2. They have a song with lyrics that go something like this: "I'm ready to let go of the steering wheel."

"That's right," I agreed out loud. "It's time for *me* to let go of the steering wheel—of *my life*."

That was a real crossroads for me—and gave me great peace. I was actually able to pray with genuine conviction: "I can head in another career direction if that's what's meant to be. I've put in tons of time and effort at medical school. But fear can have no place in my life now. I just have to move ahead and quit doubting and asking questions. My life is in God's hands now and totally out of my control—and I'm okay with that."

I laughed for the first time in a long time—maybe two years or so—and I felt truly free. When I arrived home, I immediately called my girlfriend, and I could tell she was relieved. Then I pulled out my journal and recorded my final conclusion about medical school: if I made it through, that was fine. If I didn't, I could be sure that God had something else more important for my life. In the end, that gave me all the perspective and peace I needed.

So how did it all end?

Despite my lack of preparation for medical school, I finally passed the exam and completed medical school and the requirements for my

(continued)

medical degree. I then went on to complete my internship in Virginia and earned a Masters of Public Health at the Harvard School of Public Health with close to an A average. The year after that, I finished my residency in preventive medicine at the University of South Carolina.

I'm also beginning to feel the power of the same solid philosophical base deep in my psyche—a base like the one that has transformed my father into a consummate risk taker, a medical adventurer who has not only lived his great dream but who has also changed the practice of preventive medicine. As for me, God has given me the gift of complete freedom from the stresses of striving for earthly success. Now I honestly do not care if anyone thinks I'm a "success."

As icing on the cake, I was impressed by what a great, supportive person that particular girlfriend had been during the greatest crisis of my life. And now I'm married to Angela Cooper.

Learning to deal effectively with stress is an extremely important step in developing a mind-set that will position you to stay with your fitness program for the rest of your life—for at least one overriding reason: no matter how strong you start, at some time in the future you are likely to encounter one or more catastrophic events that will upset you emotionally and mentally—and threaten to derail your program completely. Learning to push through such crises is the essence of Finishing Strong.

Part Three

Strategies for Finishing Strong

Fourteen

■ It's Time to
■ Finish Strong

To finish strong means to maintain maximum energy, mental acumen, and physical function until the very end of life. It means to "square off the curve of life," right up to the last moment. Yet to achieve this goal, you really don't have to move beyond the seven start-ups described in Part Two. All that's necessary is to *continue* with those strategies as you age.

In other words, your Finish Strong program should comprise a series of seven finish-ups that mirror the seven start-ups that have gone before:

Finish-up #1: Undergo regular gold-standard physical exams on a regular basis for the rest of your life—as indicated in Chapter 5.

Finish-up #2: Continue with a regular fitness regimen, as outlined in Chapters 6–8. Spend at least half of your days on aerobic activity, and the rest on strength work. To firm up your fitness habit, your goal should be to do something physically active every day of the week.

Finish-up #3: Pursue a low-fat, calorie-controlled "one-thing" diet—using the principles described in Chapter 9.

Finish-up #4: Follow a wise supplement program, observing the guidelines established in Chapter 10.

Finish-up #5: Eliminate smoking from your life—especially side-stream, or passive, smoke. Refer to Chapter 11 if you need to refresh your memory and find a little inspiration.

Finish-up #6: Counter creeping substance abuse—including alcohol, prescription medications, and performance-enhancing substances. Chapter 12 will be as instructive later in the program as it was in the beginning.

Finish-up #7: Develop a strong mind-spirit program to counter stress. This area of medicine is constantly developing, but the strategies suggested in Chapter 13 have proven highly effective and scientifically solid over the past few decades.

By incorporating start-ups as finish-ups—and making them a permanent part of your life—you'll greatly lower your risk of being derailed by the various health challenges of aging. In other words, you'll be much less likely to suffer from such debilitating conditions as:

- cardiovascular disease, including heart attacks and strokes;
- osteoporosis, the devastating bone thinning that often accompanies aging;
- eye problems such as macular degeneration;
- erectile dysfunction;
- memory and mental deterioration;
- adult-onset diabetes;
- advanced, life-threatening cancers; and
- a host of other complaints.

Of course, there is no guarantee that with the Start Strong, Finish Strong program you'll avoid all of these and other health problems. But as scientific studies continue to emphasize, you'll greatly lower the odds that you'll suffer from them.

Now, in an attempt to suggest ways that some of the principles we've already considered can be related to the ongoing Finish Strong phase of your program, we invite you to engage in a series of "doc-to-doc dialogues" with us.

A Doc-to-Doc Dialogue on Finishing Strong

The Start Strong, Finish Strong message can stay with you for life, spanning every generational passage you experience, in at least three ways:

- You can *start* your fitness program at any age;
- You can *continue* your program as you age; and
- You can *adjust* your program to meet your changing needs and interests, as you move from one generation to the next.

To help you bridge the major fitness generation gaps you'll encounter as you grow older, we'd like for you to join us now in some doc-to-doc dialogues. These head-to-head discussions—in which we don't always agree, by the way—will introduce you to some traps and pitfalls you may encounter as you start your program. In the process, you may also pick up some tips that may help you prevail when the going gets rough.

Each of these short interchanges begins with a common question that's on many people's minds. Then one or both of us will give you our best shot at an answer. Some of these dialogues are just reminders or summaries of important points that you encountered in the start-up phase, but that you really need to keep in the front of your mind as your program matures. Other dialogues will provide you with new information you'll need to truly "finish strong."

DOC-TO-DOC DIALOGUES

Question: How should you balance strength and aerobic training as you get older?

Ken: The basic rule of thumb, which has already been described in Chapter 7, is that both aerobic and strength components should always be part of your fitness routine, but that the precise balance will vary, depending on your age. To reiterate what we said earlier:

- If you're forty years old or younger, aerobics should compose 80 percent of your workout time; strength training, 20 percent.
- If you're forty-one to fifty years old, you do 70 percent aerobics and 30 percent strength.
- If you're fifty-one to sixty, it's 60 percent aerobics and 40 percent strength.
- If you're over sixty, split your time this way: 55 percent aerobics, 45 percent strength.

Tyler: I agree with this approach, and, in fact, my own workout schedule conforms to the forty-and-under recommendation. I typically run six or seven times a week, for a total of twenty-five to forty miles. But I also play an hour or so of basketball two to three times a week as part of an informal basketball league.

In addition, I spend a couple of days a week doing strength work on the weight-training machines at the Cooper Aerobics Center. I'll usually do this strength work on days when I've had a relatively light running or basketball workout. I use a trainer when I do the strength work, not because I don't know how to manage my resistance work, but because the trainer becomes a hot button for me: In other words, I'm more likely to do the strength work regularly and not skip sessions if I know I'm accountable for showing up at a certain time and place with my trainer.

Also, more often than not, I'll work out in some way every day in a given week. That's not so much to firm up habits that I've already developed as it is to *feel good*. Although I rely on a number of motivational triggers, probably my main motivational hot button is the Feel-Good Hot Button.

Question: What's the main requirement for those in their thirties and forties who want to *start* strong—with the healthiest lifestyle possible?

Tyler: Decide what's most important in your life—identify your two or three major goals. For example, you may determine that you want to be energetic enough to put in ten hours at the office, but then to have plenty of steam left for your family when you get home. Or you may be a parent in your forties, fifties, or sixties who still wants to be able to compete athletically with your kids (or grandkids!).

Then, proceed to make the seven health start-ups in Part Two a permanent part of your life. This program will give you the high levels of energy and stamina necessary to realize your goals.

Question: What's the main requirement for those in their fifties or older who want to *finish* strong—with high-functioning, maximum longevity?

Ken: Basically, I would agree with what Tyler has said—and expand on it a little.

First, know what you want to accomplish in your remaining years. Maybe you want to continue to work well into your seventies or eighties—an age range when many people are slowing down markedly or become incapacitated. Or maybe you want to devote as much time to your favorite charitable work as you have been to your regular job. As you continue to work in your retirement years, you'll find that the frequency of incapacitating diseases decreases, along with the cost of your health care.

Then, focus on maximizing your physical powers to realize these objectives. A special goal of older people should also be to avoid the dozen or so years that most spend in states of incapacity—as a result of such health issues as neurological and heart problems, bad backs, broken hips, porous bones, or weak muscles.

Question: **Once you've set your priorities, what are the most powerful motivational factors to help you stick to your guns and achieve your priorities?**

Tyler: In my age group, I find one of the most common motivators is a network of straight-talking friends who will remind and advise me when I get off track. The best friends to support a fitness effort are those who are ready to join me in a workout.

Ken: In my generation, especially among those with a managerial or executive background, important motivations are a desire to be disciplined, work hard, and succeed in achieving professional or charitable goals.

Also, when you pass fifty, and certainly when you move into your sixties and seventies, countering the process of aging becomes an increasingly important motivation. If I had to pick a decade that would make the biggest impression on most people, it would be the period from fifty-five to sixty-five. When you reach this age, just *looking* at yourself in the mirror—examining that expanding waistline or seeing the muscle tone disappearing from arms, legs, and abdomen—may be enough to light a fire under you.

Question: **What's the biggest emotional barrier to starting and finishing strong?**

Ken and Tyler: Stress—especially out-of-control stress.

Question: **Name one or two major causes you've noticed for destructive stress at different age levels.**

Tyler: For young people, stress arises from uncertainty about their careers, their own future, and the future of their children. Divorce or another personal relationship problem is another big factor that may add to the pressure.

Ken: For older people, stress most commonly arises from financial pressures and worries about health problems, the direction children are taking in their lives, and retirement. Also, many marriages break up as couples move into the "empty nest" phase, with their children gone from home.

Question: **What's the best way to reduce or manage bad stress as we grow older?**

Tyler: Get philosophical or spiritual perspective on your pressures—understand that there will always be a tomorrow to deal with today. Draw support from personal relationships. Take time off from work.

Among those in the thirty-five to forty-five age range, striking a balance between your work and personal life is critical—including wise management of responsibilities related to job, spirituality, family, friends, and fun. "Work hard, play hard" may be a cliché, but I believe in it.

Ken: Cultivate your spiritual life, and exercise at the end of the day. But keep working. Now in my midseventies, I still work twelve hours a day. For me, taking time off just pushes today's tasks to tomorrow—and increases stress.

Most younger people aren't thinking about what they'll be doing after they pass sixty, but my advice would be this: *definitely don't retire!* I'm not saying you shouldn't take some time off to smell the roses as you grow older. Certainly, Millie and I spend as many weeks as we can every year at our mountain home in Colorado, on cruises, or on other extended breaks from the daily routine. But actually, most of my holidays are working holidays.

I'll typically give lectures on cruises, and I'll spend time writing and doing research as part of my routine in Colorado. Also, I'll always include a fitness routine as part of my daily schedule, whether it's walking or mountain-biking in the Rockies, or walking the decks and doing strength work in the gym of a cruise ship.

My main objective is not to reinforce my natural workaholic tendencies, but to keep my mind and body active. That's the only way to hold off the inevitable wear and tear of aging.

Question: **What are the top health habits to maximize longevity?**

Tyler: Start at a young age with a good diet and fitness habits; begin regular wellness exams; choose personal risks wisely. Feel free to eat steaks and sweets—but in moderation. Also, be realistic with the goals you place on yourself. If you expect too much of yourself, you're more likely to become discouraged and give up.

As I age, I hope to follow the example of my father—who goes mountain-biking and skiing on black-diamond slopes. I want to do those things when I'm seventy-five.

Ken: To have the best chance of getting to seventy-five and beyond, I'd focus on four things: don't smoke, eliminate obesity, avoid inactivity, and control stress.

Question: **If you're only thirty-five and in good health, do you really need a complete medical exam?**

Tyler: Yes—to establish a baseline of health measurements. That way, your physician can readily see changes over time in blood pressure, coronary artery plaque, fitness, and cholesterol.

Also, having a complete exam acts as a great motivator. When you know the levels of every component of your blood, your precise coronary artery calcification, and your stress-test fitness classification, you know exactly where you're weak and where you're strong. The results of the exam challenge you with a clear-cut set of goals you need to achieve.

Question: **How often does a fifty-year-old need a complete medical exam?**

Ken: Annually, though your physician will order special tests, such as colonoscopies, less often.

I concur completely with Tyler about the fitness exams being a great motivational device. One of the most effective hot buttons to help you begin and stick with a fitness regimen is the annual exam—and I mean a *comprehensive* preventive-medicine exam, with such features as stress tests, which will allow you to compare your performance with that of other people the same age and gender. That's a real motivator.

Question: **How useful are the futuristic "virtual" diagnostic tools used at the Cooper Clinic—such as the virtual colonoscopy, the ultra-fast CT scan, and the new CT angiography (CTA)?**

Ken and Tyler: Extremely useful—and they should begin in your forties or fifties. They're noninvasive and increasingly accurate in helping us identify major problems early, such as pulmonary, pancreatic, and liver cancer, and the buildup of plaque or obstructions in the coronary arteries. These new tests can greatly reduce the odds that physicians will overlook a life-threatening condition. So play it smart and resolve to find out about any health problems while you can still do something about them.

Question: **How much do you have to pay for a "super" medical exam—with such features as a fast CT scan, stress test, colonoscopy, and blood work for "emerging risk factors" like levels of homocysteine and C-reactive protein? Is it worth the cost?**

Ken and Tyler: It's not cheap, but a complete exam can be invaluable in giving your doctors a head start in finding and treating various cancers and heart problems. Currently, plan to pay $1,500 to $3,500 for a complete workup.

What if your insurance doesn't cover this outlay? In fact, many types of health insurance may not pay for preventive-medicine benefits, or may pay only a small portion of the tab. But it's best to think about the payment in another way: actually, you should look at this annual payment as a *part* of your regular health insurance coverage. In other words, traditional health insurance is really *disease* insurance (just as life insurance is really *death* insurance). In contrast, payment for a complete preventive-medicine examination is insurance against getting sick and dying prematurely—and, as such, is *the best health insurance and life insurance you can buy.*

Question: Are there certain fitness or other health "land mines" that we should be alert to at different ages?

Tyler: Those people I know in their thirties and forties have to watch for several health traps that can undercut health or fitness efforts. Some important ones include:

- *A sense of immortality.* In other words, there's a prevailing notion among many young people that they'll "live forever" and therefore don't have to worry about establishing good health and fitness habits. They think to themselves, "I'll eat better or start working out when I'm older." But too often these young people find that when they get older, they have run out of time. They may develop a serious health condition earlier than they had expected. Or sedentary living, overeating, and other negative health habits may have become so ingrained that it may seem impossible to change them.

- *Drug abuse, including marijuana use.* A person may get into a drug habit and begin to experience temporary psychological or emotional benefits, which quickly wear off and usually lead to *negative* addiction—as opposed to the positive addiction afforded by aerobic exercise.

- *Smoking.* The widely circulated medical evidence about how smoking leads to heart disease and cancer should impress smokers so much that they quit. But, usually, younger people consider themselves immortal. They think, "Others may die from smoking, but that won't happen to me." And they may point to some ninety-year-old they know who has been smoking all his or her life.

Unfortunately the chances are excellent that they won't become that exception, and they will pay a terrible price for the habit.

- *Alcohol abuse.* The college binge drinker can easily turn into the middle-aged binge drinker. And by most definitions, binge drinkers are one type of alcoholic. Alcohol abuse is often rampant among my age group, accounting not only for occupational and relationship problems, but also for devastating auto accidents that often hurt the nondrinkers more than the drinkers. As the person ages, the problem just gets worse, unless steps are taken to deal with it.
- *Sexually transmitted disease (STD) and sexual addiction.* Those of us in the younger generation have grown up in a culture that places few, if any, restraints on extramarital sexual activity. As a result, we are facing a huge number of cases of STDs and other problems among many in their forties or younger.

Ken: Perhaps the worst problem I run into among those fifty and older is *a tendency for people to give up on a fitness program before they even make a start.*

When you finally wake up and realize what bad shape you're in, there may be a tendency to say, "What's the point in trying to do anything? I'm too old and too far gone."

Men may be the most inclined to give up. Many will take a good look at their oversize belly and decide that they would prefer to live with their obesity and rely on prescription medication or even surgery to correct cardiovascular or other risk factors. An older woman may have a similar response, but I find that women are typically more willing to make an effort to recover some of their lost youth than are many men.

On the other hand, there are plenty of older men, as well as women, who aren't quitters and who embrace their poor condition as a challenge rather than an early death sentence. What gets them moving? The one thing that most often causes patients of both genders to embark on a program is a bad report on a complete physical exam.

When you see in black and white the report on your high cholesterol, low fitness status from a treadmill test, or calcified arteries, the first response may be shock and fear. But when you hear that it's possible to improve those numbers, you'll almost certainly want to do something about them. Many people are fascinated when they learn that you can grow healthier as you grow older—and not necessarily the reverse. And who determines your future? *You* do, by eliminating cigarette smoking, inactivity, obesity, and stress—in that order.

Of course, many motivating factors, such as the Numbers-Game Hot Button and the Fear-of-Death Hot Button, may also come into play with the medical exam. Or for some, the Physical-Function and Mental-Function Hot Buttons may trump all others. The greatest fear expressed by many older patients is that they cannot stand the thought of spending a decade or more confined to a wheelchair, or in some other predicament with impaired physical or mental faculties. And that brings us to our final topic in Part One—the importance of "squaring off the curve" of life.

Fifteen

The Secret to
Maintaining Motivation

A t some point in life, most people who make a strong start on a personal health and fitness program run into some problem, event, or issue that threatens to derail the whole process—and put them back at square one in their development. In our combined decades of practicing preventive medicine, we've identified at least three reasons a strong start may turn into a weak finish:

- ***You may become discouraged by the natural aging process.***

At one time or another, it happens to everybody. No matter how well-conditioned you are physically after you pass fifty or sixty, it's virtually impossible to look at a picture of your younger self and then gaze into the mirror and not think, "I really look older." Or, "I've lost that youthful shape." Or, "I've really gone downhill."

The next step for many people is to think, "What's the point in working out or watching my diet? Isn't my effort just a finger in the dike? Why not eat, drink, and be merry?"

The key to avoiding this pitfall is to remember that the whole point of your effort is to hold off or delay aging as long as possible—a goal that medical research says is quite possible. Remember the objective of "squaring off the curve": your Start Strong, Finish Strong program is designed to help you maintain a high level of physical and mental functioning as long as possible. But even though the curve of life will eventually be squared for all of us, there's no reason to be discouraged. There is every reason to be realistic, however, and to make the most of the years that may well lie far out into the future.

- *You may become bored with your program—or neglect it for other reasons.*

This trap is quite common, especially among those who haven't quite developed a firm fitness habit or whose way of life changes radically in some way.

For example, it's easy to lapse into mental and physical complacency or paralysis after a divorce, a job change, a major move, or some other highly dislocating and stressful event. It's important to expect events like these to occur—and to establish a "personal policy" well ahead of their appearance that you will forge ahead with your program, despite the distraction or resistance. In fact, some of our patients have found that resorting to a fitness program with renewed vigor is just the antidote they need to make it past a particularly devastating life crisis.

Another problem that plagues many exercisers is staging a "comeback" after a holiday or vacation that involves a lot of sitting around and overeating. Some people have actually abandoned their entire program permanently after such a break. To protect against this pitfall, it's a good idea to schedule an exercise time during your time off—and especially during a lengthy vacation. In fact, vacations are a *great* time to *increase* your level of exercise, especially if you've planned an active or athletic time away from your regular daily life.

Finally, if you just feel yourself getting bored with your program, try varying it. If you're a jogger, for instance, you might inject a game sport like tennis or basketball into your program. See the suggestions in Chapter 3 for finding a hot button that really turns on your motivation once again.

• *You may suffer a serious injury or illness.*

No matter how hard you work out or how much care you take with your diet or other aspects of your lifestyle, you may face your greatest challenge when you're hit with an unexpected injury or illness. Broken hips in particular are notorious for ending the physical mobility and vigor of older people—often for the rest of their lives.

In such situations, you may find that you have no choice but to lay off your regular exercise program for weeks or even months. How can you cope with this sort of challenge—and return in the end to finish strong?

Ken: When the Strong Become Weak

To understand the importance of finishing life strong, it's important to grasp just how weak you really are—as I was forced to do when I was on the verge of celebrating my seventy-fourth birthday.

I had fallen into the habit of regarding myself as practically invulnerable. Even when I had a bad cold or some other health complaint, I would still come to work. The reason, I must confess, was in part so that I could point out to my family, colleagues, and lecture audiences that "I have not missed a day of work due to illness since 1956!"

But still, I had to admit privately to myself that the signs of age were beginning to creep up on me. For a couple of years, for instance, I had noticed that when I was jogging, I'd occasionally lose strength for a second or so in my right leg. A specialist who checked me out with an MRI (magnetic resonance imaging scanner, which takes three-dimensional pictures of internal body parts) diagnosed the problem as a torn cartilage and the buildup of fluid in my right knee.

The condition had been developing over many years, probably beginning with a basketball injury in high school and with intense workouts as an intercollegiate miler at the University of Oklahoma. The problem worsened during decades of daily running, including training for marathons and other competitive distance events—and finally began to affect my mobility. As a result of the knee problem, I eventually had to limit my daily workouts to race-walking instead of jogging, and I even found I was having difficulty going up and down stairs.

But as concerned as I was about my leg, I refused to give up on a family ski vacation we had planned in Beaver Creek, Colorado. So after returning from Boston, we headed off to our place in the snowy mountains. Immediately after we arrived, I headed for the intermediate-level Blue slopes at Vail. After skiing all day, I went home feeling pretty confident. But just to be safe, I made an appointment the next morning to see orthopedic surgeon Dr. Richard Steadman. Richard had worked with the U.S. Olympic team and is generally regarded as one of the best in his specialty of sports medicine.

After he looked at my MRI scans, he said, "You've torn a cartilage in that knee, and you have some scar formation, which is the result of trauma over the years."

I thought about all those races and workouts over the last few decades—but my most pressing concern was, "What does this mean for my holiday?"

"I think you can keep on skiing this week, so long as you take it easy," he finally concluded. "Then I'll see you next summer, and we'll do an arthroscopic procedure. That should repair the problem and may even get you running again."

That sounded fine to me, especially the part about my being able to continue skiing on this vacation. So early the next day, I was back on the same easy slopes with my wife, Millie, and some friends of ours—though I looked longingly after Tyler and Angie, who had decided to head for one of the more difficult black diamond runs.

I really didn't have anything to complain about. The conditions were great, with clear blue skies and crisp, if thin, air at an 11,000-foot altitude. But around midmorning, I began to get a little bored. I kept thinking about Tyler and how much fun I knew he was having on the more advanced slopes.

"Couldn't be any harm in trying a little harder slope," I thought.

So I decided to take a shot at the Centennial slope, which is definitely not recommended for beginners. "But I'm not a beginner," I reminded myself. "So there's no problem."

That was my first big mistake.

Because Millie and our other companions had decided not to join me, I found myself skiing alone on the Centennial run in snow conditions that weren't exactly ideal. I had to work my way around a lot of rocks and sticks that were protruding through a light covering of snow, and even though I started out fairly slowly, before long I began to pick up speed.

As I swept down the slope, the distractions of these natural obstacles made me miss a four-foot mogul. I lost my balance, shot off the main run, and slammed down on my back. Finally, I slid to a stop, with my legs twisted under me, a dozen or so yards below the mogul.

Even as I lay there, half-stunned among the rocks and sticks and spotty snow, I could tell I had hurt my already damaged knee. How much, I wasn't sure. But it's easy for an avid skier to go into denial if he thinks there's any chance he'll have to interrupt his fun. As I labored for about fifteen minutes to retrieve my skis and put them on again, the thought crossed my mind that maybe I should wait for the ski patrol to pick me up. But I had never had to resort to the ski patrol before—and I could already hear Tyler and the others ragging me about getting old and soft. Also, even though my knee hurt, I could stand on it. So I figured I would tough it out.

That was my second big mistake.

Looking down the mountain, I could see I was well over halfway to the bottom. So I got back onto the main run and headed downhill, carving my way back and forth through the snow among several other moguls. But the knee pain not only failed to go away, it started to get worse.

When I finally reached a flat area near the restaurant at the bottom of the slope, I found I could hardly stand by myself. Tyler, who was relaxing in the restaurant after finishing his runs, saw me struggling through the snow and rushed out to give a hand. He then accompanied me to the chairlift so that I could go to the base of the mountain, but I refused his offer. I didn't want to admit to myself that I was really hurt.

That was my third mistake.

When I arrived home, no one else was there—and our driveway is quite steep. It was also extremely slippery as a result of a light coating of ice. So I had to struggle by myself down the entire incline, all the while putting even more stress on my injured knee. When Millie arrived home, she found me lying on our bed in excruciating pain.

"I have a real problem," I said.

I could tell from her expression that she knew there was big trouble because I never complained of pain or injury or illness. With her help, I started icing the knee to reduce the swelling, and I also started taking some prescription painkillers that I had at the house. But the pain continued to build during the rest of that day and into night. Without a doubt, that was the worst night of pain I'd ever endured.

The next day, I went in to see Dr. Steadman, who put me through a battery of tests, including both CT (computerized tomography) and MRI scans. After evaluating my situation, he confirmed that I had indeed ripped up the cartilage and tendons, and broken the tibia plateau in my right knee. So he scheduled me for surgery the following day.

I was placed under general anesthesia for a two-and-a-half-hour operation, during which the surgical team bolted together the shattered pieces of my right knee. After the operation, they kept me in the hospital for an extra day just to avoid the danger of a staph infection or some other postoperative problem. Immediately upon my release, I plunged into a week of physical therapy, which involved several hours a day of rehabilitative movement, including stretching and pumping both my legs to prevent withering of the muscles and tendons.

At the end of that week, we flew home to Dallas. Now, you might think that even if I had smashed up my knee, I still had it pretty nice, at least compared to most people in that situation. After all, I was vacationing in a posh Colorado mountain resort, and my physician was the best orthopedic sports surgeon in the business. On top of all that, I'm a person who knows as much about preventive medicine as anyone, and I've seen every conceivable injury or medical condition imaginable. Finally, when I returned to Dallas and the Cooper Clinic, I could expect to have access to some of the best rehabilitative specialists in the world.

So how could anyone in my position possibly have any concerns or worries?

Actually, given the seriousness of my injury, it was easy to be worried. One big problem was that I found myself sinking into a postoperative depression immediately after my surgery. I had seen this happen to many of my patients after they had suffered debilitating injuries, including leg, knee, and hip fractures. But somehow, I had never imagined it could happen to me. Being an extremely self-reliant person, I had always figured that I would quickly gain perspective on any situation and bounce back effortlessly.

But that didn't happen.

As I fell into a funk contemplating my predicament, my resting heart rate accelerated. My blood pressure readings increased. And feelings of anxiety and nervousness began to overwhelm me. Dr. Steadman, who actually lectures on this postoperative depression phenomenon, told me, "Expect it. Understand that it's the normal thing."

He also explained—and I already knew, at least intellectually—that I was almost certainly experiencing physiologic withdrawal from regular aerobic exercise. Before the accident, my daily workouts had flooded my body with morphinelike endorphins and other neurotransmitters that promote feelings of well-being. But when I turned off that internal faucet of secretions, my body and emotions responded with withdrawal-like symptoms that triggered depression, confusion, and anxiety.

So I *knew* what was happening to me medically and biologically, and I *understood* the usual emotional response. But knowledge and understanding don't necessarily produce a cure. So I remained depressed immediately after my surgery.

Then within the next ten days, I settled into a more general, ongoing state of depression as I started using crutches and contemplated just how restricted my life and movements had become. The down mood intensified as Dr. Steadman's instructions sank in about how I had to care for myself in the ensuing weeks.

"Your leg shouldn't bear weight for about eight weeks," he had said.

For me, that was almost like a death sentence. I was used to lengthy race-walking workouts every evening after work. Now, I couldn't walk at all. Even my prayer life changed. I still spent a half hour or so every morning with my Bible open in front of me on my desk, but the injury caused me to struggle more with my devotions and to focus more on prayers of personal healing. I explored how high-tech, contemporary medicine might be combined with spiritual disciplines, such as prayer.

But no quick spiritual solution emerged, no magic elixir lifted the depression. Even when I'd have a reasonably good day, at least in comparison with all the bad days I'd been experiencing, I wouldn't automatically say to myself, as I had in the past: "Ah, there's light at the end of this tunnel."

Instead, I'd think, "Maybe that light is a train!"

But then, as time inched along during this early period of recovery, I began to consider that, even though I would never have chosen this path, there might be good reasons or a positive outcome for my debilitating injury. For one thing, I was being forced to reflect extensively, from an internal, empathetic vantage point, on the difficult medical problems confronted by many of my patients. Bit by bit, I began to see *their* problems from *their* perspective—and not just from mine, as the objective medical observer and healer. I discovered increasingly that I could literally *feel* their fears, their anxieties, their depressions—and their frustrated questions:

How long will it take this thing to heal?
Why doesn't the process move faster?
Will it *ever* heal?
Will I be one of those older patients who suffers an injury that impairs his functioning for the rest of his life?

It was frightening to consider that, as a result of that accident on that ski slope, it was indeed possible that I might be transformed from a man preparing to square off the curve of good health, fitness, and functioning in the last part of life, to one who would be relegated to a slow decline in total well-being. In fact, it was one of the worst nightmares imaginable for me, as the person widely recognized as the "father of aerobics." After all, the *Encyclopaedia Britannica* had traced the invention of the concept of aerobic exercise directly back to me, and I had provided the *Oxford English Dictionary* with its classic definition of the word. So how could I bear the idea of possibly spending the rest of my life on crutches, in a wheelchair, or in some other disabled state? What would my patients and followers think? Would my failure to stay healthy and fit doom the future of the movement I had worked so hard to establish?

Yet even as I wrestled with these internal specters, I found I was starting to look at my patients in a new light. While I sat there in my office going over their charts, I'd meditate long and hard on Mary's broken hip, John's chronic back injury, Sam's recent bypass surgery. In particular, I'd ponder in new, fresh ways how each might be feeling about his or her particular health struggle. And I was able to say, "I understand now. I can feel those feelings. I know those emotions intimately."

As I was forced into a slow-motion mode of recovery, I also found myself appreciating more than ever before the "support troops" that keep a clinic going and a patient like me on track toward maximal recovery. With new eyes, I saw how much my own success depended on my executive secretary, Cynthia Grantham, and other staff members.

My physical therapist, Dale Smith, pushed me to work out even when I didn't feel like doing the exercises necessary to keep my affected muscles, tendons, and ligaments from tightening up or atrophying. I slept with a CPM, or "continuous passive motion machine," which kept my injured leg moving back and forth, up and down at night. I also learned how important it was for me to exercise both legs, not just the injured one. The reason? Physiologically, exercising the good leg actually works synergistically to promote improvement in the bad leg.

But in the end, knowing that my improvement was up to me, I always tried to do more than what was required. When the therapist told me to do twenty leg lifts, I'd do thirty. When I was cautioned not to put weight on my bad leg, I'd negotiate with my orthopedic specialist in Dallas, Dr. Jim Montgomery, to put twenty-five to thirty pounds on it, then forty, and then fifty. From my own research, I knew that bones are likely to grow more quickly if they are subjected to regular weight-bearing exercise.

Warning: Even though I sometimes pushed to go beyond what my physician had prescribed, I always monitored my body responses closely and cleared any unusual departures from his recommendations before I tried them. In any event, if you find yourself in a situation similar to mine, I would strongly recommend that you follow closely the instructions of your physician or other medical professional. It's always better to proceed a little more slowly than you'd like with your recovery than to move too quickly and risk another injury.

Although I knew I was sometimes pressing too hard, my body always signaled danger with a thrust of pain that told me it was time to let up. Also, I found early on that I had to respect the natural healing process: all bones heal slowly. I learned that if I tried to push myself beyond what was reasonable—if I neglected the all-important principles of periodic rest and progressive improvement—I would pay a price in pain and risk setbacks that would delay my goal of swift recovery.

But I stuck to my rehabilitation plan, and about eight weeks after my injury, I was walking on my own again. In short order, I could cover more than a mile every day, and I regularly increased the distance and intensity of my exercise outings. My leg muscles remained weak for a while longer but now they are almost back to normal due not only to walking but also to cycling and a weight-training program. Equally important has been my emotional healing—the depression is gone.

On balance, then, I know that my accident on the Colorado slopes has made me a more sensitive, understanding—and humble—health-care giver. And I'll never again boast that I've never missed a day of work because of a personal health problem.

Finally, if you're ever tempted to give up on your program *for any reason,* I want to leave you with the memory of a true story that should immediately get you back on track. Frankly, I have yet to run into anyone with as much reason as Rick Salewske had to avoid or quit a program.

Rick's Story: Making the Impossible Possible

It may be that something is still holding you back from getting started on a life-changing program—or from continuing with your original resolve. Maybe you're just recovering from a major debilitating illness or injury and you can't imagine how you could return to any semblance of your healthy youthful self. Or perhaps you're so far out of shape that you think you're without hope.

So what are the outer limits of what the Start Strong, Finish Strong strategy might do for you? To see how you can make the impossible possible, consider the astonishing real-life saga of our friend Rick Salewske.

THE POSSIBILITIES: THE LONGEVITY DIET IN ACTION

When big-boned, nineteen-year-old Rick Salewske moved from Michigan to Dallas in 1981, he stood six foot one and weighed about 220. He thought he actually looked a little skinny. But because this was the first time he had been away from his family, things quickly careened out of control in his life, especially his daily eating habits.

"I was young, single, and on my own for the first time in my life—and I didn't hesitate to start drinking and wolfing down junk food," he recalls. "That got me into a very bad lifestyle."

Predictably, his weight began to shoot up. Within three years, he had gained about sixty pounds. In fact, the only thing that seemed to keep him from gaining more was his cigarette habit.

"I was smoking two packs a day," he confesses.

Still, his weight continued to climb until he hit 320 pounds in 1990.

"Being alone much of the time, I got a little depressed, so I turned to food to comfort myself," he explains. "After a bad day at work, I'd feast on ice cream, fast foods like burgers, and peanut butter and jelly sandwiches. I'd eat three sandwiches at one sitting, plus a big bag of chips."

Then, in 1990, he quit his cigarette smoking. "I went cold turkey," he says.

Even though not smoking improved his risk status for heart disease and cancer, this positive health step operated as a double-edged sword: Rick began to eat even more, and his weight skyrocketed higher than he had ever imagined possible. By the mid-1990s, he topped four hundred pounds.

A Seating Crisis: "When I hit the low four hundreds, my life really changed," he says. "For the first time, it became extremely difficult just to live a normal life. I couldn't sit in ordinary chairs because my waist was sixty inches. I couldn't go to sporting events because I couldn't fit into the stadium seats. And airline travel gradually became impossible."

After he passed four hundred, he started having to use two seats in planes because he couldn't fit into just one. "I was really lucky at first because there always seemed to be an extra seat, usually in the back part of the plane," he recalls. "But then I took a flight where all the seats were filled except one. I asked the guy sitting next to that empty seat if he could take my assigned seat so that I'd have two. If he hadn't agreed, I'd have been kicked off the plane."

Then on a subsequent trip Rick found that, despite having two seats, he couldn't fasten his seat belt. "It may have been the most embarrassing moment of my life," he admits, as he watched the people in nearby seats staring at him.

He told the flight attendant, "This belt won't reach around my stomach. What can I do?"

"I'll get you an extension," she replied.

Rick had no idea what an extension was until she explained that it was the unattached belt she used when she gave her little lecture to passengers to show them how the seat belts worked. She said that she could actually attach that demonstration belt to a regular belt to give overweight passengers a little more stomach room.

"So the last few times I flew, I had to face the embarrassment of asking the flight attendant to give me one of those extensions," he says.

Finally, as flights became increasingly crowded around 1995, he gave up flying altogether because, even though he could get seat-belt extensions, he couldn't count on finding an empty second seat.

An All-time High: Through the late 1990s, Rick's weight continued to climb toward the five-hundred-pound mark. And increasingly, he attracted stares and gibes.

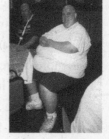

"In the grocery store, kids stared at me and tugged at their parents, saying, 'Look at how fat that guy is,'" he remembers. "Once in a restaurant, a kid poked his dad and pointed toward me. The father grabbed the kid and took him toward the bathroom, all the while hollering at him. I felt bad. After all, he was just a little kid."

Finally, by the year 2000, Rick reached his all-time-high weight of 538. "You hit a point where life becomes so difficult that you just don't feel like doing anything but eating and drinking," he says. "All I did was go to work, and then at the end of the day I'd head for a bar, where I'd drink. Finally, I'd go home, where I'd eat a lot of food."

Rock Bottom: People still invited him over for special occasions, such as Thanksgiving. But he began to make excuses because he felt he didn't have anything nice to wear anymore, and it was so hard to get up when he took a seat. "I actually broke a couple of chairs in people's homes," he says.

Even driving became an onerous task. He already had one of the biggest cars available, a Chevrolet Caprice, and adjusted the seat as far back as it would go. But the steering wheel still rubbed against his stomach to the point that he wore holes in the fabric in front of several pairs of pants. Also, he had to lower the windows before he got into the car because he couldn't reach over to lower them after he was seated. To make matters even more intolerable, whenever he bent over, his stomach compressed his torso and lungs, so that he felt out of breath.

Becoming more and more depressed, Rick tried some ad hoc positive-thinking ploys in a fruitless effort to cheer himself up. "I said to myself, 'I'm a good person. I work. I have a house. I love my parents. I don't smoke. I don't do drugs. So why do I have to lose weight?' Yet I was defiant. I said, 'The world should change for Rick!'" Down deep, he knew the world had not been made for a five-hundred-pound person.

When it became obvious that the world would not change, he became more depressed—until finally, a series of events brought him to a critical juncture in his weight-and-health saga.

First, because he was now unable to fly, he drove home to Michigan to see his family for Christmas of 1999. Over breakfast, his parents put the issue to him directly: "Your sisters have been crying because they think you're going to die."

Rick didn't argue. Instead, he replied, "I know they care about me." Furthermore, the message began to work on his mind as he drove back to Dallas.

Then in the spring of 2000, a recruiter offered him a job back in his hometown in Michigan, but there was a catch that made Rick hesitate. "The recruiter didn't know my weight," he recalls. "He never saw me, just contacted me and arranged for me to be hired over the phone."

The first thought that came to Rick was, "Okay, so am I really going to walk into that place of business weighing 538 pounds? What happens if a chair they offer has arms and I can't get into it? Or what if it breaks? How will the other employees react to me?"

So he leveled with the rep from the new company who had offered him the job: "I have to tell you something. I weigh more than five hundred pounds."

"Can you do your job?" the man replied.

"Yeah, I can do it."

"Then that's okay. We'll hire you."

But Rick still had misgivings—doubts that deepened when he got an invitation to his twentieth high school class reunion, which was scheduled for the summer of 2000. The more he thought about that event, the more intimidated he became at the possible problems he might face: "People will freak out when they see me. I'll never get a suit that fits right. What am I going to do?"

Finally, he made up an excuse. He said he wouldn't be able to attend the reunion because he had just bought a house and would be closing on it. Also, he turned down the job from the Michigan company, and he thought that was the end of the matter. But then, he got a call that turned his life upside down.

The Turning Point: Rick had worked for Clark Steel Framing for nineteen years and had risen to the position of manager of the receiving department. The CEO, who made a special trip to Dallas from the company headquarters in Ohio, immediately set up a dinner meeting with Rick.

After they got settled at the restaurant, the CEO pulled out a copy of an e-mail he had received indicating that Rick had been offered the job in Michigan. "I appreciate that you turned this down," he said. "But, Rick, I'm selfish. I want you to work for me for the next twenty years. Yet if you don't lose that extra weight, you won't last that long. What can we do to help you? How about surgery?"

"I don't want to have surgery," Rick replied.

"So how are you going to lose that weight?" the CEO countered.

"If I start eating healthy and exercise, the weight will come off," Rick said, rather weakly. "I just have to burn more calories than I take in—for the rest of my life."

"That's the most difficult way of doing it," the CEO said, and fell silent. It was obvious that the chief executive wasn't at all convinced by Rick's reply. But what the CEO couldn't be expected to fathom was the change that was just beginning inside his employee's head.

"I saw that this man cared about me and believed in me," Rick says. "And somehow that made me *begin* to think that maybe I really could achieve what both of us desired—the loss of hundreds of extra pounds. You could say that I started to *want* to change and to *believe* I could change—but I still wasn't quite sure how to go about it."

Then, after they had finished their meal and were walking out of the restaurant, the answer to Rick's dilemma began to emerge. Unexpectedly, the CEO said, "I'll make you a deal. If you can find a program to lose weight, we'll pay up to two thousand dollars for it. But the deadline for finding the program is three months from now."

He even suggested that Rick try a specific program at the Cooper Aerobics Center. So Rick got online and found the "Cooper Lean Program" at the Cooper Clinic. Then he used four hundred dollars of his boss's money to pay for ten sessions with a dietician and ten sessions with a trainer over a three-month period.

Rick's Start-up Medical Exam: Before he embarked on any diet or exercise program, Rick followed medical advice to get checked out thoroughly by a physician. He decided to consult with his regular doctor, who arranged for a complete battery of tests, including a stress test and a comprehensive set of blood tests.

These showed that his heart was healthy but that his cholesterol was high at 250 mg/dl. So his physician prescribed Lipitor to get it down. Also, because his blood pressure was elevated at 170/95, the doctor put him on a diuretic. But overall, the exam confirmed that Rick was ready to begin his downward journey from his all-time-high weight of 538 pounds.

It Really Does Begin in Your Head: Next, Rick responded to a nagging sense that he wasn't quite ready "upstairs" to make his best effort with a fitness program. "I knew I had to do something to change my terrible attitudes and habits—and to get rid of those feelings I always got into my head when I passed a McDonald's," he says. "I had to fix what was above my neck if I hoped to alter the rest of my body."

His solution was to take another seven hundred dollars from his boss's gift to pay for eight one-hour sessions at a hypnotism and mental training clinic. During the initial mental training sessions, the therapists put him in a room in a big, reclining chair, with soothing music in the background. When he was comfortable, a therapist would begin to talk to him in a low voice until she had determined that he was "totally released" from his normal, everyday thoughts. Then, she began to recite statements, which he repeated, emphasizing principles that he had decided he wanted to believe in:

I'll crave healthy foods.
I won't eat red meat.
Water is my beverage of choice.
I won't beat up on myself.
I'll get right back on the program if I slip.
I'll start liking myself.

"I wasn't actually hypnotized during these sessions," he explains. "I stayed fully conscious. But I did begin to *believe* that I could train myself to eat better. I remembered that when I quit smoking, I really became convinced I had the power to overcome that craving. It was similar with food. The mental training gradually gave me a certainty that I could cut back on my eating and lose 300 pounds—or go from 538 to 238."

The Search for "Motivational Foods": Rick then huddled with his dietician at the Cooper Clinic to design a meal plan.

"We worked hard to find good foods that I could enjoy," he recalls. "I had never eaten breakfast, but the dietician said, 'You've got to start eating breakfast!'"

So they settled on a breakfast consisting of bran cereal, bananas, strawberries, orange juice, and 1 percent fat milk. Rick had made it clear that he really liked fruit, and so they also identified a set of fruit-oriented snack foods: bananas, apples, grapes, and oranges.

For lunch, he decided he liked the Lean Cuisine meals—and also he was allotted more fruit, maybe three to four pieces. A snack later in the day would also consist of a piece of his favorite fruit.

"Won't all this fruit give me too much sugar?" he asked the dietician.

Her answer: "Don't worry about it—your blood glucose level and other readings show you're okay with the fruit."

She assured him that the Cooper Clinic would continue to monitor his blood sugar and triglycerides, just to be sure that the fruit didn't upset his blood balance. But subsequent tests showed that he didn't have a problem with sugar, no matter how much fruit he ate. Also, after adding up his total intake of calories, the dietician demonstrated clearly that he was still taking in many fewer calories with the fruit than he had been with his peanut butter sandwiches, ice cream, and other snacks.

But for dinner, Rick says, "I knew I had a problem. I like fast food. I really needed to pick a food I could enjoy that was healthy."

So he told the dietician, "I can't go from McDonald's to carrots and broccoli. What about a turkey sandwich? Can I have two of them?"

"Sure," she said, "and extra fruit as well. But no salt, okay? Your blood pressure is still too high, and we want to do everything we can to bring that down."

A major objective in these discussions and negotiations had been to find a set of healthy foods that Rick really liked and could substitute for higher-calorie offerings that were a threat to his weight and health. In other words, he needed to pick "motivational foods," which would entice him to eat the right way, rather than the wrong way.

All in the Numbers: Finally, with Rick's meal plan set, the dietician ran all of his chosen foods through our database and found that his new diet consisted of only about 1,500 to 1,800 calories per day, versus the 3,000-plus calories that he had been consuming daily in the past. Because 3,500 calories amounted to one pound of fat, he should be losing nearly a half-pound of fat per day.

"For the first two weeks of the program, those two turkey sandwiches a day curbed my craving for fast foods," he says. "It's all in your head. You start craving it, and you give in. But if you head off the craving before it hits, you can conquer it. Also, the longer you stay away from bad foods, the more likely it is that you can avoid them permanently. After just two weeks, the turkey helped me break the fast-food habit. Then, I started experimenting with other foods. Also, remember that all this time I was doing serious mental training."

More Mind Games: In addition to his other mental training, the therapist suggested a visualization exercise. "Imagine you see a figure in the distance," she said. "It's fuzzy, not quite clear. That figure is you, but at your ideal weight. You can't see yourself yet. But as time goes on, that picture will come more into focus. One day, you'll see yourself clearly at your ideal weight."

As Rick recalls, "I was totally relaxed during those sessions and totally open. Completely alert, but highly suggestible."

Soon, he found that the effect of these relaxing sessions carried over to his stressful workweek. Instead of turning to a high-calorie soft drink or a candy bar when he was under heavy pressure, he told himself it was all in his head. He knew that when he got home that night he would eat something healthy, and so all he had to do was make it to the evening.

Proof in the Pounds: Although Rick attended these mental training sessions for only about three months, he learned quickly that he had the power to control various facets of his life that he had assumed were out of his control. In the process he became totally convinced that he had control over his weight and fitness.

Also, he felt a strong, growing attraction to the mental training therapy center—and later to the exercise facilities at the Cooper Aerobics Center—because he found compelling support groups in both places. "I liked everybody I encountered or worked with," he notes. "I'm really big on support groups. A huge reason that I lost weight—and continued to lose—was that it was nice to have upbeat, encouraging people to talk to, first in the mental therapy sessions and later in the gym and workout rooms at the Cooper facilities. Even my mom sent me a card every week for encouragement."

The environment that he had helped create for himself paid off immediately: he lost nineteen pounds in the first week of his program. "I know a lot of that loss was probably due to the diuretic, the water pill I was taking for my blood pressure," he admits. "But still I had drastically cut my calories—almost in half. So I was optimistic that the weight loss would continue."

Sure enough, he lost eight pounds the second week, and then six pounds the following week. Also, he began to walk short distances regularly, about a quarter of a mile three to five times a week. Even though he had been on his program for only two months, by Christmas 2000, he had lost a total of sixty pounds.

"But a powerful feeling had gripped me that *it was really going to happen!*" he says. "I knew I had a long ways to go, and I had to tackle my program day by day. But as the mental trainer had suggested, that fuzzy figure I had pictured in my first session was becoming a little clearer. I was actually beginning to get an idea of what it might be like to lose three hundred pounds."

But even so, the next big challenge for Rick was exercise. "I knew this was a major thing—and that without an exercise component, I would fail," he declares.

The Aerobic Challenge: Rick called the personal trainer whose fees had been part of the initial package he had bought with his boss's money. The trainer said she could see him three times a month, and Rick settled with her on a regimen that involved exercising at the Cooper Aerobics Center. In addition, he continued to walk short distances on his own.

As often happens in situations like this, Rick's strong motivation to exercise was immediately reinforced by the exercise itself. After riding on a stationary bike one day, Rick remembers, he sat in his car basking in the physical sense of well-being that enveloped him.

"I must have gotten my heart rate up high enough so that those endorphins* were kicking in. It was magical. I felt so good—I was energized, even though I had worked hard at the office all day. Now, I was really believing it. Exercise really did make me feel better."

The exercise regimen he settled on was rather simple and straightforward. He began by walking on the outdoor track only about a quarter of a mile, two to three times a week. Then, as his endurance increased and his leg muscles grew stronger, he worked his way up to walking three miles a day, five to six days a week. Also, he started lifting weights two to three times a week. By the summer of 2001, less than a year after he had started his fitness program, he had lost 150 pounds.

During this period, his personal support system grew steadily. He began to go to the gym and outdoor track more often, about four times a week. Soon he was receiving all sorts of kudos from other athletes: "Hey, Rick, you're looking great!" . . . "How much have you lost now!" . . . "When's your first marathon?"

---

*Morphinelike neurotransmitters associated with a sense of well-being and released during aerobic exercise.

As his fitness steadily improved, with his weight now down to around 320, he frequently sensed that during the last quarter mile of his three-mile walk, he wanted to walk faster and faster.

"Years before, I had given up on the idea of running," he recalls. "But then I felt my feet kind of leave the ground, and I was jogging. Not walking anymore, but actually jogging. When I finally stopped after about an eighth of a mile, I just shook my head, I was so happy."

As he was walking back into the gym after his workout, a club member pulled him aside and asked, "Hey, Rick, did I actually see you run out there?"

"Yeah," he replied.

"Amazing, Rick. Just amazing."

The next time out, he ran a quarter of a mile. Then, he pushed the distance up to a half mile and then to three-quarters. Finally, in July 2001, he ran one whole mile.

"As I was walking to cool down, it hit me: I actually just ran a full mile!" Rick says. "You can't imagine what that did to my confidence. I was on top of the world."

He immediately looked for his trainer and told her the good news: "I just ran a mile."

"You know," she said, "I bet we can do a half marathon in November."

"What?" he responded, not quite comprehending what she was suggesting.

"That's right—thirteen miles."

"But that's only four months from now!" Rick protested.

"I think we can do it," she insisted.

So from July to October 2001, Rick and his trainer prepared for the event. He regularly ran a little farther each day than he had the day before and mixed running in with walking. By late October, he was able to run seven miles without stopping.

"Coincidentally, that was the exact day that Dr. Cooper put me on his radio show for the first time," he says. "'What did you do today, Rick?' Dr. Cooper asked me, unaware of what I had just accomplished. 'I ran seven miles,' I said. 'What?' he almost shouted. He couldn't quite believe what he was hearing. Also, I was now down to 308, having lost a total of 230 pounds in exactly one year."

The next weekend, Rick and his trainer ran the first eight miles of his first half-marathon without stopping. Then they walked a mile, ran another mile, walked another mile, and ran the final two miles to the finish line. In other words, Rick ran a total of eleven out of the thirteen miles at his then-current weight of 308.

After that milestone, Rick's weight loss predictably slowed down. That's usually what happens when you try to lose weight, whether your goal is only in the range of ten to twenty pounds, or prodigious amounts such as those Rick took off. In other words, the last pounds are always the toughest to shed.

But Rick was prepared, mentally and physically, for this final challenge. His transformed attitude constantly whispered, "You can do it, you can do it, you *know* you can do it!"

And his inner conviction became outer reality. During the next year, from October 2001 to October 2002, he lost a total of seventy additional pounds, usually at the rate of about a pound a week. By October 2002, or exactly two years after he had embarked on his great quest, Rick achieved his ultimate goal: a loss of 300 pounds and a new body weight of 238 pounds. Furthermore, his body fat percentage became a highly athletic 12 percent of his total body weight. Just as encouraging, his blood tests improved so much that he was able to discontinue all his cholesterol and blood pressure medications.

"Now, all I take daily is vitamins, a folic acid supplement, omega-3 fish-oil supplements, and a baby aspirin," he says.

Rick's Hot Buttons: Feeling Good and Competition with Himself: "The hardest part is the beginning," he has concluded. "And the key to the entire thing is training your mind. You have to *learn* to *want* to experience a big physical change—and you have to begin to believe that a personal revolution is possible—that you can actually translate your inner desires into outer reality."

To illustrate, he poses a hypothetical case: "Let's say I want to run four miles. Well, the first mile, I almost always want to quit. So my main goal is just to get through that first mile, just keep on going. Then, the second mile is a little easier. To help motivate myself, I may think, 'I'm halfway there.'

"Then, when I finish the third mile, my mental state always improves a lot because I know I'm almost done. Physically, I go into high gear, sometimes accelerating the pace. I almost always start feeling really great. And at the end of the run I usually sense I could easily go another half mile."

It's the same with losing weight, he says. "You just keep telling yourself you *can* do it. You *can* lose one pound and then another pound. And you keep thinking those mind-changing thoughts: 'I'll crave healthy foods. . . . Water is my beverage of choice.' Before you know it, you've actually accomplished your entire goal. For me, that goal was a total of three hundred pounds, on a pound-by-pound, day-by-day basis."

Perhaps most important, Rick has learned to believe firmly in a principle that we have long advocated here at the Cooper Clinic: *Exercise is the best tranquillizer.* Here's how he translates the concept into his own experience:

"I might have a stressful day at work, and then I'll head for the gym for a workout. It's like a drug because when I'm finished, I feel so much better. I've learned I can work all day, yet still have plenty of energy left over for my personal life—so long as I exercise almost every day. I've reached the point where my body *wants* the exercise. To feel right, I have to give in to these strong physical and mental urges to work out."

In other words, in the language of exercise physiology and psychology, Rick has experienced *positive addiction,* or habit-forming conditioning that leads to healthful and constructive results.

As part of this positive addiction, Rick also has developed an increased tendency to push himself while running. "I find myself running faster and faster miles, from twelve minutes, to eleven, to ten, to nine.

Occasionally I'll even run an eight-minute mile, and recently I actually ran the distance in six minutes and forty seconds."

To keep up his drive to exercise regularly—and to expand his developing physical skills and fitness level—he's included one to one and a half hours of basketball in his program several times a week.

"This helps expand the support group that reinforces my motivation to exercise and stay fit," he says.

Tyler's Partnership

Rick and I met during one of those basketball games, not only because we like to play hoops, but also because we both affirm the importance of establishing a "fellowship of the fit," which help reinforce our individual commitments to exercise and weight control.

Icing on the Weight–Loss Cake: Rick's exciting story goes on and on. Although he had never really dated anyone since high school, he met Kelley, his future wife, in November 2002, just after he had succeeded in taking off those three hundred pounds. Then, after a whirlwind courtship, he ended up proposing to her before a national television audience in his second appearance on the *Oprah Winfrey Show.* Their first child, a son, Owen, was born in December 2005—just before Rick was featured in *People* magazine.

You might expect us to wrap up such an extraordinary account with a fairy-tale ending: "And so Rick Salewske lived happily ever after."

But as Rick himself would tell you, his kind of success story, which has been repeated in other versions in our offices, doesn't just close like some feel-good movie. In fact, the most heroic part of Rick's saga continues even now, on a mundane, day-to-day basis, as he regularly applies sound exercise and dietary principles to *maintain* his fitness and good health. To be sure, he started strong with his program. But now he recognizes that he must *continue to finish strong*. That means daily and weekly monitoring of his personal motivation, diet, and exercise regimen—and also regularly setting new goals for himself.

Tyler, for example, has been pacing Rick to prepare him to run a sub-two-hour half marathon. Through this arrangement, Rick is availing himself of at least three of the motivational hot buttons we described in Chapter 3: 1) The Numbers-Game Hot Button: striving to improve measurements of personal health, such as treadmill times or cholesterol read-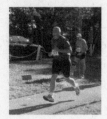ings; 2) the Please-the-Doctor (or Trainer) Hot Button: becoming answerable to a kind of "trainer" in the person of Tyler; and 3) the Sociability Hot Button: enjoying the sociability of working out with a friend (e.g., Tyler).

As part of his training, Rick recently ran his personal best for the two-mile distance—a time of thirteen minutes, forty-four seconds. Also, when we timed Rick on the Balke treadmill stress test, he walked for a total of twenty-seven minutes, thirty-one seconds, a remarkable accomplishment that placed him in the top 5 percent level of fitness for men who were twelve years younger. The latest news is even more impressive: In December 2006, Rick entered the Dallas White Rock Half-Marathon, a run of 13.1 miles. In that event, Tyler paced Rick to a time of one hour, forty-seven minutes, or a rate of just a little more than eight minutes per mile. That was truly an amazing performance for a forty-two-year-old man who had managed to shed a massive amount of fat to reach a "fighting weight" of 238 pounds.

Unlike Rick, you may not need to lose three hundred pounds, but you may still feel your situation is hopeless. You may be physically weak, lacking in endurance, or fifty pounds overweight. Or you may be suffering through the healing of a broken leg or recovery from a heart attack or a lengthy illness. Whatever your current situation, the message of the Start Strong, Finish Strong way of life is this: there is hope. The seemingly impossible really is possible.

Sixteen

■ Your Fitness Future
■ Is *Now*

Maud, who is going on ninety-two, lives alone in her home in a rural town in southwestern Georgia. She had to give up her driver's license a few years back and has had periodic health concerns, such as aches in her legs, a minor stroke, and high cholesterol. But even so, Maud cooks for herself, manages occasional household help, and even delivers her newspaper to a friend a couple of doors away who has her own health problems.

Some might say, "Too bad. She rarely sees her family. She has to fend for herself. Where are her children? At her age, she should have someone to care for her."

In fact, her children—two sons and a daughter, who live in distant parts of the country—have offered her other options, including spare rooms in their homes or, if she prefers, a spot in a nearby assisted-living facility with regular access to many old friends. As an alternative, they have urged her to make extended visits to their homes and have even sometimes pressed her to the point that she has become exasperated with them.

Maud's children have argued, "Mom, what happens if you fall and break a hip, and no one finds you on the floor for several days?"

She responded by agreeing to wear an emergency signal device around her neck.

They said, "You have so many medications to take. What if you mix them up and have a bad drug interaction?"

She responded by showing them that she could organize her pills accurately in a daily pill dispenser.

They even warned, "What if you have a health crisis? A big stroke or heart attack?"

Her response: "I'd rather take that risk than give up my independence."

In the end, Maud has made it abundantly clear that she will continue to live on her own, and further investigation reveals that she's quite happy about her situation. She "holds court," as they say in her part of Georgia, with frequent visitors from the community who drop by to say hello and see how she's doing. She has arranged to be driven regularly to deposit her Social Security check, pay her bills, and have her hair done once a week by a friend. (This friend, who is five years her senior and has also insisted on her independence, still not only sees beauty parlor clients, but also does calisthenics daily.)

Now resigned that Maud will never move or otherwise change her living situation, her children maintain regular contact by talking to her several times a week on the phone. Also, they and some of her grandchildren see her at various times of the year at her home, and the entire family has established the tradition of getting together in one of her son's homes once a year every January for her birthday.

The benefits of Maud's independence emerge almost daily, often in small but, to her, extremely significant ways. The son of her best friend in high school has dropped by with his wife on visits to "talk about old times." Close relatives passing through town always visit her—relatives she would never see if she were living in some other part of the country. People she has met at the local bank or supermarket drop by with gifts at Christmas or other holidays.

And there's the joy of the exciting, unexpected encounter that typically occurs only if you're operating on your own. For example, Ken, in trying to reach one of her sons, dialed Maud's number by mistake and proceeded to spend a lengthy time on the phone chatting with her. The experience was the highlight of her day. She still talks animatedly about "the conversation I had with Dr. Cooper." But most likely the interaction wouldn't have been possible if she had chosen to live in a setting where others were ready to take outside calls or shoulder most responsibilities for her.

If we each search our own minds and hearts for the way we would like to spend the "end game" of our lives, we might find many aspects of Maud's experience of independence quite appealing. But what exactly has been her secret?

First and foremost, she has been physically active most of her life. Even during most of her eighties, she walked at least an hour five to six times a week, often back and forth on the sidewalk in front of her house and the house of a neighbor. She also has done regular stretching and strength exercises. To maintain her mental agility, she not only exercises,[1] but also does crossword puzzles every day, studies the newspaper for new political and economic developments, and listens to sermons on the radio.

In addition, for decades she had gone in for regular medical checkups—at least two to three times a year. During the past two years she has undergone exams every two months, a practice that has enabled her physician and nurse practitioner to keep her on medications that have lowered her cholesterol to safe levels. At one point, the exams also led to a diagnosis of low iron levels and anemia, and a resulting adjustment in her diet and medications that normalized her body chemistry. Without this adjustment, the deterioration in her condition might have proved fatal.

But even with these successes, Maud has made mistakes. As she approached ninety, she began to neglect her regular exercise routine, with the result that she started to lose energy and endurance. But some encouragement and advice from her children, including instructions in less demanding stretching and strength exercises, have helped her recover some of her old vitality, and she continues to improve.

Given her current advanced age and ability to remain highly functional and independent, despite certain health challenges, Maud seems to have placed herself in a good position to finish strong. Who knows? If she continues with her exercise program and other essential fitness "start-ups," she might even begin to push the outer limit of that maximum biblical life span of 120 years.[2] More and more, we're coming to understand that such a limit is not due to some "design deficiency" in our bodies and minds, but rather to the way we abuse and mistreat them.

As you consider Maud's story, how do *you* stand right now, given your present age and health-and-fitness habits?

We hope that you've already started putting into practice some of the principles you've learned. But acquiring the know-how and making a good beginning are only the first part of the challenge. The danger that confronts us all is the tendency to blast off to a strong start and then get off the track, even as Maud did a year or so ago with her exercise routine.

Regardless of your current age or fitness level, you should always remember this basic fact: *you can't "store up" fitness.* If you slack off or quit your program, the well-being, health, and longevity benefits you have achieved may continue for a short time. But sedentary living, unhealthy eating, or other poor health practices will soon take their toll on your body, your mind, and your spirit. To square off the curve of your life, you must think not about what you hope the future will hold, but what you can do now to shape that future.

You may find it fascinating to know that whether you're thirty-five or seventy-five you can actually grow healthier as you grow older, and not necessarily the reverse. But to start strong *and* finish strong, you must *continue* strong, beginning *right now.* With a firm commitment today and then tomorrow and the next day, you're likely to find that at some distant time—perhaps when you're ninety or even older—your mind and body are as agile as they where when you started your program. But don't wait. Your future, indeed, is now.

APPENDIX

THE COOPER CALCIFICATION SCORES

Based on EBT Scans in Patients with No Known Clinical Cardiovascular Disease

The two charts on the following pages, one for men and one for women, are keyed to the percentiles in which the calcification scores will place you in the population tested at the Cooper Clinic. The higher your calcification score and percentile, the more your risk rises for plaque blockage of the coronary arteries—and for heart attacks and other cardiovascular disease. The 50th percentile is the normal, expected calcification score for both men and women who are aging normally.

You can also use this chart to determine your arterial age. For example, if you are a man forty-nine years of age with a coronary artery calcification score of zero, your chronological and arterial age are the same. But if you are forty-nine years of age and have a coronary calcification score of 120, this would give you an arterial age of sixty to sixty-four.

A similar kind of analysis works for women. So if you are a woman fifty years of age and have a calcification score of 35, your arterial age is actually seventy to seventy-four. But you'll also notice that a man up to forty-nine years of age should have zero coronary artery calcification, while, in contrast, a woman up to sixty-four years of age should have zero calcification. This difference is probably the reason women have heart attacks much later than do men.

THE COOPER CALCIFICATION SCORES

Men

n	age	5th	10th	25th	50th	60th	70th	75th	80th	90th	95th	99th
422	<35	0	0	0	0	0	0	0	0	1	12	128
1,367	35–39	0	0	0	0	0	0	0	0	8	37	227
3,226	40–44	0	0	0	0	0	0	2	5	46	132	509
3,733	45–49	0	0	0	0	2	10	23	43	141	294	1,079
4,191	50–54	0	0	0	6	25	65	101	152	409	757	2,144
3,436	55–59	0	0	0	46	101	191	254	346	741	1,326	2,879
2,248	60–64	0	0	7	120	221	383	491	666	1,338	2,132	4,469
1,422	65–69	0	0	36	256	442	706	897	1,175	1,970	2,931	5,615
799	70–74	0	2	92	459	665	1,051	1,325	1,555	2,691	3,868	7,685
346	75–79	4	22	176	765	1,102	1,491	1,784	2,123	3,354	4,491	7,335
162	80+	28	93	352	1,003	1,244	1,654	1,927	2,598	4,328	5,771	7,689

n = number of participants in the study. The total was 21,190.

Women*

n	age	5th	10th	25th	50th	60th	70th	75th	80th	90th	95th	99th
173	<35	0	0	0	0	0	0	0	0	0	0	2
515	35–39	0	0	0	0	0	0	0	0	0	0	10
1,295	40–44	0	0	0	0	0	0	0	0	0	5	94
1,817	45–49	0	0	0	0	0	0	0	0	2	34	198
2,303	50–54	0	0	0	0	0	0	0	0	29	106	442
1,849	55–59	0	0	0	0	0	2	9	25	115	282	960
1,250	60–64	0	0	0	0	1	20	45	79	206	442	1,157
843	65–69	0	0	0	8	29	77	113	157	436	831	2,340
427	70–74	0	0	0	35	91	182	263	348	746	1,236	2,643
312	75+	0	0	11	143	271	467	632	891	1,516	2,197	3,031

* The total number of participants was 10,784.

THE COOPER FITNESS CATEGORIES

Based on the Balke Treadmill Protocol

If you undergo the treadmill stress test using the Balke Treadmill Protocol (described on page 107), here is how your performance would measure up to the standards we use at the Cooper Clinic. As you can see, the six fitness categories, ranging from "very poor" to "superior," are keyed to gender and age.

FITNESS CATEGORIES

Males

	15-19	20-29	30-34	35-39	40-44	45-49
Very Poor	<17:29	<14:59	<14:29	<13:59	<13:23	<12:00
Poor	17:30-20:59	15:00-17:59	14:30-17:18	14:00-16:59	13:24-16:13	12:01-14:59
Fair	21:00-24:59	18:00-21:59	17:19-21:04	17:00-20:59	16:14-20:09	15:00-18:59
Good	25:00-27:36	22:00-25:59	21:05-24:59	21:00-24:12	20:10-23:59	19:00-22:15
Excellent	27:37-29:59	26:00-29:30	25:00-27:29	24:13-27:02	24:00-26:59	22:16-25:29
Superior	30:00	29:31	27:30	27:03	27:00	25:30

	50-54	55-59	60-64	65-69	70-79
Very Poor	<11:01	<9:59	<8:51	<6:59	<6:10
Poor	11:02-13:59	10:00-12:59	8:52-11:29	7:00-10:04	6:11-8:59
Fair	14:00-17:30	13:00-16:09	11:30-14:59	10:05-13:59	9:00-12:29
Good	17:31-20:59	16:10-19:59	15:00-18:59	14:00-16:59	12:30-16:01
Excellent	21:00-24:14	20:00-23:14	19:00-21:59	17:00-20:39	16:02-19:59
Superior	24:15	23:15	22:00	20:40	20:00

< less than
> greater than

Females

	15–19	20–29	30–34	35–39	40–44	45–49
Very Poor	<11:54	<10:59	<10:04	<9:29	<8:59	<7:59
Poor	11:55–14:24	11:00–13:59	10:05–12:40	9:30–11:59	9:00–11:29	8:00–10:30
Fair	14:25–17:59	14:00–17:59	12:41–16:16	12:00–15:29	11:30–14:59	10:31–13:59
Good	18:00–21:11	18:00–21:01	16:17–19:59	15:30–19:00	15:00–18:00	14:00–17:00
Excellent	21:12–25:01	21:02–24:29	20:00–22:25	19:01–22:01	18:01–21:02	17:01–20:10
Superior	25:02	24:30	22:26	22:02	21:03	20:11

	50–54	55–59	60–64	65–69	70–79
Very Poor	<7:00	<6:44	<5:59	<5:24	<3:59
Poor	7:01–9:49	6:45–8:59	6:00–8:08	5:25–6:59	4:00–6:06
Fair	9:50–12:29	9:00–11:59	8:09–10:59	7:00–9:32	6:07–8:33
Good	12:30–15:06	12:00–14:29	11:00–13:29	9:33–11:59	8:34–12:00
Excellent	15:07–17:59	14:30–17:04	13:30–15:45	12:00–14:32	12:01–16:29
Superior	18:00	17:05	15:46	14:33	16:30

< less than
> greater than

NOTES

Chapter 1: How to Jump-start a Stubborn Body

1. Tara Parker-Pope. "Top Secrets of Successful Aging: What Science Tells Us About Growing Older—and Staying Healthy." *The Wall Street Journal,* June 20, 2005. Personal Health (A Special Report), R1.
2. S. N. Blair; H. W. Kohl; R. S. Paffenbarger Jr.; D. G. Clark; K. H. Cooper; and L. W. Gibbons. 1989. "Physical Fitness and All-Cause Mortality: A Prospective Study of Healthy Men and Women." *Journal of the American Medical Association,* 262 (17): 2,395–2,401. See also Tedd Mitchell, USA Weekend Online. March 19, 2000.
3. Oscar H. Franco; Chris de Laet; Anna Peeters; Jacqueline Jonker; Johan Mackenbach; and Wilma Nusselder. 2005. "Effects of Physical Activity on Life Expectancy with Cardiovascular Disease." *Archives of Internal Medicine,* 165 (20): 2,355–2,360.
4. Gary E. Fraser and David J. Shavlik. 2001. "Ten Years of Life. Is It a Matter of Choice?" *Archives of Internal Medicine,* 161 (13): 1,645–1,652.
5. *Research Digest, President's Council on Physical Fitness and Sports,* December 1997.
6. Martha Clare Morris; Denis A. Evans; Christine C. Tangney; Julia L. Bienias; and Robert S. Wilson. "Fish Consumption and Cognitive Decline with Age in

a Large Community Study." 2005. *Archives of Neurology,* 62 (12): 1,849–1,853.

7. Jennifer Weuve; Jae Hee Kang; JoAnn E. Manson; Monique M. B. Breteler; James H. Ware; and Francine Grodstein. 2004. "Physical Activity, Including Walking, and Cognitive Function in Older Women." *Journal of the American Medical Association,* 292 (12): 1,454–1,461.

8. A. J. Vita; R. B. Terry; H. B. Hubert; and J. F. Fries. 1998. "Aging, Health Risks, and Cumulative Disability." *New England Journal of Medicine,* 338 (15): 1,035–1,041.

9. Antonia Trichopoulou; Tina Costacou; Christina Bamia; and Dimitrios Trichopoulos. 2003. "Adherence to a Mediterranean Diet and Survival in a Greek Population." *New England Journal of Medicine,* 348 (26): 2,599–2,608.

10. Ibid.

11. Dariush Mozaffarian; Anouk Geelen; Ingeborg A. Brouwer; Johanna M. Geleijnse; Peter L. Zock; and Martijn B. Katan. 2005. "Effect of Fish Oil on Heart Rate in Humans: A Meta-Analysis of Randomized Controlled Trials." *Circulation,* 112: 1,945–1,952.

12. E. G. Giltay; M. H. Kamphuis; S. Kalmijn; F. G. Zitman; and D. Kromhout. 2006. "Dispositional Optimism and the Risk of Cardiovascular Death." *Archives of Internal Medicine,* 166 (4): 431–436.

13. Andrew T. Chan; Edward L. Giovannucci; Jeffrey A. Meyerhardt; Eva S. Schernhammer; Gary C. Curhan; and Charles S. Fuchs. 2005. "Long-term Use of Aspirin and Nonsteroidal Anti-inflammatory Drugs and Risk of Colorectal Cancer." *Journal of the American Medical Association,* 294 (8): 914–923.

14. "Cancer Prevention & Early Detection Facts and Figures 2006," publication of American Cancer Society 2006. See also Texas Medical Association letter, March 3, 2005.

15. *Wall Street Journal,* April 6, 2006, p. D4.

16. B. Fries; J. F. Fries; D. P. Lubeck. "Aerobic Exercise and its Impact on Musculoskeletal Pain in Older Adults." 2005. *Arthritis Research and Therapy,* 6 (7): 1,263–1,270. See also WashingtonPost.com, Oct. 4, 2005, "Don't Run Away from Jogging."

17. Charles Emery. "Study of Older Adults Suffering from Osteoarthritis of the Knee." *American Psychosomatic Society,* Denver, March 7, 2005. See also Scripps Howard News Service, March 2, 2006.

18. Cited in *AARP Bulletin,* February 2006.

19. Cited in *New York Times,* March 7, 2006, p. D6.

20. *MSN Health and Fitness* online, July 13, 2005.

21. Robert John Petrella; Chastity Nina Lattanzio; Amy Demeray; Vincent Varallo; and Rachel Blore. 2005. "Can Adoption of Regular Exercise Later in Life Prevent Metabolic Risk for Cardiovascular Disease?" *Diabetes Care,* 28: 694–701.

22. *Parade* and Research America survey. *Parade* magazine, Feb. 5, 2006, p. 15.

Chapter 2: Squaring Off the Curve of Your Life

1. Kenneth H. Cooper. *Faith-Based Fitness* (Nashville: Thomas Nelson, 1995), 234 ff.

2. *Obesity Policy Report Weekly,* March 3, 2005, Vol. 3.

3. Kenneth H. Cooper. Personal notes at American Heart Association Meeting, Orlando, Nov. 9–12, 2003.

4. S. Jay Olshansky; Douglas J. Passaro; Ronald C. Hershow; Jennifer Layden; Bruce A. Carnes; Jacob Brody; Leonard Hayflick; Robert N. Butler; David B. Allison; and David S. Ludwig. 2005. "Potential Decline in Life Expectancy in the United States in the 21st Century." *New England Journal of Medicine,* 352 (11): 1,138–1,145.

5. June Stevens; Jianwen Cai; Elsie R. Pamuk; David F. Williamson; Michael J. Thun; and Joy L. Wood. 1998. "The Effect of Age on the Association Between Body-Mass Index and Mortality." *New England Journal of Medicine,* 338 (1): 1–7.

6. *Obesity Policy Report Weekly.* Jan. 20, 2005, Vol. 3.

7. Centers for Disease Control and Prevention publications, cited in *Journal of the American Medical Association* and the Associated Press, April 5, 2006.

8. Ibid.

9. B. McKay. "Here's the Skinny: Study Finds a 30-Year Upswing in Amount Americans Eat." *Wall Street Journal,* February 6, 2004, B1, B3.

10. Ali H. Mokdad; James S. Marks; Donna F. Stroup; and Julie L. Gerberding. 2004. "Actual Causes of Death in the United States, 2000." *Journal of the American Medical Association,* 291 (10): 1,238–1,245.

11. Reports on years 1999–2001, Centers for Disease Control and Prevention in Atlanta and the National Center for Health Statistics.

12. Reuters report, Aug. 9, 2005.

13. S. N. Blair; H. W. Kohl; R. S. Paffenbarger Jr.; D. G. Clark; K. H. Cooper; and L. W. Gibbons. 1989. "Physical Fitness and All-Cause Mortality. A Prospective Study of Healthy Men and Women." *Journal of the American Medical Association,* 262 (17): 2,395–2,401.

14. Ibid. Also, see Tedd Mitchell. USAWeekend Online, March 19, 2000.

15. J. D. Wright; J. Kennedy-Stephenson; C. Y. Wang; M. A. McDowell; and C. L. Johnson. 2005. "Trends in Intake of Energy and Macronutrients—United States 1971–2000." 2005. *National Health and Nutrition Examination Survey,* 80 (2). See also Medscape.com, December 11, 2003.

16. S. Wild; G. Roglic; A. Green; R. Sicree; and H. King. "Global Prevalence of Diabetes." *Diabetes Care,* 27 (5): 1,047–1,053. See also *New York Times,* January 9, 2006, p. 1.

17. Connie Tyne report, Cooper Wellness Program.

18. Cited in WebMDHealth, webmd.com, July 31, 2002.

19. *Health Affairs,* January 2004. Cited in Associated Press report, Jan. 8, 2004.

20. Ibid.

21. *President's Council on Physical Fitness and Sports: Research Digest,* December 2004, 1.

22. *Cooper Health: The Cooper Clinic Magazine,* Spring 2006, 8–10.

23. American Cancer Society, 2005 annual report.

Chapter 3: What's Your Hot Button?

1. J. Agostino. "Once an Athletic Star, Now an Unheavenly Body." *New York Times,* July 6, 2006, G1.

2. Dr. R. Brown; Y. Wang; A. Ward; C.B. Ebbeling; L. Fortlage; E. Puleo; H. Benson; and J. M. Rippe. 1995. "Chronic Psychological Effects of Exercise and Exercise Plus Cognitive Strategies." *Medical Science, Sports, and Exercise,* 765–775. H. Benson; T. Dryer; and L. H. Hartley. 1978. "Decreased VO_2 Consumption during Exercise with Elicitation of the Relaxation Response." *Journal of Human Stress,* 4: 38–42. H. Benson and W. Proctor. *The Breakout Principle* (New York: Scribner, 2003, 2004), 182–209.

3. Proverbs 13:18 (NIV).

4. J. W. Worden and W. Proctor. *PDA-Personal Death Awareness.* (Englewood Cliffs, N.J.: Prentice-Hall, 1976), 1ff.

5. W. Shakespeare. *Measure for Measure,* Act III, Scene 1, 1604 (1623), line 76.

6. Ernest Becker. *The Denial of Death* (New York: Free Press, 1973), 15.

7. Tara Parker-Pope. 2005. "The Secrets of Successful Aging: What Science Tells Us About Growing Older—and Staying Healthy." *Wall Street Journal,* June 20, 2005, Personal Health (A Special Report), R1.

8. S. N. Blair; H. W. Kohl; R. S. Paffenbarger; D. G. Clark; K. H. Cooper; and L. W. Gibbons. 1989. "Physical Fitness and All-Cause Mortality: A Prospective Study of Healthy Men and Women." *Journal of the American Medical Association,* 262 (17): 2,395–2,401.

9. *Parade* and *Research America* survey. *Parade* magazine, February 5, 2006, p. 15.

10. U.S. Public Health Service. Prevention Report. October 1991. World Health Organization, press release, June 4, 2000. "WHO Issues New Healthy Life Expectancy Rankings."

11. National Survey. "America Speaks Poll Data Summary." *Research America,* March 2006.

12. D. M. Landers. 1997. "The Influence of Exercise on Mental Health." *PCPFS Research Digest,* 2 (12) (December): 1ff.

13. Jennifer Weuve; Jae Hee Kang; JoAnn E. Manson; Monique M. B. Breteler; James H. Ware; and Francine Grodstein. 2004. "Physical Activity, Including Walking, and Cognitive Function in Older Women." *Journal of the American Medical Association,* 292 (12): 1,454–1,461. See also Stanley J. Colcombe; Kirk I. Erickson; Paige E. Scalf; Jenny S. Kim; Ruchika Prakash; Edward McAuley; Steriani Elavsky; David X. Marquez; Liang Hu; and Arthur F. Kramer. 2006. Special Section: "Aerobic Exercise Training Increases Brain Volume in Aging Humans." *The Journals of Gerontology Series A: Biological Sciences and Medical Sciences,* 61: 1,166–1,170. Also cited in *The Wall Street Journal,* November 16, 2006, "Personal Journal," p. 1.

14. M. T. Sturman; M. C. Morris; C. F. Mendes de Leon; J. L. Bienias; R. S. Wilson; and D. A. Evans. 2005. "Physical Activity, Cognitive Activity, and Cognitive Decline in a Biracial Community Population." *Archives of Neurology,* 62: 1,750–1,754.

15. See Genesis 1:31; 1 Timothy 4:4. (HCSB)

16. See 1 Corinthians 3:16–17; 6:19. (HCSB)

17. H. Benson and W. Proctor. *The Breakout Principle* (New York: Scribner, 2003, 2004), 257–282.

18. *New York Times,* www.nytimes.com, August 15, 2006.

19. For further information, see K. H. Cooper. *Controlling Cholesterol the Natural Way* (New York: Bantam, 1999).

20. John Tyndall. *Fragments of Science.* Vol. II, "An Address to Students."

Chapter 4: The Science of Starting and Finishing Strong

1. Publilius Syrus. Maxims, no. 305. Trans. by Darius Lyman.

2. William James. *Principles of Psychology* (New York: Henry Holt and Co., 1890), 80.

3. Ibid.

4. Ibid., 81.

5. Ibid., 82.

6. Ibid.

7. Much of the historical information in the following paragraphs draws upon the account of Eugene I. Taylor, "The Connection between Mind and Body." *Harvard Medical School Bulletin,* Winter 2000, 40–47.

8. K. H. Cooper. *Can Stress Heal?* (Nashville: Thomas Nelson, 1997).

9. J. E. Brody. "Forget the Second Helpings. It's the First Ones That Supersize Your Waistline," *New York Times,* July 11, 2006.

10. Taylor, "Mind and Body."

11. H. Benson; B. A. Rosner; B. R. Marzetta; and H. M. Klemchuk. 1974. "Decreased Blood Pressure in Pharmacologically Treated Hypertensive Patients Who Regularly Elicited the Relaxation Response." *Lancet:* 289–291. H. Benson; J. F. Beary; and M. P. Carol. 1974. "The Relaxation Response." *Psychiatry,* 37: 37–46. J. F. Beary and H. Benson. 1974. "A Simple Psychophysiologic Technique Which Elicits the Hypometabolic Changes of the Relaxation Response." *Psychosomatic Medicine,* 36: 115–120.

12. Scientific support for the following discussion can be found in the following research articles: J. A. Dusek; B. Chang; G. Jacobs; J. Zaki; S. Lazar; A. Deykin; G. G. Stefano; A. L. Wohlheuter; P. L. Hibberd; and H. Benson. 2005. "Association between Oxygen Consumption and Nitric Oxide Production During the Relaxation Response." *Medical Science Monitor.* 11: CR1–10. S. W. Lazar; C. Kerr; R. H. Wasserman; J. R. Gray; D. Greve; M. Treadway; M. McGarvey; B. T. Quinn; J. A. Dusek; H. Benson; S. L. Rauch; C. I. Moore; and B. Fischl. 2005. "Meditation Experience Is Associated with Increased Cortical Thickness." *NeuroReport,* 16 (Nov. 28): 1,893–1,897. S. W. Lazar; G. Bush; R. L. Gollub; G. L. Fricchione; G. Khalsa; and H. Benson. 2000. "Functional Brain Mapping of the Relaxation Response and Meditation." *NeuroReport,* 11: 1,581–1,585. G. B. Stefano; G. L. Fricchione; B. T. Slingsby; and H. Benson. 2001. "The Placebo Effect and the Relaxation Response: Neural Processes and Their Coupling to Constitutive Nitric Oxide." *Brain Research Reviews,* 35: 1–19.

13. See J. A. Dusek; B. Chang; G. Jacobs; J. Zaki; S. Lazar; A. Deykin; G. G. Stefano; A. L. Wohlheuter; P. L. Hibberd; and H. Benson. 2005. "Association between Oxygen Consumption and Nitric Oxide Production During the Relaxation Response." *Medical Science Monitor,* 11: CR1–10.

14. H. Benson; T. Dryer; and L.H. Hartle. 1978. "Decreased VO_2 Consumption During Exercise with Elicitation of the Relaxation Response." *Journal of Human Stress.* 4: 38–42. Dr. R. Brown; Y. Wang; A. Ward; C. B. Ebbeling; L. Fortlage; E. Puleo; H. Benson; and J. M. Rippe. 1995. "Chronic Psychological

Effects of Exercise and Exercise Plus Cognitive Strategies." *Medical Science, Sports, and Exercise,* 765–775.

15. S. W. Lazar; G. Bush; R. L. Gollub; G. L. Fricchione; G. Khalsa; and H. Benson. 2000. "Functional Brain Mapping of the Relaxation Response and Meditation." *NeuroReport,* 11 (2000): 1,581–1,585.

16. See H. Prast and A. Philippu. 2001. "Nitric Oxide as Modulator of Neuronal Function." *Progress in Neurobiology,* 64 (2001): 51–68. Benson and Proctor, *The Breakout Principle,* 50.

17. Peter Sterling. "Principles of Allostasis: Optimal Design, Predictive Regulation, Pathophysiology and Rational Therapeutics," in J. Schulkin, *Allostasis, Homeostasis, and the Costs of Adaptation.* Cambridge: MIT Press, 2003: 29.

18. S. W. Lazar; C. Kerr; R. H. Wasserman; J. R. Gray; D. Greve; M. Treadway; M. McGarvey; B. T. Quinn; J. A. Dusek; H. Benson; S. L. Rauch; C. I. Moore; and B. Fischl. 2005. "Meditation Experience is Associated with Increased Cortical Thickness." *NeuroReport,* 16 (November 28): 1893–1,897.

19. Richard Benyo. "Exercise Addiction—When More Is Less." *Online FootNotes,* Press release from Road Runners Club of America. See also Jim Parker. "Total Recovery: A Guide to Balancing Body and Mind, Heart and Soul in Chemical Dependency Recovery." Pamphlet published by *Do It Now Foundation,* February 1999.

20. See K. H. Cooper. *The Antioxidant Revolution* (Nashville: Thomas Nelson, 1994), 96.

21. Sterling, "Principles of Allostasis," 15–16.

22. J. O. Prochaska. *Systems of Psychotherapy: A Transtheoretical Analysis.* Pacific, Calif: Brooks-Cole, 1979. J. O. Prochaska and C. C. DiClemente. 1982. "Transtheoretical Therapy Toward a More Integrative Model of Change." *Psychotherapy: Theory, Research and Practice,* 19 (3) (1982), 276–87. J. O. Prochaska; J. C. Norcross; and C. C. DiClemente. *Changing for Good* (New York: William Morrow, 1994).

23. Modern Library Giant Edition, trans. by John Dryden, rev. by Arthur Hugh Clough. *Rules for Preservation of Health,* 18.

24. Montaigne, *Essays,* Book III, Chapter 10.

Chapter 5: Start-up #1—Don't Put Off Your Gold-Standard Physical Exam

1. Kenneth H. Cooper. *Running Without Fear* (New York: M. Evans and Company, 1985).

2. J. Fixx. *The Complete Book of Running* (New York: Random House, 1977).

3. Nove K. Kalia; Loren G. Miller; Khurram Nasir; Roger S. Blumenthal; Nisha Agrawal; and Matthew J. Budoff. 2006. "Visualizing Coronary Calcium Is Associated with Improvements in Adherence to Statin Therapy." *Atherosclerosis*, 185 (2): 394–399.

4. Press release, The Los Angeles Biomedical Research Institute at Harbor-UCLA Medical Center (LA BioMed).

5. Steve Halligan; Douglas G. Altman; Stuart A. Taylor; Susan Mallett; Jonathan J. Deeks; Clive I. Bartram; and Wendy Atkin. 2005. "CT Colonography in the Detection of Colorectal Polyps and Cancer: Systematic Review, Meta-Analysis, and Proposed Minimum Data Set for Study Level Reporting." *Radiology*, 237 (3): 893–904. R. M. Summers; J. Yao; P. J. Pickhardt; M. Franaszek; I. Bitter; D. Brickman; V. Krishna; and J. R. Choi. 2005. "Computed Tomographic Virtual Colonoscopy Computer-Aided Polyp Detection in a Screening Population." *Gastroenterology*, 129 (6): 1,832–1,844. M. L. Kochman and B. Levin. 2004. "Expert Commentary—Virtual Colonoscopy: Utility as a Screening Test for Colorectal Cancer?" *Medscape General Medicine*, 6 (1).

6. Robert L. Barclay; Joseph J. Vicari; Andrea S. Doughty; John F. Johanson; and Roger L. Greenlaw. 2006. "Colonoscopic Withdrawal Times and Adenoma Detection During Screening Colonoscopy." *New England Journal of Medicine*, 355 (24): 2,533–2,541.

7. Benson and Proctor. *The Breakout Principle*, 212.

8. S. M. Grundy; Scott M. Grundy; James I. Cleeman; C. Noel Bairey Merz; H. Bryan Brewer, Jr.; Luther T. Clark; Donald B. Hunninghake; Richard C. Pasternak; Sidney C. Smith, Jr.; and Neil J. Stone. 2004. "Implications of Recent Clinical Trials for the National Cholesterol Education Program Adult Treatment Panel III Guidelines." *Circulation*, 110: 227–329. Mike Mitka. 2004. "Guidelines: New Lows for LDL Target Levels." *Journal of the American Medical Association*, 292 (8): 911–913.

9. S. M. Grundy. 2004. "Metabolic Syndrome: A Growing Clinical Challenge." *Medscape Cardiology*, 8 (2). S. M. Grundy, et al. 2004. "Clinical Management of Metabolic Syndrome." *Circulation*, 109: 551–556.

10. U. N. Khot; M. B. Khot; C. T. Bajzer; S. K. Sapp; E. M. Ohman; S. J. Brener; S. G. Ellis; A. M. Lincoff; and E. J. Topol. 2003. "Prevalence of Conventional Risk Factors in Patients with Coronary Heart Disease." *Journal of the American Medical Association*, 290 (7): 898–904.

Chapter 6: Start-up #2—The Active Mind-set: Focus on the Amazing Benefits of Fitness

1. S. N. Blair et al. *JAMA,* 1989.
2. News release, American College of Sports Medicine, March 2, 2004 on the position paper, "Exercise and Hypertension" published in the March 2004 issue of *Medicine & Science in Sports & Medicine.*
3. S. N. Blair; N. N. Goodyear; L. W. Gibbons; and K. H. Cooper. 1984. "Physical Fitness and Incidence of Hypertension in Healthy Normotensive Men and Women." *Journal of the American Medical Association,* 252: 487–490. See also Jirayos Chintanadilok and D. T. Lowenthal. 2002. "Exercise in Treating Hypertension: Tailoring Therapies for Active Patients." *The Physician and Sportsmedicine,* Vol. 30 (March): 11–23.
4. Marvin Moser. 2004. Editorial: "Effective Treatment of Hypertension Without Medication: Is It Possible?" *Journal of Clinical Hypertension,* 6 (5): 219–221.
5. Jirayos Chintanadilok and David T. Lowenthal. 2002. "Exercise in Treating Hypertension."
6. D. G. Vidt. *Hypertension Q & A,* www.ConsultantLive.com.
7. N. Haapanen; S. Miilunpalo; I. Vuori; P. Oja; and M. Pasanen. 1997. "Association of Leisure Time Physical Activity with the Risk of Coronary Heart Disease, Hypertension and Diabetes in Middle-aged Men and Women." *International Journal of Epidemiology,* 26 (4): 739–747.
8. M. Tanasescu; M. F. Leitzmann; E. B. Rimm; W. C. Willett; M. J. Stampfer; and F. B. Hu. 2002. "Exercise Type and Intensity in Relation to Coronary Heart Disease in Men." *Journal of the American Medical Association,* 288 (16): 1,994–2,000.
9. Q and A section. *Environmental Nutrition,* December 1998:7.
10. David M. Pober; Barry Braun; and Patty S. Freedson. 2004. "Effects of a Single Bout of Exercise on Resting Heart Rate Variability." *Medicine & Science in Sports & Exercise,* 36 (7): 1,140–1,148.
11. "Poster Abstracts—The Association of Fitness and C-Reactive Protein in Males Aged 60 Years and Older." The Cooper Institute Conference Series, Physical Activity: Preventing Physical Disablement in Older Adults, Program and Abstract Book, October 17–19, 2002: 18.
12. Jennifer Weuve; Jae Hee Kang; JoAnn E. Manson; Monique M. B. Breteler; James H. Ware; and Francine Grodstein. 2004. "Physical Activity, Including Walking, and Cognitive Function in Older Women." *Journal of the American Medical Association,* 292 (12): 1,454–1,461.

13. Stanley J. Colcombe; Kirk I. Erickson; Paige E. Scalf; Jenny S. Kim; Ruchika Prakash; Edward McAuley; Steriani Elavsky; David X. Marquez; Liang Hu; and Arthur F. Kramer. 2006. "Special Section: Aerobic Exercise Training Increases Brain Volume in Aging Humans." *The Journals of Gerontology Series A: Biological Sciences and Medical Sciences,* 61:1,166–1,170. Also cited in the *Wall Street Journal,* November 16, 2006, "Personal Journal," 1.

14. Andrea L. Dunn; M. H. Trivedi; J. B. Kampert; C. G. Clark; and H. O. Chambliss. 2005. "Exercise Treatment for Depression: Efficacy and Dose Response." *American Journal of Preventive Medicine,* 28 (1): 1–8. See also *President's Council on Physical Fitness and Sports: Research Digest,* December 1997: 1. Amy Forliti. "Exercise May Help in Treating Depression." Associated Press, March 18, 2005.

15. Kenneth H. Cooper. *Can Stress Heal?* (Nashville: Thomas Nelson, 1997), 85.

16. James A. Blumenthal; Andrew Sherwood; Michael A. Babyak; Lana L. Watkins; Robert Waugh; Anastasia Georgiades; Simon L. Bacon; Junichiro Hayano; R. Edward Coleman; and Alan Hinderliter. 2005. "Effects of Exercise and Stress Management Training on Markers of Cardiovascular Risk in Patients With Ischemic Heart Disease. A Randomized Controlled Trial." *Journal of the American Medical Association,* 293 (13): 1,626–1,634.

17. H. Chen; S. M. Zhang; M. A. Schwarzschild; M. A. Hernán; and A. Ascherio. "Physical Activity and the Risk of Parkinson's Disease." 2005. *Neurology,* 64: 664–669.

18. Katherine Esposito; Francesco Giugliano; Carmen Di Palo; Giovanni Giugliano; Raffaele Marfella; Francesco D'Andrea; Massimo D'Armiento; and Dario Giugliano. 2004. "Effect of Lifestyle Changes on Erectile Dysfunction in Obese Men." *Journal of the American Medical Association,* 291 (24): 2,978–2,984.

19. Reported in Reuters news release, June 13, 2005, www.reuters.com.

20. Reported by Reuters Health. Charnicia E. Huggins. "Exercise Key to Longevity for Type 2 Diabetics," www.reuters.com.

21. L. C. Shackelford; A. D. LeBlanc; T. B. Driscoll; H. J. Evans; N. J. Rianon; S. M. Smith; E. Spector; D. L. Feeback; and D. Lai. 2004. "Resistance Exercise as a Countermeasure to Disuse-Induced Bone Loss." *Journal of Applied Physiology,* 97(1): 119–129. Reported in *The Physician and Sportsmedicine,* 2005, 33: 8–9.

22. "Poster Abstracts—Exercise and Dietary Weight Loss in Overweight and Obese Older Adults with Knee Osteoarthritis: The Arthritis, Diet, and Activity Promotion Trial (ADAPT)." The Cooper Institute Conference Series, Physical

Activity: Preventing Physical Disablement in Older Adults, Program and Abstract Book, October 17–19, 2002.

23. "Poster Abstracts—Novel Exercise Training Improves Perceived and Actual Balance Among the Elderly." The Cooper Institute Conference Series, Physical Activity: Preventing Physical Disablement in Older Adults, Program and Abstract Book, October 17–19, 2002, 17.

24. David C. Nieman; Dru A. Henson; Melanie D. Austin; and Victor A. Brown. "Immune Response to a 30-Minute Walk." 2005. *Medicine & Science in Sports & Exercise*, 37: 57–62.

25. American Heart Association 2004 Scientific Sessions: Abstract 3826. Presented November 10, 2004. See also *Medscape Medical News*, 2004.

26. Michelle D. Holmes, M.D.; Wendy Y. Chen; Diane Feskanich; Candyce H. Kroenke; and Graham A. Colditz. 2005. "Physical Activity and Survival after Breast Cancer Diagnosis." *Journal of the American Medical Association*, 293 (20): 2,479–2,486. See also American Cancer Society News Center, article date: May 25, 2005.

27. Deborah Franklin. "The Consumer: Ankle Sprains: New Remedies but Still Little Sympathy." *New York Times*, July 18, 2006.

28. Bruce D. Beynnon; Pamela M. Vacek; Darlene Murphy; Denise Alosa; and David Paller. 2005. "First-Time Inversion Ankle Ligament Trauma. The Effects of Sex, Level of Competition, and Sport on the Incidence of Injury." *The American Journal of Sports Medicine*, 33: 1,485–1,491. See also University of Vermont Communications. July 19, 2006. "Ankle Injury Risk Factors Different in Young Men and Women."

29. Blair et al. *JAMA*, 1989.

30. University of Pittsburgh Medical Center News Bureau, June 8, 2005, report. "Secrets of Successful Aging May Be Found in Senior Olympics Athletes, Say University of Pittsburgh Researchers." See also "Scientists Eye Older Athletes for Insights." Associated Press, June 8, 2005, www.newsday.com.

31. Ibid.

32. Stanley J. Colcombe et al., *Journals of Gerontology*, 2006.

Chapter 7: Start-up #2—Your Basic Exercise Program: Launch a Personal Plan

1. Blair et al. *JAMA*, 1989.

2. Ibid.

3. These values have been calculated from a number of sources, including

Kenneth H. Cooper. *The Aerobics Program for Total Well-Being* (New York: M. Evans, 1982), 118.

4. Reports in the *Journal of the American Dietetic Association,* quoted in *Bottom Line Health,* September 1998: 6.

5. *President's Council on Physical Fitness and Sports: Research Digest,* December 2004: 2.

Chapter 8: Start-up #2—Advanced Fitness: Explore Your Physical Potential

1. Blair et al. *JAMA,* 1989.

2. Ibid.

3. Carl D. Paton. "Combining Explosive and High-Resistance Training Improves Performance in Competitive Cyclists." 2005. *The Journal of Strength and Conditioning Research,* 19 (4): 826–830. See also *Journal of Science and Medicine in Sport* 2006. 9 (June): 249–255.

Chapter 9: Start-up #3—Go on a One-Thing Weight-Loss Eating Plan

1. Kenneth F. Adams; Arthur Schatzkin; Tamara B. Harris; Victor Kipnis; Traci Mouw; Rachel Ballard-Barbash; Albert Hollenbeck; and Michael F. Leitzmann. "Overweight, Obesity, and Mortality in a Large Prospective Cohort of Persons 50 to 71 Years Old." *New England Journal of Medicine,* 355 (8): 763–778. Sun Ha Jee; Jae Woong Sull; Jungyong Park; Sang-Yi Lee; Heechoul Ohrr; Eliseo Guallar; and Jonathan M. Samet. 2006. "Body-Mass Index and Mortality in Korean Men and Women." *New England Journal of Medicine,* 355 (8): 779–787.

2. Guijing Wang; Zhi-Jie Zheng; Gregory Heath; Carol Maceraa; Mike Pratt; and David Buchner. "Economic Burden of Cardiovascular Disease Associated with Excess Body Weight in U.S. Adults." 2002. *American Journal of Preventive Medicine,* 23 (1): 1–6.

3. Frank B. Hu and Walter C. Willett. 2002. "Optimal Diets for Prevention of Coronary Heart Disease." *Journal of the American Medical Association,* 288 (20): 2,569–2,578.

4. André Nkondjock; Daniel Krewski; Kenneth C. Johnson; and Parviz Ghadirian. "Dietary Patterns and Risk of Pancreatic Cancer." 2005. *International Journal of Cancer,* 114 (5): 817–823.

5. Presentation at a 2005 meeting of the American Association for Cancer Research in Anaheim, California, and reported by Reuters Health, April 19, 2005.

6. Ann Chao; Michael J. Thun; Cari J. Connell; Marjorie L. McCullough; Eric J. Jacobs; W. Dana Flanders; Carmen Rodriguez; Rashmi Sinha; and Eugenia E. Calle. "Meat Consumption and Risk of Colorectal Cancer." 2005. *Journal of the American Medical Association,* 293 (2): 172–182.

7. Eric N. Taylor; Meir J. Stampfer; and Gary C. Curhan. "Obesity, Weight Gain, and the Risk of Kidney Stones." 2005. *Journal of the American Medical Association,* 293 (4): 455–462.

8. Katherine Esposito; Alessandro Pontillo; Carmen Di Palo; Giovanni Giugliano; Mariangela Masella; Raffaele Marfella; and Dario Giugliano. "Effect of Weight Loss and Lifestyle Changes on Vascular Inflammatory Markers in Obese Women. A Randomized Trial." 2003. *Journal of the American Medical Association,* 289 (14): 1,799–1,804.

9. Gill M Price; Ricardo Uauy; Elizabeth Breeze; Christopher J Bulpitt; and Astrid E. Fletcher. "Weight, Shape, and Mortality Risk in Older Persons: Elevated Waist-Hip Ratio, Not High Body Mass Index, Is Associated with a Greater Risk of Death." 2006. *American Journal of Clinical Nutrition,* 84 (2): 449–460.

10. A. Heather Eliassen; Graham A. Colditz; Bernard Rosner; Walter C. Willett; and Susan E. Hankinson. "Adult Weight Change and Risk of Postmenopausal Breast Cancer." 2006. *Journal of the American Medical Association,* 296 (2): 193–201.

11. The information that follows is based on research that can be found in the following journals: W.C. Willett and A. Ascherio. "Trans Fatty Acids: Are the Effects Only Marginal?" 1994. *American Journal of Public Health,* 84 (5): 722–724; R. P. Mensink and M. B. Katan. "Effect of Dietary Trans Fatty Acids on High-Density and Low-Density Lipoprotein Cholesterol Levels in Healthy Subjects." 1990. *New England Journal of Medicine,* 323 (7): 439–445; A. H. Allen. "Translating the Mixed Signals of Trans Fat," November 1995, FoodProductDesign.com. Alice H. Lichtenstein; Lynne M. Ausman; Susan M. Jalbert; and Ernst J. Schaefer. "Effects of Different Forms of Dietary Hydrogenated Fats on Serum Lipoprotein Cholesterol Levels." 1999. *New England Journal of Medicine,* 340 (25): 1,933–1,940.

12. U.S. Department of Agriculture publications say that if food is cooked in partially hydrogenated vegetable oils, there are 3.6 grams of trans fat in one standard serving of fast-food French fries, and 3.8 grams of trans fat in a doughnut.

13. Pauline Koh-Banerjee; Nain-Feng Chu; Donna Spiegelman; Bernard Rosner; Graham Colditz; Walter Willett; and Eric Rimm. 2003. "Prospective study of the association of changes in dietary intake, physical activity, alcohol consump-

tion, and smoking with 9-y gain in waist circumference among 16,587 U.S. men." *American Journal of Clinical Nutrition,* 78 (4): 719–727. See also Sally Squire, "Small Lifestyle Changes Could Have Big Impact on Health," *Washington Post,* Nov. 17, 2003.

14. See Skarnulis, Leanna. "With New Labeling, Trans Fats Should Be Easier to Spot, But Are They Truly?" *WebMD* feature, September 2006.

15. Martha Clare Morris; Denis A. Evans; Christine C. Tangney; Julia L. Bienias; and Robert S. Wilson. "Fish Consumption and Cognitive Decline with Age in a Large Community Study." 2005. *Archives of Neurology,* 62 (12): 1,849–1,853.

16. Dariush Mozaffarian; Anouk Geelen; Ingeborg A. Brouwer; Johanna M. Geleijnse; Peter L. Zock; and Martijn B. Katan. 2005. "Effect of Fish Oil on Heart Rate in Humans. A Meta-Analysis of Randomized Controlled Trials." *Circulation,* 112: 1,945–1,952.

17. See studies cited at www.benecol.com.

18. See studies cited at www.takecontrol.com.

Chapter 10: Start-up #4—Follow a Wise Supplement Strategy

1. Jacob Selhub; Paul F. Jacques; Andrew G. Bostom; Ralph B. D'Agostino; Peter W. F. Wilson; Albert J. Belanger; Daniel H. O'Leary; Philip A. Wolf; Ernst J. Schaefer; and Irwin H. Rosenberg. 1995. "Association between Plasma Homocysteine Concentrations and Extracranial Carotid-Artery Stenosis." *New England Journal of Medicine,* 332 (5): 286–291. C. J. Boushey; S. A. Beresford; G. S. Omenn; and A. G. Motulsky. 1995. "A Quantitative Assessment of Plasma Homocysteine as a Risk Factor for Vascular Disease. Probable Benefits of Increasing Folic Acid Intakes." *Journal of the American Medical Association,* 274 (13): 1,049–1,057. H. I. Morrison; D. Schaubel; M. Desmeules; and D. T. Wigle. 1996. "Serum Folate and Risk of Fatal Coronary Heart Disease." *Journal of the American Medical Association,* 275 (24): 1,893–1,896.

2. J. A. Reiffel and A. McDonald. 2006. "Antiarrhythmic Effects of Omega-3 Fatty Acids." *American Journal of Cardiology,* 98 (4A): 50i–60i. R. Jabbar, T. Saldeen. 2006. "A New Predictor of Risk for Sudden Cardiac Death." *Upsala Journal of Medical Science,* 111 (2): 169–177. T.A. Jacobson. 2006. "Secondary Prevention of Coronary Artery Disease with Omega-3 Fatty Acids." *American Journal of Cardiology,* 21: 98 (4A): 61i–70i. G. Schwalfenberg. 2006. "Omega-3 Fatty Acids: Their Beneficial Role in Cardiovascular Health." *Canadian Family Physician,* 52: 734–740.

3. Z. Kurugol; M. Akilli; N. Bayram; and G. Koturoglu. 2006. "The Prophylactic and Therapeutic Effectiveness of Zinc Sulphate on Common Cold in Children." *Acta Paediatrica,* 95 (10): 1,175–1,181. G. A. Eby. 2004. "Zinc Lozenges: Cold Cure or Candy? Solution Chemistry Determinations." *Bioscience Reports,* 24 (1): 23–39. R. Silk and C. LeFante. 2005. "Safety of Zinc Gluconate Glycine (Cold-Eeze) in a Geriatric Population: A Randomized, Placebo-Controlled, Double-Blind Trial." *American Journal of Therapeutics,* 12 (6): 612–617. D. J. Hulisz. 2004. "Efficacy of Zinc Against Common Cold Viruses: An Overview." *American Pharmaceutical Association,* 44 (5): 594–603.
4. M. Gleeson. 2006. "Can Nutrition Limit Exercise-Induced Immunodepression?" *Nutrition Review,* 64 (3): 119–131. U. Singh; S. Devaraj; and I. Jialal. 2005. "Vitamin E, Oxidative Stress, and Inflammation." *Annual Review of Nutrition,* 25: 151–174. S. N. Meydani; L. S. Leka; B. C. Fine; G. E. Dallal; G. T. Keusch; M. F. Singh; and D. H. Hamer. 2004. "Vitamin E and Respiratory Tract Infections in Elderly Nursing Home Residents: A Randomized Controlled Trial." *Journal of the American Medical Association,* 292 (7): 828–836. S. N. Meydani; S. N. Han; and D. H. Hamer. 2004. "Vitamin E and Respiratory Infection in the Elderly." *Annals of the New York Academy of Sciences,* 1,031: 214–222. H. Hemila and R. M. Douglas. 1999. "Vitamin C and Acute Respiratory Infections. *International Journal Tuberculosis and Lung Disease,* 3 (9): 756–761. H. Hemila. 2004. "Vitamin C Supplementation and Respiratory Infections: A Systematic Review." *Military Medicine,* 169 (11): 920–925. S. Sasazuki; S. Sasaki; Y. Tsubono; S. Okubo; S. M. Hayashi; and S. Tsugane. 2006. "Effect of Vitamin C on Common Cold: Randomized Controlled Trial." *European Journal of Clinical Nutrition,* 60 (1): 9–17.
5. Conrad P. Earnest; Kherrin A. Wood; and Timothy S. Church. 2003. "Complex Multivitamin Supplementation Improves Homocysteine and Resistance to LDL-C Oxidation." *Journal of the American College of Nutrition,* 22 (5): 400–407.
6. J. M. Seddon; U. A. Ajani; R. D. Sperduto; R. Hiller; N. Blair; T. C. Burton; M. D. Farber; E. S. Gragoudas; J. Haller; and D. T. Miller. 1994. "Dietary Carotenoids, Vitamins A, C, and E, and Advanced Age-Related Macular Degeneration. Eye Disease Case-Control Study Group." *Journal of the American Medical Association,* 272 (18): 1,413–1,420.
7. P. F. Jacques; A. Taylor; S. E. Hankinson; W. C. Willett; B. Mahnken; Y. Lee; K. Vaid; and M Lahav. "Long-Term Vitamin C Supplement Use and Prevalence of Early Age-Related Lens Opacities." 1997. *American Journal of Clinical Nutrition,* 66: 911–916.

8. G. D. Plotnick; M. C. Corretti; and R. A. Vogel. 1997. "Effect of Antioxidant Vitamins on the Transient Impairment of Endothelium-Dependent Brachial Artery Vasoactivity Following a Single High-Fat Meal." *Journal of the American Medical Association,* 278: 1,682–1,686.

9. See Kay-Tee Khaw; Sheila Bingham; Ailsa Welch; Robert Luben; Nicholas Wareham; Suzy Oakes; and Nicholas Day. 2001. "Relation Between Plasma Ascorbic Acid and Mortality in Men and Women in EPIC-Norfolk Prospective Study: A Prospective Population Study." *The Lancet,* 357 (9257). 3 March 2001. Pages 657–663. Tetsuji Yokoyama; Chigusa Date; Yoshihiro Kokubo; Nobuo Yoshiike; Yasuhiro Matsumura; and Heizo Tanaka. 2000. "Serum Vitamin C Concentration Was Inversely Associated with Subsequent 20-Year Incidence of Stroke in a Japanese Rural Community: The Shibata Study." *Stroke,* 31: 2,287–2,294.

10. Cedric F. Garland; Frank C. Garland; Edward D. Gorham; Martin Lipkin; Harold Newmark; Sharif B. Mohr; and Michael F. Holick. 2006. "The Role of Vitamin D in Cancer Prevention." *American Journal of Public Health,* 96 (February): 252–261.

11. A. Hartmann; A. M. Niess; M. Grunert-Fuchs; B. Poch; and G. Speit. 1995. "Vitamin E Prevents Exercise-Induced DNA Damage." *Mutation Research,* 346 (4): 195–202.

12. See evaluation at www.CooperAerobics.com.

13. J. V. Woodside; J. W. Yarnell; D. McMaster; I. S. Young; D. L. Harmon; E. E. McCrum; C. C. Patterson; K. F. Gey; A. S. Whitehead; and A. Evans. 1998. "Effect of B-group Vitamins and Antioxidant Vitamins on Hyperhomocysteinemia: A Double-Blind, Randomized, Factorial-Design, Controlled Trial." *American Journal of Clinical Nutrition,* 67: 858–866. [published erratum appears in *American Journal of Clinical Nutrition* 1998. 68 (3): (September): 758]

14. Killian Robinson; Kristopher Arheart; Helga Refsum; Lars Brattström; Godfried Boers; Per Ueland; Paolo Rubba; Roberto Palma-Reis; Raymond Meleady; Leslie Daly; Jacqueline Witteman; and Ian Graham. 1998. "Low Circulating Folate and Vitamin B_6 Concentrations: Risk Factors for Stroke, Peripheral Vascular Disease, and Coronary Artery Disease." *Circulation,* 97: 437–443.

15. G. D. Plotnick et al., *JAMA,* 1997.

16. Edward Giovannucci; Meir J. Stampfer; Graham A. Colditz; David J. Hunter; Charles Fuchs; Bernard A. Rosner; Frank E. Speizer; and Walter C. Willett. 1998. "Multivitamin Use, Folate, and Colon Cancer in Women in the Nurses' Health Study." *Annals of Internal Medicine,* 129 (7): 517–524.

17. J. V. Woodside et al., *American Journal of Clinical Nutrition*, 1998.

18. L. C. Clark; G. F. Combs Jr.; B. W. Turnbull; E. H. Slate; D. K. Chalker; J. Chow; L. S. Davis; R. A. Glover; G. F. Graham; E. G. Gross; A. Krongrad; J. L. Lesher Jr.; H. K. Park; B. B. Sanders Jr.; C. L. Smith; and J. R. Taylor. 1996. "Effects of Selenium Supplementation for Cancer Prevention in Patients with Carcinoma of the Skin. A Randomized Controlled Trial. Nutritional Prevention of Cancer Study Group." *Journal of the American Medical Association*, 276: 1,957–1,963.

19. P. K. Whelton; J. He; J. A. Cutler; F. L. Brancati; L. J. Appel; D. Follmann; and M. J. Klag. 1997. "Effects of Oral Potassium on Blood Pressure. Meta-analysis of Randomized Controlled Clinical Trials." *Journal of the American Medical Association*, 277: 1,624–1,632.

20. H. Langsjoen; P. Langsjoen; R. Willis; and K. Folkers. 1994. "Usefulness of Coenzyme Q_{10} in Clinical Cardiology: A Long-term Study." *Molecular Aspects of Medicine*, 15, (Supplement 1): s165–s175.

21. Edward Giovannucci; Alberto Ascherio; Eric B. Rimm; Meir J. Stampfer; Graham A. Colditz; and Walter C. Willett. 1995. "Intake of Carotenoids and Retino in Relation to Risk of Prostate Cancer." *Journal of the National Cancer Institute*, 87: 1,767–1,776.

22. J. M. Seddon et al. *JAMA*, 1994.

23. Mitchell S. Buckley; Angela D. Goff; and Walter E. Knapp. 2004. *Annals of Pharmacotherapy*, 38: 50–53. Y. Nagakawa; H. Orimo; M. Harasawa; I. Morita; K. Yashiro; and S. Murota. 1983. "Effect of Eicosapentaenoic Acid on the Platelet Aggregation and Composition of Fatty Acid in Man: A Double-Blind Study." *Atherosclerosis*, 47 (1): 71–75.

24. Megan N. Hall, Hannia Campos, Haojie Li, Howard D. Sesso, Meir J. Stampfer, Walter C. Willett, and Jing Ma. 2007. "Blood Levels of Long-Chain Polyunsaturated Fatty Acids, Aspirin, and the Risk of Colorectal Cancer." *Cancer Epidemiology, Biomarkers and Prevention.* 16: 314–321.

25. P. M. Ridker; N. R. Cook; I. M. Lee; D. Gordon; J. M. Gaziano; J. E. Manson; C. H. Hennekens; and J. E. Buring. 2005. "A Randomized Trial of Low-Dose Aspirin in the Primary Prevention of Cardiovascular Disease in Women." *New England Journal of Medicine*, 352: 1,293–1,304. Published at www.nejm.org on March 7, 2005.

26. Timothy E. McAlindon; Michael P. LaValley; Juan P. Gulin; and David T. Felson. 2000. "Glucosamine and Chondroitin for Treatment of Osteoarthritis: A Systematic Quality Assessment and Meta-analysis." *Journal of the American Medical Association*, 283: 1,469–1,475.

27. Daniel O. Clegg; Domenic J. Reda; Crystal L. Harris; Marguerite A. Klein; James R. O'Dell; Michele M. Hooper; John D. Bradley; Clifton O. Bingham III; Michael H. Weisman; Christopher G. Jackson; Nancy E. Lane; John J. Cush; Larry W. Moreland; H. Ralph Schumacher, Jr.; Chester V. Oddis; Frederick Wolfe; Jerry A. Molitor; David E. Yocum; Thomas J. Schnitzer; Daniel E. Furst; Allen D. Sawitzke; Helen Shi; Kenneth D. Brandt; Roland W. Moskowitz; and H. James Williams. 2006. "Glucosamine, Chondroitin Sulfate, and the Two in Combination for Painful Knee Osteoarthritis." 2006. *New England Journal of Medicine,* 354 (8): 795–808.

28. A. F. Tallia and D. A. Cardone. 2002. "Asthma Exacerbation Associated with Glucosamine-Chondroitin Supplement." *Journal of the American Board of Family Practice,* 5: 481–484.

29. Tatu A. Miettinen; Pekka Puska; Helena Gylling; Hannu Vanhanen; and Erkki Vartiainen. 1995. "Reduction of Serum Cholesterol with Sitostanol-Ester Margarine in a Mildly Hypercholesterolemic Population." *New England Journal of Medicine,* 333 (20): 1,308–1,312.

30. J. A. Weststrate and G. W. Meijer. 1998. "Plant Sterol-Enriched Margarines and Reduction of Plasma Total- and LDL-Cholesterol Concentrations in Normocholesterolaemic and Mildly Hypercholesterolaemic Subjects." *European Journal of Clinical Nutrition,* 52 (5): 334–343.

31. P. Rampal; N. Moore; E. Van Ganse; J. M. Le Parc; R. Wall; H. Schneid; and F. Verriere. 2002. "Gastrointestinal Tolerability of Ibuprofen Compared with Paracetamol and Aspirin at Over-the-Counter Doses." *Journal of International Medical Research,* 30 (3): 301–308. T. Suenobu; T. Yoshioka; S. Maruta; and H. Shimoji. 2006. "Post-Marketing Surveillance of Acetylcysteine Oral Solution 17.6% 'SENJU' for the Antidote to Acetaminophen Overdose—Use—Results Surveillance." *Chudoku Kenkyu,* 19 (4): 383–394.

Chapter 11: Start-up #5—Do Serious Smoke Control

1. This was the conclusion reached by British researcher Richard Doll, who studied nearly 35,000 British physicians over a fifty-year period, from 1951 to 2001. The study, which has been published in the *British Medical Journal,* is continuing. See Richard Doll, Richard Peto, Jillian Boreham, and Isabelle Sutherland. 2004. "Mortality in Relation to Smoking: 50 Years' Observations on Male British Doctors." *British Medical Journal,* 328 (7,455): 1,519. Also, see Richard Doll and A. Bradford Hill. 2004. "The Mortality of Doctors in Re-

lation to Their Smoking Habits: A Preliminary Report." *British Medical Journal*, 328 (7,455): 1,529–1,533.

2. See the Associated Press news report, Aug. 31, 2006, and a *New York Times* editorial, Aug. 31, 2006.

3. Peter A. Andersen; David B. Buller; Jenifer H. Voeks; Ron Borland; Donald Helme; Erwin P. Bettinghaus; and Walter F. Young. 2006. "Predictors of Support for Environmental Tobacco Smoke Bans in State Government." *American Journal of Preventive Medicine*, 30 (4): 292–299.

4. See surveys cited by Memorial Sloan-Kettering Cancer Center in New York City in the *New York Times*, "Personal Health," March 21, 2006.

5. American Cancer Society, *Cancer Facts and Figures*, 2002 (Atlanta: American Cancer Society, 2002).

6. Medical News & Perspectives, *Journal of the American Medical Association*, 2003, 289: 163.

7. Release from the American Heart Association, Oct. 30, 2002.

8. A study by Northwestern University researchers, presented at a meeting of cancer specialists in Chicago, and reported by Reuters on Jan. 27, 2005.

9. Naomi M. Gades; Ajay Nehra; Debra J. Jacobson; Michaela E. McGree; Cynthia J. Girman; Thomas Rhodes; Rosebud O. Roberts; Michael M. Lieber; and Steven J. Jacobsen. 2005. "Association between Smoking and Erectile Dysfunction: A Population-based Study." *American Journal of Epidemiology*, 161: 346–351.

10. J. R. Evans; A. E. Fletcher; and R. P. L. Wormald. 2005. "28,000 Cases of Age-related Macular Degeneration Causing Visual Loss in People Aged 75 Years and Above in the United Kingdom May Be Attributable to Smoking." *British Journal of Ophthalmology*, 89 (May): 550–553.

11. Jeffrey G. Johnson; Patricia Cohen; Daniel S. Pine; Donald F. Klein; Stephanie Kasen; and Judith S. Brook. 2000. "Association Between Cigarette Smoking and Anxiety Disorders During Adolescence and Early Adulthood." *Journal of the American Medical Association*, 284: 2,348–2,351.

12. Diane Baer Wilson and Paul J. Nietert. 2002. "Patterns of Fruit, Vegetable, and Milk Consumption Among Smoking and Nonsmoking Female Teens." *American Journal of Preventive Medicine*, 22 (4): 240–246.

13. Karen J. Cruickshanks; Ronald Klein; Barbara E. K. Klein; Terry L. Wiley; David M. Nondahl; and Ted S. Tweed. 1998. "Cigarette Smoking and Hearing Loss: The Epidemiology of Hearing Loss Study." *Journal of the American Medical Association*, 279: 1,715–1,719.

14. Karen Markussen Linnet; Kirsten Wisborg; Carsten Obel; Niels Jørgen Secher; Per Hove Thomsen; Esben Agerbo; and Tine Brink Henriksen. 2005. "Smoking During Pregnancy and the Risk for Hyperkinetic Disorder in Offspring." *Pediatrics,* 116: 462–467.

15. American Heart Association report, Abstracts 3631 and 3639, Nov. 18, 2002.

16. Ibid.

17. Koon K. Teo; Stephanie Ounpuu; Steven Hawken; M. R. Pandey; Vincent Valentin; David Hunt; Rafael Diaz; Wafa Rashed; Rosario Freeman; Lixin Jiang; Xiaofei Zhang; and Salim Yusuf. "Tobacco Use and Risk of Myocardial Infarction in 52 Countries in the INTERHEART Study: A Case-Control Study." *Lancet,* 368 (9,536), 19 August–25 August: 647–658. (Reported online by *Healthy Living,* copyright 2006 National News.) George Howard; Lynne E. Wagenknecht; Gregory L. Burke; Ana Diez-Roux; Gregory W. Evans; Paul McGovern; F. Javier Nieto; and Grethe S. Tell. 1998. "Cigarette Smoking and Progression of Atherosclerosis. The Atherosclerosis Risk in Communities (ARIC) Study." *Journal of the American Medical Association,* 279: 119–124.

18. Ibid.

19. See the I-ELCAP Newsletter International, p. 1. Early Lung Cancer Action Program, Weill Medical College of Cornell University, at www.ielcap.org.

20. Ibid., p. 2.

21. Dorothee Twardella; Jutta Küpper-Nybelen; Dietrich Rothenbacher; Harry Hahmann; Bernd Wüsten; and Hermann Brenner. 2004. "Short-term Benefit of Smoking Cessation in Patients with Coronary Heart Disease: Estimates Based on Self-reported Smoking Data and Serum Cotinine Measurements." *European Heart Journal,* 25: 2,101–2,108.

22. Neville Suskin; Tej Sheth; Abdissa Negassa; and Salim Yusuf. 2001. "Relationship of Current and Past Smoking to Mortality and Morbidity in Patients with Left Ventricular Dysfunction." *Journal of the American College of Cardiology,* 37: 1,677–1,682.

23. Daniel Menzies; Arun Nair; Peter A. Williamson; Stuart Schembri; Mudher Z. H. Al-Khairalla; Martyn Barnes; Tom C. Fardon; Lesley McFarlane; Gareth J. Magee; and Brian J. Lipworth. 2006. "Respiratory Symptoms, Pulmonary Function, and Markers of Inflammation Among Bar Workers Before and After a Legislative Ban on Smoking in Public Places." *Journal of the American Medical Association,* 296: 1,742–1,748.

24. See the I-ELCAP Newsletter International, p. 2. Early Lung Cancer Action Program, Weill Medical College of Cornell University, at www.ielcap.org. Also,

see the June 24, 2003, report in the *Wall Street Journal* and the Web site of the Cancer Research and Prevention Foundation, www.preventcancer.org.

25. Michael C. Fiore; Dorothy K. Hatsukami; and Timothy B. Baker. 2002. "Effective Tobacco Dependence Treatment." *Journal of the American Medical Association,* 288: 1,768–1,771.

26. M. Fennessy; D. S. Moneley; J. H. Wang; C. J. Kelly; and D. J. Bouchier-Hayes. 2003. "Taurine and Vitamin C Modify Monocyte and Endothelial Dysfunction in Young Smokers." *Circulation,* 107: 410–415.

27. From www.mdconsult.com and *USA Today,* May 20, 2002.

28. Reported by the *Washington Post* online, January 19, 2004. The device is manufactured by Nymox Corp. of Maywood, N.J.

29. Michael C. Fiore et al. *JAMA,* 2002.

30. Nina S. Godtfredsen; Eva Prescott; and Merete Osler. 2005. "Effect of Smoking Reduction on Lung Cancer Risk." *Journal of the American Medical Association,* 294: 1,505–1,510.

31. Mary Shaw; Richard Mitchell; and Danny Doirling. 2000. "Time for a Smoke? One Cigarette Reduces Your Life by 11 Minutes." *British Medical Journal,* 320 (7,226): 53.

32. Shu-Hong Zhu; Christopher M. Anderson; Gary J. Tedeschi; Bradley Rosbrook; Cynthia E. Johnson; Michael Byrd; and Elsa Gutiérrez-Terrell. 2002. "Evidence of Real-World Effectiveness of a Telephone Quitline for Smokers." *New England Journal of Medicine,* 347 (14): 1,087–1,093.

33. Bess H. Marcus; Anna E. Albrecht; Teresa K. King; Alfred F. Parisi; Bernardine M. Pinto; Mary Roberts; Raymond S. Niaura; and David B. Abrams. 1999. "The Efficacy of Exercise as an Aid for Smoking Cessation in Women: A Randomized Controlled Trial." *Archives of Internal Medicine,* 159: 1,229–1,234.

34. Cary P. Gross; Benny Soffer; Peter B. Bach; Rahul Rajkumar; and Howard P. Forman. 2002. "State Expenditures for Tobacco-Control Programs and the Tobacco Settlement." *New England Journal of Medicine,* 347 (14): 1,080–1,086.

35. Frederick P. Rivara; Beth E. Ebel; Michelle M. Garrison; Dimitri A. Christakis; Sarah E. Wiehe; and David T. Levy. 2004. "Prevention of Smoking-related Deaths in the United States." *American Journal of Preventive Medicine,* 27 (2): 118–125.

Chapter 12: Start-up #6—Counteract Substance Surprises

1. C. A. Camargo Jr.; C. H. Hennekens; J. M. Gaziano; R. J. Glynn; J. E. Manson; and M. J. Stampfer. 1997. "Prospective Study of Moderate Alcohol Consumption and Mortality in U.S. Male Physicians." *Archives of Internal Medicine,* 157: 79–85.

2. Janne Tolstrup; Majken K. Jensen; Anne Tjønneland; Kim Overvad; Kenneth J. Mukamal; and Morten Grønbæk. 2006. "Prospective Study of Alcohol Drinking Patterns and Coronary Heart Disease in Women and Men." *British Medical Journal,* 332 (7552): 1,244–1,248.

3. Stefan Kiechl; Johann Willeit; Gregor Rungger; Georg Egger; Friedrich Oberhollenzer; and Enzo Bonora. 1998. "Alcohol Consumption and Atherosclerosis: What Is the Relation? Prospective Results From the Bruneck Study." *Stroke,* 29: 900–907.

4. Meir J. Stampfer; Jae Hee Kang; Jennifer Chen; Rebecca Cherry; and Francine Grodstein. 2005. "Effects of Moderate Alcohol Consumption on Cognitive Function in Women." *New England Journal of Medicine,* 352 (3): 245–253.

5. Denis A. Evans and Julia L. Bienias. 2005. Editorial: "Alcohol Consumption and Cognition." *New England Journal of Medicine,* 352: 289–290.

6. Chris Power; Bryan Rodgers; and Steven Hope. 1998. "U-shaped Relation for Alcohol Consumption and Health in Early Adulthood and Implications for Mortality." *Lancet,* 352 (9131): 877. Timothy S. Naimi; David W. Brown; Robert D. Brewer; Wayne H. Giles; George Mensah; Mary K. Serdula; Ali H. Mokdad; Daniel W. Hungerford; James Lando; Shapur Naimi; and Donna F. Stroup. 2005. "Cardiovascular Risk Factors and Confounders Among Nondrinking and Moderate-Drinking U.S. Adults." *American Journal of Preventive Medicine,* 28 (4): 369–373.

7. Luc Djoussé; Daniel Levy; Emelia J. Benjamin; Susan J. Blease; Ana Russ; Martin G. Larson; Joseph M. Massaro; Ralph B. D'Agostino; Philip A. Wolf; and R. Curtis Ellison. 2004. "Long-Term Alcohol Consumption and the Risk of Atrial Fibrillation in the Framingham Study." *The American Journal of Cardiology,* 93 (6): 710–713.

8. *National Masters News,* August 2001, posted Aug. 14, 2001, on www.masterstrack.com.

9. Steve Boman and Sean Callahan. "What Makes Supergran Run?" www.salon.com.

10. R. E. Emptage and T. P. Semla. 1996. "Depression in the Medically Ill Elderly: A Focus on Methylphenidate." *Annals of Pharmacotherapy,* 30: 151–157. See also Helen Lavretsky; Susan Park; Prabha Siddarth; Anand Kumar; and Charles F.

Reynolds III. 2006. "Methylphenidate-Enhanced Antidepressant Response to Citalopram in the Elderly: A Double-Blind, Placebo-Controlled Pilot Trial." *American Journal of Geriatric Psychiatry,* 14: 181–185.

11. June announcement from the FDA, reported in July 1, 2005, issue of the *New York Times.*

12. Reported in Reuters online, Dec. 1, 2005.

13. Rob M. van Dam and Frank B. Hu. 2005. "Coffee Consumption and Risk of Type 2 Diabetes: A Systematic Review." *Journal of the American Medical Association,* 294: 97–104.

14. J. V. Higdon and B. Frei. 2006. "Coffee and Health: A Review of Recent Human Research." *Critical Review of Food Science and Nutrition,* 46 (2): 101–123. See also Pierre Philip; Jacques Taillard; Nicholas Moore; Sandrine Delord; Cédric Valtat; Patricia Sagaspe; and Bernard Bioulac. 2006. "The Effects of Coffee and Napping on Nighttime Highway Driving: A Randomized Trial." *Archives of Internal Medicine,* 144 (11): 785–791.

15. Lene Frost Andersen; David R Jacobs, Jr.; Monica H. Carlsen; and Rune Blomhoff. 2006. Consumption of coffee is associated with reduced risk of death attributed to inflammatory and cardiovascular diseases in the Iowa Women's Health Study. *American Journal of Clinical Nutrition,* 83: 1,039–1,046.

16. Mehdi Namdar; Pascal Koepfli; Renate Grathwohl; Patrick T. Siegrist; Michael Klainguti; Tiziano Schepis; Raphael Delaloye; Christophe A. Wyss; Samuel P. Fleischmann; Oliver Gaemperli; and Philipp A. Kaufmann. 2006. "Caffeine Decreases Exercise-Induced Myocardial Flow Reserve." *Journal of the American College of Cardiology,* 47: 405–410.

17. Quoted in the *New York Times,* Jan. 24, 2006, "Vital Signs" column.

18. Reported in the *New York Times,* www.nytimes.com, March 14, 2006, "Vital Signs" column.

19. See Kenneth H. Cooper, *Advanced Nutritional Therapies* (Nashville: Thomas Nelson, 1996), 133–137.

Chapter 13: Start-up #7—Combat Stress with Mind-Spirit Strength

1. J. L. Boone and J. P. Anthony. 2003. "Evaluating the Impact of Stress on Systemic Disease: The MOST Protocol in Primary Care." *Journal of the American Osteopathic Association,* 103: 239–246.

2. For extensive discussions of the negative impact of stress on health, see Kenneth H. Cooper, *Can Stress Heal?* (Nashville: Thomas Nelson, 1997); Herbert

Benson, *Timeless Healing* (New York: Fireside/Simon & Schuster, 1996), 146–148, 228–229; Herbert Benson and William Proctor, *The Breakout Principle* (New York: Scribner, 2003, 2004), 58, 223.

3. M. A. Mittleman and M. Maclure. 1997. "Mental Stress During Daily Life Triggers Myocardial Ischemia." *Journal of the American Medical Association,* 277: 1,558–1,559. See also Ilan S. Wittstein; David R. Thiemann; Joao A. C. Lima; Kenneth L. Baughman; Steven P. Schulman; Gary Gerstenblith; Katherine C. Wu; Jeffrey J. Rade; Trinity J. Bivalacqua; and Hunter C. Champion. 2005. "Neurohumoral Features of Myocardial Stunning Due to Sudden Emotional Stress." *New England Journal of Medicine,* 352 (6): 539–548.

4. Report in the *New York Times,* March 14, 2006, citing studies in D. R. Witte; D. E. Grobbee; M. L. Bots; and A.W. Hoes. 2005. "A Meta-analysis of Excess Cardiac Mortality on Monday." *European Journal of Epidemiology,* 20 (5): 401–406. See also *European Journal of Epidemiology* (2005) and C. Martyn. 2000. "Hebdomadal Rhythms of the Heart: Why Do Deaths Peak at the Start of the Week? Because We Don't Like Mondays." *British Medical Journal,* 321 (7,276): 1,542–1,543.

5. Mike Mitka. 2005. "Depression–Heart Disease Link Probed." *Journal of the American Medical Association,* 293: 283–284. See also J. L. Boone and J. P. Anthony. 2003. "Evaluating the Impact of Stress on Systemic Disease: The MOST Protocol in Primary Care." *Journal of the American Osteopathic Association,* 103: 239–246.

6. Ilan S. Wittstein; David R. Thiemann; Joao A.C. Lima; Kenneth L. Baughman; Steven P. Schulman; Gary Gerstenblith; Katherine C. Wu; Jeffrey J. Rade; Trinity J. Bivalacqua; and Hunter C. Champion. 2005. "Neurohumoral Features of Myocardial Stunning Due to Sudden Emotional Stress." *New England Journal of Medicine,* 352 (6): 539–548.

7. J. L. Boone and J. P. Anthony. 2003. "Evaluating the Impact of Stress on Systemic Disease: The MOST Protocol in Primary Care." *Journal of the American Osteopathic Association,* 103: 239–246.

8. Ibid.

9. Ibid.

10. Ibid. See also a July 28, 2005, *New York Times* report citing studies at Weill Medical College of Cornell University (2001), University of California (2001), University of Massachusetts (1998), and Johns Hopkins University (1999).

11. "Can Stress Make You Sick? Emotions and Health." *Harvard Health Letter,* April 1998, Vol. 23, No. 6.

12. Chris Cinque. 1989. "The Role of Stress in Ditka's Heart Attack." *The Physician and Sportsmedicine,* 17 (January): 40–41.

13. Leo Cohen; Rita C. Ardjoen; and Karin S. M. Sewpersad. 1997. "Type A Behaviour Pattern as a Risk Factor after Myocardial Infarction: A Review." *Psychology and Health,* 12: 619–632.

14. Philip C. Strike and Andrew Steptoe. 2005. "Behavioral and Emotional Triggers of Acute Coronary Syndromes: A Systematic Review and Critique." *Psychosomatic Medicine,* 67: 179–186.

15. Andrea L. Dunn; Madhukar H. Trivedi; James B. Kampert; Camillia G. Clark; and Heather O. Chambliss. 2005. "Exercise Treatment for Depression: Efficacy and Dose Response." *American Journal of Preventive Medicine,* 28 (1): 1–8.

16. See Herbert Benson, *Timeless Healing* (New York: Fireside–Simon & Schuster, 1995, 1996), 134–137.

17. Herbert Benson and William Proctor. *The Breakout Principle* (New York: Scribner, 2003, 2004), 19, 26ff.

18. E. J. Giltay; M. H. Kamphuis; S. Kalmijn; F. G. Zitman; and D. Kromhout. 2006. "Dispositional Optimism and the Risk of Cardiovascular Death: The Zutphen Elderly Study." *Archives of Internal Medicine,* 166: 431–436.

19. Reported in Reuters.com news release, Monday, March 7, 2005.

20. "Spatting with the Spouse Can Harden Your Heart." *Salt Lake Tribune,* March 5, 2006.

21. Raymond Niaura; John F. Todaro; Laura Stroud; Avron Spiro; Kenneth D. Ward; and Scott Weiss. 2002. "Hostility, the Metabolic Syndrome, and Incident Coronary Heart Disease." *Health Psychology,* Vol 21 (6) 588–593. Also reported on webmd.com.

22. Reported at *WebMD Medical News,* webmd.com, November 18, 2002.

23. Eva Selhub. 2002. "Stress and Distress in Clinical Practice: A Mind-Body Approach." *Nutrition and Clinical Care,* 5 (4) (July/August): 187.

24. See Thomas H. Holmes and Richard H. Rahe. 1967. "The Social Readjustment Rating Scale." *Journal of Psychosomatic Research,* 11 (2): 213–218. See also Kenneth H. Cooper, *Can Stress Heal?* (Nashville: Thomas Nelson, 1997), 29–30; Herbert Benson and William Proctor, *The Breakout Principle* (New York: Scribner, 2003, 2004); Scott Brady and William Proctor, *Pain Free for Life* (New York: Center Street/Hachette, 2006), 200–201.

25. Cited in Reuters.com report, February 17, 2005.

Chapter 16: Your Fitness Is Now

1. See Stanley J. Colcombe; Kirk I. Erickson; Paige E. Scalf; Jenny S. Kim; Ruchika Prakash; Edward McAuley; Steriani Elavsky; David X. Marquez; Liang Hu; and Arthur F. Kramer. 2006. Special Section: Aerobic Exercise Training Increases Brain Volume in Aging Humans. *The Journals of Gerontology Series A: Biological Sciences and Medical Sciences,* 61: 1,166–1,170.

2. Genesis 6:3 (NIV).

INDEX

stress test, 106–8
stretches
  fitBALL chest, 149
  kneeling back, 153–54
  lying abdominal, 152–53
  lying glute/low-back, 152
  lying hamstring, 150–51
  lying hip, 151
  lying quadriceps, 151–52
  seated back, 149
  seated groin, 150
  seated triceps, 153
stroke
  aspirin supplements and, 257
  blood pressure and, 118
  hiking on hilly terrain and, 126
  homocysteine and, 100
  metabolic syndrome and, 23
  smoking cessation and, 277
  trans fats and, 208
  vitamin C supplements and, 244
  weight loss and, 207
substance abuse
  addiction, 336
  alcohol, 290–92
  caffeine, 297–99
  creep effect, 287, 288–89, 292–93
  over-the-counter painkillers, 262
  performance enhancers, 293–96
  as stress response, 65
  threat of, 21
  wariness of, 300–301
supplements
  benefits, 235–38
  dangers, 260–62
  dosage recommendations, 238–43
  functional foods, 259–60
  over-the-counter medical supplements, 257–59, 262
  program strategies, 264–67
  purity and potency of, 262
  research on, 262–64
  for stress management, 314
  See also specific health conditions; specific supplements
Surgeon General report on smoking, 272, 276–77

Take Control, 206, 220, 260
target heart rate, 169–71
thiamine supplements, 246
30-60-90-minute exercise guidelines, 161–62, 195
tobacco. See smoking
tobacco manufacturers, 271, 284–85
trans fats, 206n, 208–11, 226
triceps stretch, seated, 153
triglyceride levels, 23n, 111, 125, 219, 256, 264
Tufts University, USDA Nutrition Center, 250

Tyndall, John, 58
type-2 diabetes. See diabetes

ubiquinone (coenzyme Q_{10}) supplements, 252
ulcers, 305
University of California at San Diego, 245
University of Illinois, Urbana, 120, 132
University of Lethbridge (Canada), 124–25
University of Maryland, 312
University of Pittsburgh Medical Center, 130, 131
University of Texas Medical Branch, Galveston, 252
University of Utah, 312–13
University of Vermont, 127
University of Western Ontario, London, 13
upper body exercises, 142–44
urinalysis, 101
U.S. government 30-60-90-minute guidelines, 195
USDA Nutrition Center at Tufts University, 250

vegetables, 217–18, 225, 227
vitamin and mineral supplement dosages, 238–43
vitamin A supplements, 243–44, 279
vitamin-B complex supplements, 246–49, 252
vitamin C supplements, 244, 314
vitamin D supplements, 123, 245
vitamin E supplements, 245–46, 314–15
vitamin K supplements, 246

waist measurement, 23n, 111, 207
Wake Forest University, 124
walking
  for basic fitness, 117–18
  bone mass and, 123
  on hilly terrain, 125–26
  immune response and, 125
  mental function and, 120
weight-bearing exercise. See strength and resistance training
weight loss and maintenance
  accident risk and, 13
  action supplement, 222–24
  erectile function and, 122
  fitness sequences and add-ons, 195–202
  options and strategies, 230–31
  pain relief and, 12
  sleep patterns and, 22
  wealth and, 13
  See also One-Thing Weight-Loss Eating Plan
weight training. See strength and resistance training
whole grains, 218, 227
Willett, Walter, 208
Williams, Redford, 313
workplace wellness programs in, 54–55
Wright, Vonda, 131

zinc supplements, 236, 250

PERSONAL PROGRESS—*START STRONG* FITNESS PROGRAM

Date	Exercise	Distance	Duration	Aerobic Points	Cumulative Points

PERSONAL PROGRESS—*START STRONG* FITNESS PROGRAM

Date	Exercise	Distance	Duration	Aerobic Points	Cumulative Points

PERSONAL PROGRESS—*START STRONG* FITNESS PROGRAM

Date	Exercise	Distance	Duration	Aerobic Points	Cumulative Points

PERSONAL PROGRESS—*START STRONG* FITNESS PROGRAM

Date	Exercise	Distance	Duration	Aerobic Points	Cumulative Points

PERSONAL PROGRESS—*START STRONG* FITNESS PROGRAM

Date	Exercise	Distance	Duration	Aerobic Points	Cumulative Points

PERSONAL PROGRESS—*START STRONG* FITNESS PROGRAM

Date	Exercise	Distance	Duration	Aerobic Points	Cumulative Points